NUTRITION AND DIET RESEARCH PROGRESS

VITAMIN C

DIETARY SOURCES, TECHNOLOGY, DAILY REQUIREMENTS AND SYMPTOMS OF DEFICIENCY

NUTRITION AND DIET RESEARCH PROGRESS

Additional books in this series can be found on Nova's website
under the Series tab.

Additional e-books in this series can be found on Nova's website
under the e-book tab.

BIOCHEMISTRY RESEARCH TRENDS

Additional books in this series can be found on Nova's website
under the Series tab.

Additional e-books in this series can be found on Nova's website
under the e-book tab.

VITAMIN C

DIETARY SOURCES, TECHNOLOGY, DAILY REQUIREMENTS AND SYMPTOMS OF DEFICIENCY

RAQUEL GUINÉ, Ph.D.
EDITOR

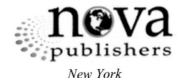

New York

For permission to use material from this book please contact us:
Telephone 631-231-7269; Fax 631-231-8175
Web Site: http://www.novapublishers.com

NOTICE TO THE READER

The Publisher has taken reasonable care in the preparation of this book, but makes no expressed or implied warranty of any kind and assumes no responsibility for any errors or omissions. No liability is assumed for incidental or consequential damages in connection with or arising out of information contained in this book. The Publisher shall not be liable for any special, consequential, or exemplary damages resulting, in whole or in part, from the readers' use of, or reliance upon, this material. Any parts of this book based on government reports are so indicated and copyright is claimed for those parts to the extent applicable to compilations of such works.

Independent verification should be sought for any data, advice or recommendations contained in this book. In addition, no responsibility is assumed by the publisher for any injury and/or damage to persons or property arising from any methods, products, instructions, ideas or otherwise contained in this publication.

This publication is designed to provide accurate and authoritative information with regard to the subject matter covered herein. It is sold with the clear understanding that the Publisher is not engaged in rendering legal or any other professional services. If legal or any other expert assistance is required, the services of a competent person should be sought. FROM A DECLARATION OF PARTICIPANTS JOINTLY ADOPTED BY A COMMITTEE OF THE AMERICAN BAR ASSOCIATION AND A COMMITTEE OF PUBLISHERS.

Additional color graphics may be available in the e-book version of this book.

Library of Congress Cataloging-in-Publication Data

ISBN: 978-1-62948-154-8

Library of Congress Control Number: 2013948788

Published by Nova Science Publishers, Inc. † New York

CONTENTS

PREFACE

Vitamin C is one of the most important components to include in a regular diet, being a powerful vitamin that provides a number of very important health benefits and that can affect multiple body processes. Because vitamin C is not produced by our body, we need to ingest daily amounts of this nutrient for our body to function properly and prevent disease. Undoubtedly, the best way to ingest vitamin C is through food, and fruits and vegetables are particularly rich in this vitamin. Citrus fruits, for example, are famous for including generous dosages of vitamin C. However, cooking or processing will deplete some of the vitamin C that needs to be ingested by the body.

Vitamin C is a cofactor in at least eight enzymatic reactions, including several collagen synthesis reactions that, when dysfunctional, cause the most severe symptoms of scurvy. Vitamin C is also known to help prevent colds and flu, but it is much more than that, it is a potent antioxidant, that fights free radicals in the body thus preventing premature aging, gives strength to bones and teeth, strengthens blood capillaries, fights infections, strengthens the immune system, it also helps reduce the level of triglycerides and bad cholesterol in the blood, and even helps in the absorption of iron, preventing anemia. Furthermore, the antioxidants in vitamin C help warding off inflammation, infections, and viruses, and, by helping to build proteins in various types of cellular constructions, vitamin C also protects against heart attacks and strokes, promoting in general a better vascular health and longevity. Studies suggest that vitamin C may even be important in preventing Alzheimer's disease or autoimmune problems, as well as atherosclerosis.

This book is aimed at gathering valuable information about this important vitamin, including sources of this nutrient with so important biological properties, the effects of processing and a number of different approaches to the roles of this powerful vitamin in the human body.

By preparing this book I intended to give an updated contribution to the knowledge about this vitamin and I truly believe that the updated information that is provided here will help people in general and professionals in particular.

I wish to thank all the authors for their valuable contributions and the reviewers for their precious help on improving the contents of each chapter. I also wish to thank Nova Science Publishers for the opportunity to produce this book, that I hope you may find interesting and most of all useful.

Raquel P. F. Guiné

LIST OF CONTRIBUTORS

Ana Rodríguez-Bernaldo de Quirós
Department of Analytical Chemistry,
Nutrition and Food Science University of Santiago de Compostela,
Campus Vida s/n, 15782 Santiago de Compostela , Spain.
E-mail: ana.rodriguez.bernaldo@usc.es

Ayman EL-Meghawry EL-Kenawy
Department of Molecular biology,
Genetic Engineering and Biotechnology Inst.,
University of Menofia,
Sadat City, Egypt.
Temporary address: Saudi Arabia- Taif – College of Medicine -Taif University.
E-mail: elkenawyay@yahoo.com

Bréhima Diawara
Département Technologie Alimentaire /IRSAT/CNRST
03 BP 7047 Ouagadougou 03 Burkina Faso, Tel: (00226) 70898243
Email: b.diawara@yahoo.fr

Challaghatta Seenappa Shiva Shankar Reddy
Laboratory of Gerontology, Department of Zoology
Bangalore University, Bangalore 560 056, India
E-mail: ssreddy6@gmail.com

Charles Parkouda
Département Technologie Alimentaire /IRSAT/CNRST
03 BP 7047 Ouagadougou 03 Burkina Faso,
Tel: (00226) 70308930
Email: cparkouda@yahoo.fr

Daniel Prá
Laboratório de Nutrição Experimental – Universidade de Santa Cruz do Sul - UNISC
Programa de Pós Graduação Promoção da Saúde- UNISC
(Prédio 42, sala 4206;
Prédio 31, Sala 3137)
Av. Independência, 2293 Santa Cruz do Sul/RS, 968215-900, Brazil.
E-mail: dpra@unisc.br

Daniela Leffa
Laboratório de Biologia Celular e Molecular,
Universidade do Extremo Sul Catarinense – UNESC,
Av. Universitária, 1105 (Bloco S, Sala 21), Criciúma/SC, 88806-000, Brazil
E-mail: daniela_leffa@yahoo.com.br

Edite Teixeira de Lemos
Department of Food Industry, Polythecnic Institute of Viseu, Portugal, and
IBILI – Institute for Biomedical Imaging and Life Sciences, Faculty of Medicine,
University of Coimbra, Portugal
Quinta da Alagoa, Estrada de Nelas
3500-606 Viseu, Portugal.
E-mail: etlemos2@gmail.com

Goreti Botelho
Food Science and Technology Department,
CERNAS Research Unit,
Coimbra College of Agriculture,
Polytechnic Institute of Coimbra,
Bencanta, 3040-316 Coimbra, Portugal.
E-mail: goreti@esac.pt

Hosam Eldin Osman
Department of Anatomy, faculty of medicine, Al Azhar University,
Cairo, Egypt
Temporary address: Saudi Arabia- Taif – College of Medicine -Taif University.
E-mail: semsemcairo61@yahoo.com

Hyeonho Yun
Department of Marine Bio-materials and Aquaculture
Department of Fisheries Biology (Graduate)
Feeds and Foods Nutrtion Research Center (FFNRC)
Pukyong National University
Busan 608-737, Korea
yun841007@nate.com

Iqbal Ahmad
Department of Pharmaceutical Chemistry, Institute of Pharmaceutical Sciences,
Baqai Medical University, Toll Plaza, Super Highway,
Gadap Road, Karachi-74600, Pakistan.
E-mail: iqbal.ahmed@baqai.edu.pk

Ivana Lavanda
School of Nutrition, Faculty of Health Sciences, Maimonides University,
Hidalgo 775, Ciudad de Buenos Aires, Argentina.
E-mail: nutricion@maimonides.edu

Ivy S. C. Pires
Departamento de Nutrição, Faculdade de Ciências Biológicas e da Saúde,
Universidade Federal dos Vales do Jequitinhonha e Mucuri.
Rodovia MGT 367 - Km 583, n° 5000 - Alto da Jacuba, Diamantina, 39100-000.
Minas Gerais, Brasil.
E-mail: ivycazelli@gmail.com

Jan Svejgaard Jensen
Planting and Landscape Majsmarken 1
7190 Billund, Denmark Tel: (0045) 40213410
Email: jsj@plantningoglandskab.dk

Julia López-Hernández
Department of Analytical Chemistry,
Nutrition and Food Science University of Santiago de Compostela,
Campus Vida s/n, 15782 Santiago de Compostela, Spain.
E-mail: julia.lopez.hernandez@usc.es

Juliana da Silva
Laboratório de Genética Toxicológica, Universidade Luterana do Brasil - ULBRA,
Av. Farroupilha, 8001 (Prédio 22, Quarto Andar, Sala 22),
Canoas/RS, 92425-900, Brazil.
E-mail: juliana.silva@ulbra.br

Koji Yashiro
Department of Chemistry, Fujita Health University School of Medicine,
Toyoake, Japan
E-mail: yashiro@fujita-hu.ac.jp

Kumar Katya
Department of Marine Bio-materials and Aquaculture
Department of Fisheries Biology (Graduate)
Feeds and Foods Nutrtion Research Center (FFNRC)
Pukyong National University
Busan 608-737, Korea; kumarkatya85@gmail.com

Luís Pedro Teixeira de Lemos
Faculty of Medicine, University of Coimbra, Portugal
Polo III - Health Sciences Campus
Azinhaga Santa Comba, Celas
3000-548 Coimbra | PORTUGAL
lupelemos@gmail.com

Marcela A. Leal
School of Nutrition Director, Faculty of Health Sciences, Maimonides University,
Hidalgo 775, Ciudad de Buenos Aires, Argentina.
E-mail: leal.marcela@maimonides.edu

Marcia N. C. Harder
Department of Agroindustry, Technology College of Piracicaba "Dep. Roque Trevisan",
FATEC Piracicaba,
Av. Diácono Jair de Oliveira, 651, Santa Rosa, 13.417-155 Piracicaba, Brazil.
E-mail: marcia.harder@fatec.sp.gov.br

Marco Aguiar
PhD student at Sport Sciences Department,
University of Trás-os-Montes e Alto Douro, 5000-911 Vila Real, Portugal.
E-mail: mvdaguiar@gmail.com

Maria João Reis Lima
Department of Food Industry, Polythecnic Institute of Viseu,
and
Educational Technologies and Health Study Center
Quinta da Alagoa, Estrada de Nelas 3500-606 Viseu, Portugal
E-mail: mjoaolima@esav.ipv.pt

Marisa Nunes
Laboratório de Genética Toxicológica, Universidade Luterana do Brasil - ULBRA,
Av. Farroupilha, 8001 (Prédio 22, Quarto Andar, Sala 22), Canoas/RS, 92425-900,
Brazil.
E-mail: marisafernanda@dermakos.com.br

Marium Fatima Khan
Department of Pharmaceutics, Institute of Pharmaceutical Sciences,
Baqai Medical University,
Toll Plaza, Super Highway, Gadap Road, Karachi-74600, Pakistan.
E-mail: marium87@gmail.com

Milton C. Ribeiro
Pós Graduação Profissional em Ensino e Saúde,
Faculdade de Ciências Biológicas e da Saúde,
Universidade Federal dos Vales do Jequitinhonha e Mucuri.
Rodovia MGT 367 – Km 583, nº 5000 - Alto da Jacuba, Diamantina,
39100-000. Minas Gerais, Brasil.
E-mail: miltoncribeiro@gmail.com

Muhammad Ali Sheraz
Department of Pharmaceutics, Institute of Pharmaceutical Sciences,
Baqai Medical University,
Toll Plaza, Super Highway, Gadap Road, Karachi-74600, Pakistan.
E-mail: ali_sheraz80@hotmail.com

Paula B. Arthur
Department of Radiobiology and Enviroment,
Center of Nuclear Energy in Agriculture, University of São Paulo, CENA/USP
Av. Centenário, 303, São Judas, 13.400-000 Piracicaba, Brazil.
E-mail: paula.arthur@hotmail.com

Roberta Nunes
Laboratório de Genética Toxicológica, Universidade Luterana do Brasil - ULBRA,
Av. Farroupilha, 8001 (Prédio 22, Quarto Andar, Sala 22),
Canoas/RS, 92425-900, Brazil.
E-mail: robertaulbra@gmail.com

Said Said Elshama
Department of Forensic Medicine and Clinical Toxicology - College of Medicine
Suez Canal University, Ismailia, Egypt.
Temporary address: Saudi Arabia- Taif – College of Medicine -Taif University.
E-mail:saidelshama@yahoo.com

Sambe Asha Devi
Laboratory of Gerontology, Department of Zoology
Bangalore University, Bangalore 560 056, India
E-mail: sambe.ashadevi@gmail.com

Silvia Isabel Rech Franke
Laboratório de Nutrição Experimental – Universidade de Santa Cruz do Sul - UNISC
Programa de Pós Graduação Promoção da Saúde- UNISC
(Prédio 42, sala 4206; Prédio 31, sala 3137)
Av. Independência, 2293 Santa Cruz do Sul/RS, 968215-900, Brazil.
E-mail: silviafr@unisc.br

Sofia Ahmed
Department of Pharmaceutics, Institute of Pharmaceutical Sciences,
Baqai Medical University,
Toll Plaza, Super Highway, Gadap Road, Karachi-74600, Pakistan.
E-mail: sofia.ahmed@baqai.edu.pk

Suely S. H. Franco
Department of Radiobiology and Enviroment,
Center of Nuclear Energy in Agriculture, University of São Paulo, CENA/USP
Av. Centenário, 303, São Judas, 13.400-000 Piracicaba, Brazil.
E-mail: gilmita@uol.com.br

Sungchul C. Bai
Department of Marine Bio-materials and Aquaculture
Department of Fisheries Biology
Feeds and Foods Nutrition Research Center (FFNRC), Pukyong National University
Busan 608-737, Korea
scbai@pknu.ac.kr

Valter Arthur
Department of Radiobiology and Enviroment,
Center of Nuclear Energy in Agriculture, University of São Paulo, CENA/USP
Av. Centenário, 303, São Judas, 13.400-000 Piracicaba, Brazil.
E-mail: arthur@cena.usp.br

Vanessa A. Ferreira
Departamento de Nutrição, Faculdade de Ciências Biológicas e da Saúde,
Universidade Federal dos Vales do Jequitinhonha e Mucuri.
Rodovia MGT 367 - Km 583, nº 5000 - Alto da Jacuba, Diamantina,
39100-000. Minas Gerais, Brasil.
E-mail: vanessa.nutr@ig.com.br

Vanessa Andrade
Laboratório de Biologia Celular e Molecular,
Universidade do Extremo Sul Catarinense – UNESC,
Av. Universitária, 1105 (Bloco S, Sala 21), Criciúma/SC, 88806-000, Brazil
E-mail: vma@unesc.net

Vivian Kahl
Laboratório de Genética Toxicológica, Universidade Luterana do Brasil - ULBRA,
Av. Farroupilha, 8001 (Prédio 22, Quarto Andar, Sala 22),
Canoas/RS, 92425-900, Brazil.
E-mail: vivian.kahl@gmail.com

Yoshiji Ohta
Department of Chemistry, Fujita Health University School of Medicine, Toyoake, Japan
E-mail: yohta@fujita-hu.ac.jp

In: Vitamin C
Editor: Raquel Guiné

ISBN: 978-1-62948-154-8
© 2013 Nova Science Publishers, Inc.

Chapter 1

VITAMIN C SUPPLEMENTATION: FAVORABLE OR NOXIOUS?

Juliana da Silva[1,*], Daniel Prá[2,†], Vivian Kahl[1,‡],
Marisa Nunes[1,§], Roberta Nunes[1,#], Vanessa Andrade[3,**],
Daniela Leffa[3,††] and Silvia Isabel Rech Franke[2,‡‡]
[1]Laboratório de Genética Toxicológica,
Universidade Luterana do Brasil - ULBRA, Canoas/RS, Brazil
[2]Laboratório de Nutrição Experimental –
Universidade de Santa Cruz do Sul – UNISC,
Programa de Pós Graduação Promoção da Saúde- UNISC,
Santa Cruz do Sul/RS, Brazil
[3]Laboratório de Biologia Celular e Molecular,
Universidade do Extremo Sul Catarinense – UNESC, Criciúma/SC, Brazil

ABSTRACT

Vitamin C (Vit C; ascorbic acid), found in fresh fruits and vegetables, is an important micronutrient, mainly required as a cofactor for enzymes involved in oxi-reduction reactions. Humans, other primates, some fish species, bats, and guinea pigs do not synthesize the Vit C. This vitamin is one of the most commonly consumed antioxidants, as a food supplement or medicinal drug, and it has been studied for its protective action against different chemical expositions and diseases. Vit C has been the subject of numerous studies due to its possible protective action against high cholesterol,

[*] E-mail: juliana.silva@ulbra.br.
[†] E-mail: dpra@unisc.br.
[‡] E-mail: vivian.kahl@gmail.com.
[§] E-mail: marisafernanda@dermakos.com.br.
[#] E-mail: robertaulbra@gmail.com.
[**] E-mail: vma@unesc.net.
[††] E-mail: daniela_leffa@yahoo.com.br.
[‡‡] E-mail: silviafr@unisc.br.

hypertension, and possibly some cancers, such as stomach, prostate, mouth and lung, and also due to its role in the improvement of vascular function in patients with vascular diseases. Mechanisms by which ascorbic acid act includes bioantimutagenic and desmutagenic activities, as well as regulation of DNA-repair enzymes. Then, Vit C has several biological effects, including: 1) action as targets for toxicants; 2) influence in drug metabolization/detoxification; and 3) effect in DNA repair and homeostasis. Moreover, Vit C can also induce oxidative stress when high doses are used. Vit C has been insufficiently studied for its ability to interact, either directly or indirectly, with mutagens, especially in view of the controversial results of its consumption on genome stabilization. Interaction between Vit C and transition metals can induce the formation of reactive oxygen species (ROS). Treatments with Vit C in some studies induce a cumulative genotoxic response and it can enhance DNA damage caused by different substances. Our research group has studied the different protective and harmful effects of vitamin C in relation to different agents, such as alkylating agents, metal sulfates, nicotine, amfepramone, as well as in relation to personal nutrition. This chapter compiles data from literature about Vit C and from our research results, which show that Vit C can be either beneficial, or noxious, for a biological system, depending of its' metabolic context.

1. INTRODUCTION

Vitamin C comprises two biologically-active vitamers, ascorbic acid and its two-electron reduction product dehydroascorbic acid (DHA). Most species of plants and animals synthesize ascorbic acid from glucose, but humans are unable to produce ascorbic acid endogenously. Vitamin C is an essential human nutrient that must be obtained in the diet (Benzie, 1999). Thus, this vitamin is a micronutrient that is acquired primarily through the consumption of fruit, vegetables, supplements, fortified beverages, and fortified breakfast or "ready-to-eat" cereals (WHO - World Health Organization, 2006). Ascorbic acid, the functional and primary *in vivo* form of the vitamin, is the enolic form of an α-ketolactone (2,3-didehydr L -threo-hexano-1,4-lactone). The two enolic hydrogen atoms give the compound its acidic character and provide electrons for its function as a reductant and antioxidant. Its one-electron oxidation product, the ascorbyl radical, readily dismutates to ascorbate and DHA, the two-electron oxidation products. Both the ascorbyl radical and DHA are readily reduced back to ascorbic acid *in vivo*. However, DHA can be hydrolyzed irreversibly to 2,3-diketogulonic acid. The molecular structure of ascorbic acid contains an asymmetric carbon atom that allows two enantiomeric forms, of which the L form is naturally occurring. The D-form, isoascorbic or erythorbic acid, provides antioxidant, as shown in Figure 1.1 (IOM, 2000a).

Vitamin C plays a role in numerous biological reactions, many of which are known in little detail. Over the years, it has been suggested that vitamin C could be used as a medicine against many diseases as different as common colds and cancers. Even today, there is considerable controversy about the exact role of this vitamin in human health and no agreement has been reached on the amount needed to be consumed for optimum wellbeing.

The biological functions of ascorbic acid are based on its ability to provide reducing equivalents for a variety of biochemical reactions as an antioxidant and enzyme cofactor. Because of its reducing power, vitamin C can reduce majority of physiologically relevant reactive oxygen species (ROS) (Buettner, 1993; Buettner & Jurkiewicz, 1996). Generally, ascorbic acid is regarded as a reducing agent; it is able to serve as an antioxidant in free radical-mediated oxidation processes. However, as a reducing agent it is also able to reduce redox-active metals such as copper and iron, thereby increasing the pro-oxidant chemistry of these metals. Thus ascorbate can act as both as a pro-oxidant and an antioxidant (Yin et al., 2012)

In addition, as an electron donor, vitamin C acts as a cofactor for 8 enzymes involved in collagen hydroxylation, biosynthesis of carnitine and norepinephrine, tyrosine metabolism and amidation of peptide hormones (Padayatty & Levine, 2001). As a reducer, it participates in biosynthesis of tetrahydrofolic acid, hyaluronic acid and prostaglandins. It also modulates the body's immunity by stimulating the production of immunoglobulins and interferons. However, while the systems themselves are diverse, the biochemical role played by vitamin C in each system appears to be mediated via its antioxidant properties (Benzie, 1999; Frei et al., 1989). Vitamin C is easily and reversibly oxidized into dehydro-L-ascorbic acid, creating a redox system, which allows it to act as an antioxidant. It deactivates multiple ROS: superoxide anion (O_2•-), hydrogen peroxide (H_2O_2), hydroxylradical (OH•), singlet oxygen (O_2^1), $HO_2^•$ (hydroperoxyl radical), as well as peroxides and free radicals produced with their participation.

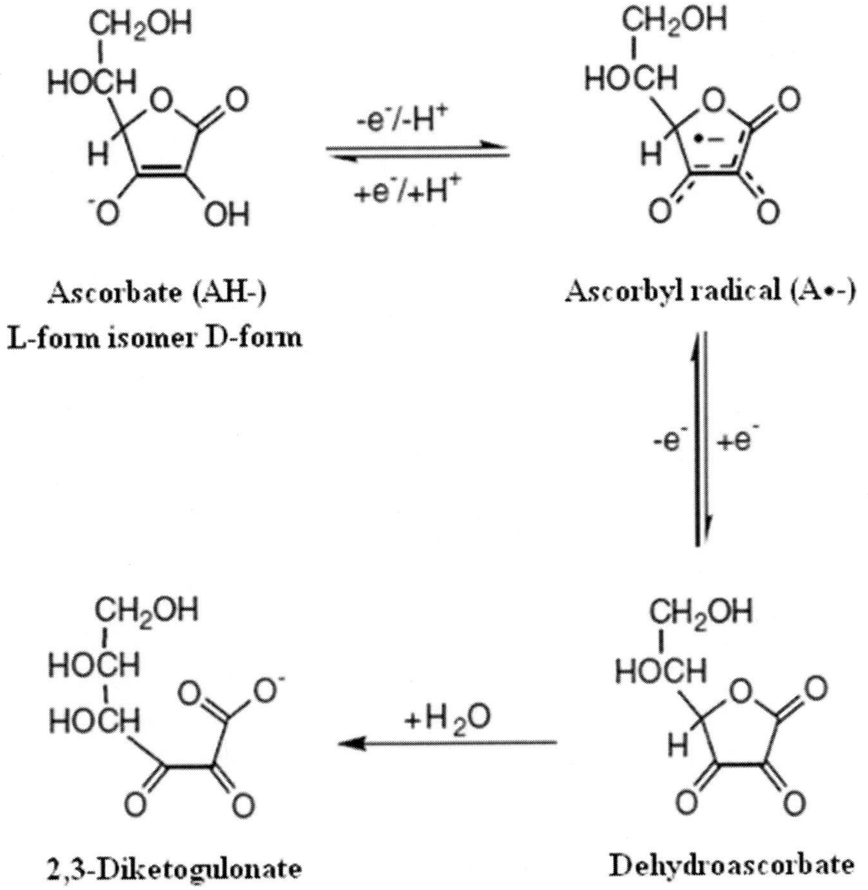

Figure 1.1. Chemical structure of ascorbic acid in relation to its redox state (IOM, 2000a).

Thanks to this it prevents reactions of these ROS with biomolecules at the stage of prevention, termination and even repair of some damages. It also regenerates vitamin E used up during similar processes. Thus, vitamin C plays an important role in eliminating oxidative stress which, in combination with its water solubility, makes it the main antioxidant of extracellular fluids. The above described processes constitute grounds for using vitamin C in prevention and therapy of diseases resulting from, or occurring with, oxidative stress. Vitamin C also takes part in detoxification of xenobiotics, contributing to the production of ROS (Rutkowski & Grzegorczyk, 2012).

Increased risk of chronic disease, including cancer, cataracts and coronary heart disease (CHD), is associated with low intake or plasma concentrations of vitamin C (Benzie, 1999; Block, 1991; Fletcher & Fairfield, 2002; Gey, 1995; Machlin, 1995; Maxwell & Lip, 1997; Riemersma, 1994). Supplementation with vitamin C is reported to decrease blood pressure and blood lipids, improve glucose metabolism and endothelial function, and to increase resistance of lipids and DNA to oxidative damage (Benzie, 1996; Frei et al., 1989; Halliwell, 1996; Levine et al., 1996; Paolisso et al., 1993; Rahman, 2007; Sweetman et al., 1997; Weber et al., 1996). However, the contribution of high intake or plasma levels of vitamin C to lowered risk of disease is difficult to assess, as other health-promoting habits generally accompany high vitamin C intake, and clinical trials have shown inconsistent and inconclusive results (Benzie, 1996; Benzie, 1999; Halliwell, 1996).

2. PHYSIOLOGICAL CONCENTRATIONS OF VITAMIN C

Vitamin C is a ubiquitous vitamin and the dietary intakes, dietary sources, bioavailability, and serum levels are described in the following subheadings.

2.1. Dietary Reference Intake (DRI) of Vitamin C

The *Dietary Reference Intakes* (DRI) are reference values that are quantitative estimates of nutrient intakes to be used for planning and assessing diets for healthy people. They set the minimum intakes to avoid symptoms of deficiency and reduce the risk of chronic diseases as well as set the maximum intake (IOM, 2000a; IOM, 200b; IOM, 2003).

The minimum intake to avoid symptoms of deficiency of vitamin C is 10 mg per day. This level is needed to prevent scurvy in adults. However, it is much lower than the level needed to promote health and wellbeing. The current DRI for vitamin C according to life stage, age, and sex are presented in Table 1.1. Recommended dietary allowance (RDA) is the daily intake used as target value for planning diets for individuals. Adequate intake (AI) is the daily intake used as target value for planning diets for individuals when there is no RDA available. The AI is based in experimental or limited epidemiological data. In the case of young infants the AI is based in gastric volume and vitamin C levels in human milk. Estimated average requirement (EAR) is the daily intake used for: (i) planning diets for groups; and (ii) assessing the prevalence of nutrition inadequacies for individuals and groups. Tolerable upper intake level (UL) is the maximum amount beyond which there is a potential risk of adverse effects for individuals and groups. UL is not used for dietary planning purposes. The symptom used to define the UL for vitamin C is diarrhea (IOM, 2000a).

It is important to take into account that the DRI are updated constantly. Health professionals must always consider the current DRI as provisional and look for their updated values when planning and assessing diets for healthy people. In the case of vitamin C, until the beginning of the 2000s, RDA for adults was 60 mg per day. At that time, higher levels were suggested for people subject to stress and for smokers. In 2000, the RDA levels were increased to 75 and 90 mg per day for adult females and males, respectively. The DRI for vitamin C was not reviewed in the time-span between 2001 and 2012. In chronic oxidative stress conditions, such as smoking, the vitamin C daily intake has to be increased by 35 mg per day, or 100 and 120 mg per day for adult females and males, respectively (Murphy & Poos, 2002).

Table 1.1. Dietary Reference Intake (DRI) of the vitamin C

Life stage group	Vitamin C (mg per day)		
	RDA or AI*	EAR	UL
Infants			
0-6 months	40*	NA	NA
7-12 months	50*	NA	NA
Children			
1-3 years	15	13	400
4-8 years	25	22	650
Males			
9-13 years	45	39	1,200
14-18 years	75	63	1,800
19-30 years	90	75	2,000
31-50 years	90	75	2,000
51-70 years	90	75	2,000
> 70 years	90	75	2,000
Females			
9-13 years	45	39	1,200
14-18 years	65	56	1,800
19-30 years	75	60	2,000
31-50 years	75	60	2,000
51-70 years	75	60	2,000
> 70 years	75	60	2,000
Pregnancy			
≤ 18 years	80	66	1,800
19-30 years	85	70	2,000
31-50 years	85	70	2,000
Lactation			
≤ 18 years	115	96	1,800
19-30 years	120	100	2,000
31-50 years	120	100	2,000

RDA: Recommended Dietary Allowance; AI: Adequate Intake; EAR: Estimated Average Requirement; UL: Tolerable Upper Intake Level; NA: not available. Source: IOM (2000a).

2.2. Dietary Sources and Bioavailability of Vitamin C

Fruits and vegetables are the richest sources of vitamin C, including several fruits such as berries and citrus fruits, followed by raw green leafy vegetables (Table 1.2). The content of vitamin C in vegetables depends on the maturity, the plant part, the seasons, and the geographic areas where they are produced (Nunes et al., 2011). Some processed or frozen foods marketed close to their source can have greater vitamin C content than unprocessed foods that travel long distances (Franke et al., 2004; Mahan et al., 2011; Peluzio & de Oliveira, 2008).

Vitamin C is the most unstable of vitamins and can be easily lost by heat, oxidation, drying, storage, alkalinity, light exposure, as well as by the interaction with transition metals. As it is water soluble, vitamin C is easily extracted and discarded in the cooking water. Sodium bicarbonate (alkaline pH), added to preserve and improve the color of cooked vegetables, also destroys vitamin C (Franke et al., 2004; Mahan et al., 2011; Peluzio & de Oliveira, 2008).

The vitamin C content of food is commonly reported as the sum of the ascorbate and its oxidized form DHA. The bioavailability of vitamin C naturally present in food and that added as supplement is the same. Some substances such as aspirin and the phenolic compound as quercetin can limit vitamin absorption (Wilson, 2005).

Table 1.2. Vitamin C level in selected fruits, fruit juices and beverages, vegetables, and spices and herbs

Food, type, portion size	mg of vitamin C
Fruit	
Acerola (West Indian Cherry), ½ cup	820
Apple, 1 medium	8
Avocado, cubes, ½ cup	8
Banana, 1 medium	10
Blackcurrants, ½ cup	100
Blueberries, ½ cup	7
Cherries, ½ cup	5
Grapefruit, ½ medium fruit	40
Guava, 1 medium fruit	126
Grapes, ½ cup	2
Kiwi fruit, 1 medium fruit	72
Lemon, 1 medium fruit	31
Mango, ½ cup	23
Melon, cantaloupe, ¼ medium fruit	51
Melon, honeydew, ⅛ medium fruit	40
Orange, 1 medium fruit	70
Papaya, cubes, ½ cup	43
Pineapple, raw, ½ cup	28
Strawberries, ½ cup	48
Tangerine or tangelos, 1 medium fruit	25
Watermelon, 1 cup	15

Food, type, portion size	mg of vitamin C
Juice (not added vitamin C)	
Apple, ½ cup	2
Grape, ½ cup	0.2
Grapefruit, ½ cup	47
Lime, ½ cup	36
Orange, ½ cup	50
Tomato, ½ cup	22
Beverages	
Cranberry juice cocktail, ½ cup	45
Vegetable juice cocktail, ½ cup	34
Vegetables	
Asparagus, cooked, ½ cup	10
Broccoli, cooked, ½ cup	51
Brussels sprouts, cooked, ½ cup	50
Purple cabbage, raw, chopped, ½ cup	20
Green cabbage, raw, chopped, ½ cup	10
Cauliflower, raw or cooked, ½ cup	25
Kale, cooked, ½ cup	55
Mustard greens, cooked, ½ cup	22
Onion, chopped, ½ cup	6
Pepper, red or green, raw, ½ cup	65
Plantains, sliced, cooked, 1 cup	15
Potato, baked, 1 medium	25
Radish, raw, ½ cup	9
Snow peas, frozen, cooked, ½ cup	20
Spinach, cooked, ½ cup	9
Sweet potato, backed, 1 medium	30
Tomato, raw, 1 medium	17
Kohlrabi, cooked, ½ cup	45
Edible pod peas, cooked, ½ cup	38
Spices and Herbs	
Parsley, raw, 1 tablespoon	5
Coriander leaf, dried, 1 tablespoon	10

Source: U.S. Department of Agriculture (2012).

2.3. Pharmacokinetics of Vitamin C

Vitamin C has 2 hydroxyl groups at positions 2 and 3 that ionize with pK values of 4.17 and 11.57. Therefore, reduced vitamin C exists predominantly as the ascorbate anion in most body fluids. DHA also occurs in biological systems. Biological systems can interconvert DHA to ascorbate and their metabolism is equivalent (Wilson, 2005).

Serum and plasma concentrations reflect the recent intake of vitamin C, while the leukocytes concentration reflects the organic reserve of the vitamin. Normal plasma concentration of vitamin C ranges from 0.8-1.4 mg/dL, whereas the leukocytes concentration ranges from 20-40 $\mu g/10^8$ cells (Tomita, 2006).

The absorption of vitamin C occurs in the intestine by facilitated diffusion and active mechanisms, several times in shared pathways with glucose (Wilson, 2005). At lower concentrations, the active transport is the predominant. At higher concentration, when the active mechanism is saturated, facilitated diffusion also occurs. The absorption of DHA is faster (about 10 times) than ascorbic acid either for intestinal or blood cells. Ascorbate absorption is downregulated by glucose transport and DHA is not. After DHA is absorbed, it is rapidly reduced to ascorbate within the intestinal cells. Due to this process, intracellular DHA is rarely found (Malo and Wilson, 2000; Tomita, 2006).

Levine et al. (1996) tested 30 to 2500 mg vitamin C in healthy volunteers and observed that no vitamin C was excreted in urine of six of seven volunteers until the 100 mg dose. At single doses of 500 mg daily and higher, bioavailability declined and the absorbed amount was excreted. Bioavailability was complete for 200 mg per day of vitamin C as a single dose. But, when vitamin C is fractionated during the day a higher absorption can occur (Tomita, 2006).

Ascorbate and DHA transport varies extensively between different cells (Tomita, 2006). Many cells have been shown to be capable of using extracellular DHA to produce intracellular ascorbate, including adipocytes, astrocytes, endothelial cells, erythrocytes, granulosa cells, hepatocytes, neutrophils, osteoblasts and smooth muscle cells. The interplay between DHA and glucose transport is not yet elucidated in biological system and deserves further attention (Wilson, 2005). Table 1.3 presents the concentration of vitamin C in key tissue and fluids.

Table 1.3. Concentration of vitamin C in key tissues and fluids

Tissue/ fluid	Concentration (mg vitamin C per 100 g)
Pituitary gland	40-50
Adrenal gland	30-40
Leukocytes	7-140
Eye (crystalline)	25-31
Brain	13-15
Liver	10-16
Spleen and pancreas	10-15
Kidney	5-15
Heart	5-15
Semen	3-10
Lungs	7
Skeletal muscle	3
Testicles	3
Cerebrospinal fluid	2-4
Thyroid gland	2
Plasma	0.3-1
Saliva	0.09

Source: Tomita (2006).

There is relatively little research on how vitamin C is transported out of cells (Franke et al., 2005a; 2005b).The excretion of ascorbate and DHA is performed by the kidneys, which maintain the homeostasis of vitamin C, but only occurs at high serum concentrations. Vitamin C is eliminated with an elimination half-life of 10 h (Malo and Wilson, 2000; Tomita, 2006).

3. EFFECTS OF VITAMIN C ON HEALTH

Vitamin C is essential to health, it plays a fundamental role in the development and regeneration of muscles, skin, teeth and bones, collagen formation, body temperature regulation, production of various hormones and metabolism in general (Gardener et al., 2000). The lack of this vitamin in the organism increases the propensity for several diseases. When the deficiency is severe the body becomes vulnerable to more serious illnesses such as scurvy. However, when consumed in high doses it may cause adverse effects such as diarrhea, abdominal pain and kidney calculus in genetically predisposed individuals (Gardener et al., 2000).

Epidemiological studies show that diets high in fruits and vegetables are associated with lower risk of cardiovascular and neurodegenerative diseases, stroke and several types of cancer (Fenech & Ferguson, 2001; Padayatty et al., 2003). The potential anticarcinogenic effects of vitamin C are related to its ability to neutralize carcinogenic substances and their antioxidant activity (Ferraz et al., 2010). The antimutagenic and anticarcinogenic mechanisms of vitamin C include bioantimutagenics and desmutagenic activities, as well as the regulation of DNA repair enzymes. In the desmutagenesis, protective agents, or antimutagenic, act directly on the compounds which induce DNA mutations, inactivating them chemically or enzymatically, inhibiting the metabolic activation of promutagenic or abducting reactive molecules. In bioantimutagenesis the antimutagenics act upon the process that leads to the induction of mutations, or repairing injuries caused to the DNA (Antunes & Araújo, 2000).

The antioxidant action mechanism attributed to vitamin C is due for its direct reaction with $O_2\bullet-$, $OH\bullet$, O_2^1, in addition to regenerate E vitamin. It also maintains thiols enzymes in their reduced states and spares glutathione peroxidase, which is an important intracellular antioxidant and enzyme cofactor (Carr & Frei, 1999). Oxidant damage might cause or exacerbate common human diseases, and due to antioxidant effect, vitamin C has been described with a protective effect (Table 1.4).

In breast carcinogenesis, ascorbic acid has its action based on the antioxidant defense (Willet, 2001). Studies have demonstrated an inverse relation between vitamin C intake and relative risk of this neoplasm kind (Gandini et al., 2000). In gastric inflammation caused by *Helicobacter pylori*, a bacterium with carcinogenic potential, vitamin C has shown an interrelation with this microorganism being capable to affect directly its growth and virulence (Correa et al., 1998; Zhang & Farthing, 2005). However, the prevention of gastric cancer does not occur only by this fact, but due to the major mechanism of vitamin C, which is the inhibition of the N-nitroso compounds and reactive oxygen metabolites inside the stomach (Bingham et al., 2002, Zhang & Farthing, 2005).

Table 1.4. The effect of vitamin C in different health conditions

Health condition	Type of research	Effects of vitamin C
Cigarette smoking	Controlled clinical trial; single oral dose (2 g)	Restores impaired coronary flow velocity reserve
Wound healing	Controlled clinical trials; oral supplementation (0.5-3 g)	Accelerated wound healing
Asthma	Double-blind, controlled trial; single oral dose (2 g)	Protective effect on airway hyperreactivity in some patients with exercise-induced asthma.
Cardiovascular disease	Controlled clinical trial; oral supplementation (2 g/day) Observational study within elderly population Double-blind, randomized, controlled, 2-waycross over trial; intraarterial administration (24 mg/min for 110 min). In vitro study; various concentrations added to human plasma	Increased fibrinolytic activity in patients with coronary artery disease. Negative correlation between serum vitamin C and total cholesterol. Improves lipid-induced impairment of endothelium-dependent vasodilation. Completely protects human plasma from lipid peroxidation.
Neurodegenerative disorders	Cross-sectional and prospective study; vitamin C end vitamin E supplementation Mouse behavioral models; intraperitoneal injection (60 and 120 mg)	Reduced prevalence and incidence of Alzheimer disease in elderly population. Memory-restorative action, particularly in aged mice.
Cancer	In vitro study; dose concentration studies and pharmacokinetic modeling In vitro human lymphoma cell study Case-control prospective study In vitro B16 murine melanoma cell study	Toxicity to various cancer cells. Action as a pro-drug to deliver hydrogen peroxide to tissues. Inverse association of gastric cancer risk with high levels of plasma vitamin C. Induces the apoptosis in melanoma cells.
Diabetes mellitus	Controlled trial; intraarterial infusion(<1g)	Improves endothelium-dependent vasodilation.
Cataract	Probability survey of Americans	Importance for the prevention of cataract among older Americans.

Source: Domitrović (2006).

The function of vitamin C in the prevention of cardiovascular diseases is currently well documented. It is believed that vitamin C protects against lipid peroxidation, besides interfering on other factors related to cardiovascular risk, such as vascular tissue integrity, vascular tone, lipid metabolism and blood pressure. Whereas ascorbic acid is an essential cofactor in collagen molecular formation and may therefore interfere in the elasticity and structural integrity of the vascular matrix. It also seems to exert a vasodilator and anticoagulant effect through relocation of prostacyclin production and other prostaglandins (Jacob, 1998).

A study conducted with 15 patients from 9 to 20 years, with familiar hyper-cholesterolemia (LDL > 130mg/dL) used vitamin E supplements (400 UI/day) and C (500 mg/day) for six weeks. The authors observed the restoration of endothelial function in dyslipidemic children with the medicated supplementation and concluded that supplementing is essential for children with dyslipidemia, since only 20% of them consume five or more servings of fruits and vegetables per day (Engler et al., 2003).

In addition, vitamin C improves the endothelial dysfunction, at an early stage of atherosclerosis among smokers (Ames, 2001). The current dietary recommendation for vitamin C considers, at least to some degree, the protective effect of vitamin C, and even indicates higher levels of intake for smokers and people with high stress levels (Ames, 2001). In type I diabetes, the association of vitamin C to good glycemic control is able to improve epithelial dysfunction present in this pathology (Ceriello et al., 2007).

Vitamin C intake may reduce the effects of aging, mainly through its antioxidant action (Pallas, 2002).It has been shown that vitamin C decreases the proteins glycation, thus slowing the aging process (Bartali et al., 2003; Krone & Ely, 2004, Nelson et al., 2003). A study on skin aging and intake of foods rich in vitamin C showed that women with the lowest intake of these foods had a more wrinkled skin, dry and withered, than women who had a good intake of foods rich in this nutrient (Cosgrove et al., 2007).

Results of studies with large amounts of vitamin C to prevent and cure common cold have been reported in the literature since the early 1970s. Since then, several studies demonstrated that vitamin C ameliorates the symptoms of colds, although placebo-effect seems to bias the conclusion (Mahan et al., 2011). A recent comprehensive meta-analysis (Hemilä & Chalker, 2007) was designed to evaluate if oral doses of 200 mg per day or more of vitamin C could be beneficial in common colds. The main conclusion was that vitamin C can reduce the incidence, duration or severity of the common cold when used as continuous prophylaxis (regularly every day) or as therapy after onset of symptoms. It also indicated a failure of vitamin C supplementation to reduce the incidence of colds in the general population. This aspect indicates that routine prophylaxis is not justified for the overall population. While the prophylaxis trials have consistently shown that vitamin C reduces the duration and alleviates the symptoms of colds, this was not replicated in the few therapeutic trials that have been carried out so far. Therefore, further therapeutic research clinical trials should be developed (Hemilä & Chalker, 2007).

Vitamin C supplementation seems to be beneficial to other respiratory illnesses. A review covering three prophylactic trials (37 cases of pneumonia in 2335 people) concluded that vitamin C supplementation may be reasonable for pneumonia patients who have low vitamin C plasma levels because its cost and risks are low. The review also indicated the need of more studies (Hemilä & Louhiala, 2007).

There are evidences that severe physical exercise decrease mucosal immunity (Bishop & Gleeson, 2009), and that vitamin C could be useful for athletes exposed to brief periods of exercises (Hemilä & Chalker, 2007). It is also important to emphasize the role that this vitamin plays in promoting the resistance against infections, which occurs due to its involvement with the immunological activity of leukocytes, interferon production, inflammatory reaction process and mucous membranes integrity (Mahan & Stump-Scott, 2005).

4. ANTIOXIDANT AND PRO-OXIDANT EFFECT OF VITAMIN C

Oxidative DNA damages are due to oxidative stress. This happens when there is an imbalance between the formation and elimination of ROS. ROS are generated as byproducts of oxidative metabolism which was a milestone in the evolution, it has generated an increased metabolic efficiency. On the other hand, also increase instability in biological systems, for 2-5% of all oxygen is converted into ROS metabolized. These reactive oxygen species are primarily responsible for the basal level of mutations (Halliwell & Guterridge, 2000). It is estimated that a person suffers about 10,000-20,000 ROS attack by free radicals and other cells per day as part of normal oxidative metabolism. For an athlete in intense training, these attacks can increase about 50% (Valko et al., 2005).

ROS include a vast number of molecules chemically derived from oxygen. The most important ROS are $O_2^{\cdot-}$, H_2O_2, nitric oxide (NO), OH• and O_2^1 (Imai & Nakagawa, 2003; Saffi & Henriques 2003; Slupphaug et al., 2003). ROS attack DNA, giving rise to many lesions, including base modifications and apurinic/apyrimidinic sites, deletions, single strand breaks, frameshifts, chromosomal rearrangements, and causing cross-linkages between DNA and proteins. The discovery that 8-hydroxy-deoxyguanosine (8-OHdG) is one of the most prevalent oxidation products has motivated studies on its role in the carcinogenic process (Cerda & Weitzman, 1997; Dizdaroglu et al., 2002; Goldman & Shields, 2003; Picada et al., 2003; Saffi & Henriques, 2003; Risom et al., 2005).

The effects of ROS depend not only on their levels but are also influenced by the chemical environment, as well as the distance between the site where damage is produced and the target tissue, considering the potential distribution and half-life of the free radicals and ROS (Halliwell & Guterridge, 2000; Linder, 2001). Thus, if ROS are not effectively eliminated, they can cause various cellular effects, such as lipid peroxidation, cytotoxicity and oxidative DNA damage (Cerda & Weitzman, 1997; Halliwell, 2001).

The oxidative modification of proteins by ROS is also associated with the source or progression of various diseases and physiological disorders. Additionally, oxidants can affect gene expression through oxidation-reduction mechanisms, which can regulate protein-protein and protein-DNA interactions (Cerda & Weitzman, 1997). Such structural change can cause partial or total inactivation of protein function (Halliwell & Guterridge, 2000).

All cells of eukaryotic organisms are endowed with antioxidant enzymes, which control the levels of ROS, and the set of them is known as enzymatic antioxidant defense mechanism (Iannitti & Palmieri, 2009; Sies, 1997). The three major antioxidant enzymes of this mechanism are superoxide dismutase (SOD), catalase (CAT) and glutathione peroxidase (GPx). As SOD is responsible for the dismutation of $O_2^{\cdot-}$, the catalase decomposes H_2O_2 into molecular oxygen and water. Glutathione, in its turn, acts as an intracellular reducing agent. There are also some secondary enzymes of this mechanism, such as glucose-6-phosphate dehydrogenase and glutathione reductase (Iannitti & Palmieri, 2009). In addition to the enzymatic defenses are still non-enzymatic antioxidants such as glutathione, vitamin E (tocopherol), vitamin C, flavonoids and other molecules such as ß-carotene and N-acetylcysteine (Borella & Varela, 2004). These antioxidants act mainly by blocking the lipid peroxidation chain, eliminating oxygen or chelating metal ions (Sies, 1993).

Vitamin C is a water soluble nutrient involved in multiple biological functions. Additionally, it is important in the absorption of dietary iron, due to its ability to reduce ferric form (Fe^{3+}) to ferrous (Fe^{2+}), providing absorption of non-heme iron in the gastrointestinal tract (Halliwell, 2001; Kagan et al., 1990; Loureiro et al., 2002). Besides the important anti-scorbutic function, vitamin C is a powerful reducing agent ($E^{o'}= -170mV$), capable of minimizing most of the physiologically relevant oxygen/nitrogen reactive species (Halliwell & Gutteridge, 2000).

In recent years, great interest has been focusing on the role of oxygen reactive species in several diseases etiology (Halliwell, 2001). Vitamin C antioxidant properties are thus attracting attention to preventive nutrition, once it protects the food constituents against oxidative damage and may also contribute to preventing major diseases such as cardiovascular disease, aging, cancer, among others.

There are several studies on vitamin C supplementation in humans by using biomarkers of oxidative damage to DNA, lipids (lipid oxidation releases mutagenic aldehydes) and proteins. Although there are studies presenting ambiguous answers, the vitamin C antioxidant activity is in agreement with those who show an antioxidant effect *in vitro*, it corroborate with the beneficial effects of this compound. It must be emphasized, however, that the pro-oxidant role of the compound may represent health risks when consumed is high levels (Paoloni-Giacobino et al., 2003).

Carr & Frei (1999) have observed the antioxidant action of the vitamin C for lipids in biological fluids, both in animals and in human beings. Several studies have also proven that foods (Alleva et al., 2012), fresh fruits (Nunes et al., 2011) and frozen fruits (Spada et al., 2008), rich in vitamin C, promote an antioxidant protection against oxidative stress in mice (Nunes et al., 2011), yeast (Spada et al., 2008) and humans (Alleva et al., 2012). Through vitamin C supplementation, the levels of 8-OHdG were significantly reduced (Cooke et al., 1998; Sram et al., 2012). The oxidative stress caused by H_2O_2 has also been significantly reduced by the administration of this vitamin in human lymphocytes *in vitro* (Harreus et al., 2005) and *ex vivo* (Collins et al., 2001). In another recent study, the intake of vitamin C presented direct correlation between longer telomeres and lower risk of breast cancer (Shen et al., 2009). Such result also demonstrates the antioxidant action of the vitamin C since the telomeric shortening is associated with the mechanism of oxidative stress (Von Zglinicki, 2002).

5. MUTAGENICITY AND ANTIMUTAGENICITY OF THE VITAMIN C

As we have discussed before, vitamin C is an important micronutrient and has been studied for its protective action against different diseases. Some studies have shown that vitamin C can display ambiguous effects. Given controversial mutagenic effects, some results from our group will be discussed below.

5.1. Effects of Vitamin C Over Transition Metals

Vitamin C can interact with transition metals. It can either reduce or increase the toxicity of the metals, depending on physicochemical aspects such as molecular structure and valence. Iron and copper are among the most relevant transition metals because they are ubiquitous and have relevant biological roles. Therefore, this section will focus on iron and copper.

Transition metals can catalyze the oxidation of vitamin C, generating both glyoxal and hydrogen peroxide (Hara et al., 2009; Shangari et al., 2007). The pro-oxidant effect of vitamin C is likely to depend upon the transition metal concentration. In line, iron-induced pro-oxidant effect was shown to be mild when dietary iron concentration was low and strong at high dietary iron (Premkumar et al., 2007).

Vitamin C is the second most-abundant antioxidant water-soluble low molecular in the human serum, after urate. Vitamin C and urate inhibit the oxidation of each other and reduce the copper-induced peroxidation *ex vivo* (Samocha-Bonet et al., 2005). Vitamin C can also modulate the level of DNA damage induced by metals. Franke et al (2005a) treated mice with a single dose of iron (33.23 mg Fe/kg) or copper (8.25 mg Cu/kg) as sulfates and, after 24 hours, treated the mice again with a single dose of vitamin C (1 or 30 mg/kg). They observed that the post-treatment with both doses increased the level of primary DNA damage induced by the metals as evaluate by the comet assay. This DNA damage increase can be interpreted in three ways: i) a pro-oxidant effect of the metals leading to DNA damage increase; ii) the alkaline version of the comet assay simultaneously detects different kinds of DNA damage, such as cross-links, strand breaks, alkali-labile and incomplete excision repair events. Thus, it is possible to detect an increase in DNA strand breaks as a consequence of a stimulus in DNA repair; iii) an increase in apoptosis (Franke et al., 2005a), i.e. reduction in the number of damaged cells and, therefore, reduction in the DNA damage captured by the assay. In favor to the DNA repair-increase hypothesis, it was shown that vitamin C stimulates some DNA repair pathways (Cooke et al., 1998).

In humans, iron supplementation (ferrous glycine sulphate equivalent to 12.5 mg iron or 0.5 mg/kg day for an average adult for 6 weeks) had no effect on the oxidative damage to DNA in female and male volunteers with high serum vitamin C (mean plasma vitamin C approximately equal to 70 micromol/L). Further studies evaluating the interplay between vitamin C and iron are needed particularly among children whose supplementation with iron can be as high as 2mg/kg/day (WHO, 2006).

There is a lack of studies evaluating the effect of copper supplementation in individuals with high serum levels of vitamin C. As copper deficiency is much rarer its supplementation is not common.

The above presented evidence indicates that further studies are needed to evaluate the interaction between vitamin C and transition metals *in vivo* in humans. The fact that humans cannot synthesize vitamin C and most rodents can limits the possibility of extrapolating results obtained with rodents to humans. The available evidence in humans indicates that vitamin C does not induce DNA damage (Crott & Fenech, 1999) itself at least when used in physiologic doses, but when at high concentrations vitamin C is pro-oxidant.

5.2. Effects of Vitamin C Over Alkylating Agents

Alkylating drugs are widely used as mutagen/carcinogen chemotherapeutic agents. Vitamin C can interact with alkylating agents, reducing their toxicity. Vitamin C was shown to modulate the level of DNA damage induced by alkylating agents. Franke et al (2005b) treated mice with methyl methanesulfonate (40 mg/kg) or cyclophosphamide (25 mg/kg) and 24 later treated the animals with a single dose of vitamin C (1 and 30 mg/kg). The authors observed a decreased in the level of primary DNA damage induced by methyl methanesulfonate, but not by cyclophosphamide at the lower vitamin C dose. Again, the potential of vitamin C to stimulate DNA repair pathways may explain the result (Cooke et al., 1998). Also, vitamin C could have acted as a target for reactive species or metabolites generated by the alkylating agents. Other studies showed that vitamin C (2-200 mg/kg) was antimutagenic against cyclophosphamide while simultaneous oral administration of Vit C with intraperitonel administration of the drug (Ghaskadbi et al., 1992) or when administered twice, one dose 24 h prior to the cyclophosphamide (51.6 mg/kg) administration and the second dose simultaneously with the cyclophosphamide (Gurbuz et al., 2009).

Vitamin C also reduced the toxicity of cyclophosphamide when liposomes containing the drug plus vitamin C were used as drug delivery system (Tohamy et al., 2012). Vitamin C was also shown to reduce the *in vivo* mutagenicity of N-ethyl-N-nitrosourea (Aidoo et al., 1994). Co-administration of Vitamin C (200 mg/kg) was capable of reducing abnormalities in the lipid profile of fibrosarcoma-bearing rats treated for 120 days with cyclophosphamide (10 mg/kg), methotrexate (1 mg/kg) and 5-fluorouracil (10 mg/kg) in combination (Muralikrishnan et al., 2001).

5.3. Effects of Vitamin C in Diabetes

There are two common types of diabetes. Type 1 diabetes affects 5-10% and type 2 diabetes affects 90-95% of the diabetic individuals. While type 1 diabetes is an autoimmunity-triggered lack of insulin production, type 2 diabetes is a decrease in body response to insulin (resistance). Type 2 diabetes is more related to inadequate lifestyle (Kloppel et al., 1985). Type 2 diabetes is a common condition that affects mainly adults, but recently has become a serious health problem also among young individuals. Diabetes prevalence is increasing more rapidly in the developing countries. It is estimated that diabetes will affect 5% of the world population by 2030. The prevalence of diabetes for all age-groups worldwide was estimated to be 2.8% in 2000 and 4.4% in 2030. This situation can be much higher among adults, particularly within those with 65 years old or more (Wild et al., 2004).

Diabetes is marked by increased oxidative stress, which leads to micro and macrovascular complications, encompassing inefficient wound-healing, vasculopathy, nephropathy and retinopathy (Selvaraju et al., 2012). The serum level of vitamin C in diabetics is lowered (Fadupin et al., 2007).

Several studies have shown that vitamin C can improve metabolic dysfunctions associated to diabetes, among other mechanism by its antioxidant potential (Afkhami-Ardekani & Shojaoddiny-Ardekani, 2007; Choi et al., 2005). There is growing evidence linking diabetes to oxidative stress. Oxidative stress has been shown to be involved in many of the micro and macrovascular complications associated to diabetes. Glucose, while in excess, auto-oxidizes and leads to oxidative stress. Besides its antioxidant action in diabetes, vitamin C has been shown to modulate glucose transport (Castro et al., 2008). Oxidative stress generates DNA damage in diabetes. In another models of oxidative stress, vitamin C modulated DNA damage and repair (Franke et al., unpublished data). Therefore, it is possible that a modulation of oxidative stress mediated by vitamin C could also occur in diabetes. In agreement, Choi et al. (2005) evaluated the relationship between fasting plasma ascorbic acid and DNA damage in lymphocytes in 427 individuals with type 2 diabetes and observed a negative correlation between DNA damage and serum ascorbic acid, indicating that vitamin C protects against DNA damage in diabetes in a dose-related manner. Additionally, our results support that intakes of vitamin C higher than 200 mg per day can reduce the level of glycated hemoglobin and DNA damage in individuals with type 2 diabetes (Franke et al., unpublished data). Although this intake is superior than the dietary recommendation for individuals with increased oxidative stress (about 120 mg/day) it is lower than the levels of vitamin C ingested by individuals with a healthy diet (i.e. at least 5 portion of fruits and vegetables daily, according to WHO and National Cancer Institute of the United States).

5.4. Effects of Vitamin C in Obesity

Obesity is a chronic disease that has become a serious public health concern worldwide. The incidence of obesity has reached epidemic proportions in industrialized and semi industrialized nations across the globe. According to the WHO, over 300 million adults world-wide were classified as obese in 2005, and this figure had risen to 500 million in 2008 (Ong et al., 2013).

This disease is a metabolic disorder associated with social and psychological factors, genetic predisposition, and dietary habits (Bartolomucci et al., 2009), and it affects all ages and social classes (Chinn & Rona, 2001). The worldwide increase in obesity is related to changes in eating patterns and the intake of hypercaloric foods (Naska et al., 2011), such as high-fat, low fiber-rich foods (Ledikwe et al., 2005; Washi & Ageib, 2010), vegetables, fruits (Boutelle et al., 2007; Washi & Ageib, 2010) and the intake of sweetened beverages (Flood et al., 2006). This eating pattern may alter micronutrient status in obese patients, since snack foods tends to be high in sugar, sodium, and fat and relatively low in vitamins and minerals (Washi & Ageib, 2010).

In addition, obesity is characterized by the excessive buildup of adipose tissue, which is associated with the development of chronic diseases, characterized by excessive oxidative stress, like cardiovascular diseases, diabetes, metabolic syndrome and cancers (Eikelis et al., 2003).

Epidemiologic and laboratory studies indicate that a high consumption of antioxidant-rich fruit and vegetables can reduce the risk of cancer (Lee et al., 2003). Vitamin C is considered to be one of the most prevalent antioxidative components of fruit and vegetables, and it could exert chemopreventive effect (Lee et al., 2003). Our recent study, evaluated different type of cells, of Swiss male mice, treated with vitamin C in association with a fat- and sugar-rich diet named cafeteria diet (CAF). During 13 weeks animals were fed with CAF or standard chow (STA). After this period the animals were divided into three groups and received treatment orally, for 4 weeks: CAF plus water, CAF plus vitamin C (1 mg/kg) and STA plus water. After, samples of blood and tissues like kidney, liver and brain were collected for DNA analyzes by comet assay and bone marrow for micronucleus (MN) test. The genotoxicity of CAF was evaluated by CA and showed that CAF group presented significantly higher damage than control group (STA) in both parameters of comet assay, damage frequency and damage index, in all tissues and peripheral blood. In addition, the CAF plus vitamin C group had DNA damage significantly higher than the STA group in blood, liver and brain. The antigenotoxic potential of ascorbic acid was evaluated and the group CAF plus vitamin C reduced significatively the high levels of DNA damage showed in the CAF group, in kidney and liver. The mutagenic effect detected by MN test was increased in the frequency of micronucleated polychromatic erythrocytes at CAF group in relation at the control group and, in this assay the ascorbic acid was not capable to reverse these damages (Leffa et al., unpublished data).

In conclusion, our results showed that CAF leads to damage to the genetic material in blood, liver, kidney, brain and bone marrow cells, probably due to increased oxidative stress. However, ascorbic acid supplementation reduces DNA damage induced by a high fat diet in kidney and liver of animals. These results suggest that vitamin C intake is efficient for alleviating oxidative stress by modulating the antioxidant system in a cafeteria diet. Further clinical studies are required to support this proposal and also to establish the beneficial and protective effects of ascorbic acid resulting from reduced DNA damage levels in obesity-related metabolic disorders.

5.5. Vitamin C and Cardiovascular Disease Risk Factors

Cardiovascular diseases (CVD) are multifactor slow-progressing pathologies (Argiles et al., 1998), which might start forming early in childhood, but manifest later in middle age and is a leading cause of death (Lloyd-Jones et al., 1999). The risk of developing CVD is related to a set of characteristics or risk factors that interact to increase the probability of developing CVD; these characteristics include metabolic and hemodynamic disturbances, as well as an unhealthy diet and physical inactivity (Wu 1999).

Several studies have demonstrated that oxidative stress can contribute to CVD progression (Wattanapitayakul & Bauer 2001). For instance, a diet rich in saturated fat and poor in micronutrients with antioxidant properties (such as vitamins A and C) may increase the formation of oxidized lipids and reduce antioxidant reactions, leading to oxidative stress thereby increasing the risk of developing CVD (Obrenovich et al., 2011; Poulsen, 2005).

Thus, the intake of antioxidant vitamins not as supplements, but within a healthy diet, reduces CVD risks (Eichholzer et al., 2001, Obrenovich et al., 2011). Despite controversies, there is evidence that antioxidant vitamins may inhibit LDL oxidation to its more atherogenic form, therefore preserving the inhibition of atherosclerotic plaque formation (Wattanapitayakul & Bauer 2001). Vitamin C is also associated with lower levels of primary and permanent DNA damage. An inverse relationship between vitamin C intake and CVD mortality has been shown (Simon, 1992), and the effect of vitamin C on DNA damage has been studied (Franke et al., 2005).

Our recent study (Kliemann et al., 2012) evaluated the association between CVD risk factors and DNA damage levels in children and adolescents. DNA damage levels were accessed by the comet assay and cytokinesis-blocked MN assays in leukocytes. A total of 34 children and adolescents selected from a population sample were divided into three groups according to their level of CVD risk. Moderate and high CVD risk subjects showed significantly higher body fat and serum CVD risk markers than low risk subjects. High risk subjects also showed a significant increase in DNA damage, which was higher than that provided by low and moderate risk subjects according to comet assay, but not according to the cytokinesis-blocked micronucleus assay. Vitamin C intake was inversely correlated with DNA damage by comet assay. The present results indicate an increase in DNA damage that may be a consequence of oxidative stress in young individuals with risk factors for CVD, indicating that the DNA damage level can be reduced with a good diet.

5.6. Effects of Vitamin C in Amfepramone Treatment

The amfepramone or diethylpropion is an anorexic drug, which acts on the Central Nervous System (CNS), by a catecholaminergic mechanism, increasing the release of catecholamines in neural terminals and/or inhibiting its recapture (Samarin & Garattini, 1993). Before the prohibition in 2011, this type of medicine was one of the most commonly used drugs for years in obesity treatment in Brazil (Planeta & De Lúcia, 1998) and its action has a psychoactive effect, suppressing appetite by voluntarily reducing food intake.

Therefore, our study aimed to evaluate the mutagenic activity of amfepramone in human beings by the micronuclei test in buccal mucosa cells and also the effect of vitamin C supplementation and its possible protective action. The study involved a total of 108 women, characterized as follows: 52 women participated in the control group and 56 women were users of amfepramone. All the study participants were assessed at two points: 1st collection, with at least one month of amfepramone consumption and 2nd collection after 30 days of concomitant use of amfepramone with vitamin C. The amfepramone doses were 120 mg/day (divided into two intakes per day) throughout the research period and vitamin C supplementation was given at a dosage of 1000 mg/daily. Results demonstrated the mutagenic activity of the drug amfepramone in humans; and individuals who consumed amfepramone and were supplemented with vitamin C for 30 days demonstrated a significant decrease in the micronucleus frequency. Based on our results and on previous reports (Snyder et al., 2009; 2010), we can suggest that the main mechanism of action of amfepramone in inducing DNA damage occurs through the formation of ROS, intercalation and topoisomerase binding, caused by the presence of a N-dialkyl group in its molecule. In addition, we can suggest that vitamin C presented an important effect in inhibiting amfepramone-induced DNA damage. This protective effect induced by the vitamin C might be related to its role as a free radical scavenger and the DNA repair enzymes regulation (Bjelakovic et al., 2012; Cooke et al., 1998; Halliwell, 2001; Lunec et al., 2002; Thomas et al., 2007).

5.7. Vitamin C and Nicotine

Nicotine is an alkaloid present in many plants, and highly expressed in tobacco leaves (*Nicotiana tabacum*), acting as a natural insecticide (Leete, 1983). The main concern about the toxic effects of nicotine present in tobacco is related to a smoking habit. Mutagenicity of nicotine has been evaluated, with various outcomes, which can be attributed to differences between genotoxicity parameters evaluated, to repair capacity between various cells types used and, furthermore, to differences on doses (Adler & Attia, 2003; Argentin & Cichetti, 2004; Attia, 2007; Guarnieri et al., 2008).

Nicotine absorption increases with the amount of contact surface, and therefore, dermal contact by tobacco farmers, with tobacco leaves, is a pathway of exposure. Hence, the larger the contact surface the greater the nicotine absorption (Da Silva et al., 2012a). When leaves are wet, or when farmers are with skin bruises, the absorption is significantly increased. Absorption is also affected by variables that influence vasodilatation as heat, temperature, alcohol consumption and smoking (Quandt et al., 2000). Nicotine is absorbed and metabolized by cytochrome P450 (CYP450), a superfamily of enzymes responsible for the metabolism of many xenobiotics. The enzyme cytochrome P450 2A6 (CYP2A6) is responsible for metabolizing 90% of nicotine (Nakajima et al., 1996; Tricker, 2003). Da Silva et al. (2012b) analyzed genetic polymorphisms and their relationship with mutagenicity in individuals exposed to nicotine from tobacco leaves in tobacco fields. Results showed that, of the various genes analyzed, the genotype *CYP2A6*9*1/*1* protected the genetic material against micronucleus generation on cells from oral mucosa, indicating a relationship between genetic susceptibility and damage caused by nicotine (Da Silva et al., 2012b). Other studies demonstrated mutagenic effect of nicotine (Adler & Attia, 2003; Arabi, 2004; Argentin & Cichetti, 2004; Da Silva et al., 2010; Munzner & Renner, 1989).

Attia (2007) and Da Silva et al. (2010) noted that antioxidants protect DNA against damages caused by nicotine, suggesting that nicotine genotoxicity may be, at least in part, mediated by a mechanism of oxidative stress. Messner et al. (2012), using humans endothelial cells incubated with the tar fraction of cigarettes found that after 5 hours of incubation occurred a significant increase in ROS, indicating high oxidative stress. Furthermore, high level of oxidative stress, observed in who exercise and smokers, are associated with high production of 8-OHdG (Huang et al., 2000). Jacobson et al. (2000) performed a study aimed to identify the possible antioxidants effects of vitamins intake (C, E and β-carotene) in smokers. First of all, they found that smokers, regardless of ingesting vitamins or placebo, showed elevated levels of 8-OHdG. Plasma levels of the three antioxidants significantly increased in the smoking group, but the DNA damage evaluated showed no statistic difference between the groups. In a recent work from our group, at a dose of 1mg/kg, as recommended by the USDA (U.S. Department of Agriculture, 2005), vitamin C showed an antigenotoxic potential related to nicotine, up to 99% when used in pre-treatment on mice (Kahl et al., 2012). The study analyzed the possible antigenotoxic and antimutagenic activities of vitamin C against DNA damage induced by nicotine in mice. At three times of blood collection after nicotine administration (2h, 4h and 24h), it was observed that starting from 4h, vitamin C in pre-treatment, protected the genetic material from blood cells of animals. Vitamin C also decreased the micronucleus frequency in reticulocytes induced by nicotine, demonstrating its antimutagenic potential (Kahl et al., 2012).

For human smokers, a seven days supplementation with vitamin C decreased significantly the micronucleus frequency, which are cytogenetic markers of mutation (Schneider et al., 2001), while DNA repair activities were increased to smokers with high levels of oxidative stress with 500mg of vitamin C daily intake for 4 weeks (Guarnieri et al., 2008). The exposure to nicotine, through the smoking habit, increases plasma levels of DNA adducts of type polycyclic aromatic hydrocarbons (PAH), which are reduced when vitamin C intake occurs (Grinberg-Funes et al., 1994). Micronutrients (Fenech & Bonassi, 2011), vegetables and fruits intake (Franke, 2006; Guarnieri et al., 2008; Riso et al., 2010), and also the influence of polymorphisms of xenobiotics (Grinberg-Funes et al., 1994; Riso et al., 2010) appear to contribute to individual differences observed with respect to human response to treatment with antioxidants such as vitamin C.

It is possible, therefore, that the nicotine genotoxic effect is mediated by an oxidative stress mechanism and that vitamin C protects the genetic material acting as antioxidant (Attia, 2007; Da Silva et al., 2010; Kahl et al., 2012). Nevertheless it is important to consider that vitamin C impact on human health and, particularly, on DNA damage, depends on both individual levels of vitamin C as individual level of exposure to xenobiotics or oxidative stress (Sram et al., 2012).

CONCLUSION

Vitamin C is the only antioxidant vitamin which intake as supplement is not associated to increased mortality among well-nourished populations (Biesalski et al., 2010; Bjelakovic et al., 2007). There is evidence that slight intake of vitamin C is enough to cause oxidative stress protection, and protection against diseases (IOM, 2000a). This fact indicates that the noxious effects of vitamin C supplementation at typical doses are likely to be very limited. Vitamin C usage must be more relevant to populations with low vitamin C status due to under-nourishment or diets with lack of fruits and vegetables.

There is suggestive evidence showed by our research group and others researchers that vitamin C may act in DNA repair. If vitamin C may stimulate DNA repair, the DRI could be increased for the general population (referred to pollution and diets deficient in micronutrients), and not just for smokers or individuals with high levels of oxidative stress, as has been advocated by dietary guidelines (IOM, 2000a). It is worth remembering that eating five servings of fruits and vegetables, recommended to the prevention of chronic degenerative diseases, can provide at least 200 mg per day of vitamin C, clearly above the DRI set in 2000 (75-90 mg vitamin C day (Franke et al., 2005b) for adult women and men, respectively).

There is evidence that higher dietary intakes of vitamin C reduces the level of DNA damage in several human conditions such as early cardiovascular risk (Kliemann et al., 2012), diabetes (Franke et al., unpublished data) and obesity (Leffa et al., unpublished data). The supplementation of vitamin C (120 mg/day) was shown to reduce DNA damage associated to anfepramone, an anorexigenic drug (Nunes, 2011). Also, vitamin C was shown to reduce the DNA damage associated with nicotine (Kahl et al., 2012).

Vitamin C supplementation did not appear to cause DNA damage under normal physiological conditions nor did it protect cells against hydrogen peroxide-induced toxicity (Crott & Fenech, 1999). This fact summed to the potential of vitamin C to act as pro-oxidant when in higher concentrations, leads to the concept that vitamin C supplementation can be suggested up to certain levels. In line, negative interaction with metals could lead to increased oxidative stress.

The levels of supplementation seem not to be any higher than 2 g/day, given the risk of renal calculi. However, further studies are needed to define the ideal intake of vitamin C to increase genome stability. Importantly, decisions regarding vitamin C supplementation should be evaluating all available evidence and weighting all probability risk against the likelihood of benefit (Mahan et al., 2011). The clinical decision must take into consideration most recently available scientific information and follow the evidence-based medicine principles.

ACKNOWLEDGEMENTS/REVISION

The present chapter has been reviewed by:

- Alexandre de B. F. Ferraz (PhD), Programa de Pós-Graduação em Biologia Celular e Molecular Aplicada à Saúde, Universidade Luterana do Brasil (ULBRA), Canoas, RS, Brazil.
- Fernanda Rabaioli da Silva (PhD), Programa de Pós-Graduação em Biologia Celular e Molecular, Universidade Federal do Rio Grande do Sul (UFRGS), Porto Alegre, RS, Brazil.

REFERENCES

Adler, I. D. & Attia, S. M. (2003). Nicotine is not clastogenic at doses of 1 or 2 mg/kg body weight given orally to male mice. *Mutation Research, 542,* 139-142.

Afkhami-Ardekani, M. & Shojaoddiny-Ardekani, A. (2007). Effect of vitamin C on blood glucose, serum lipids & serum insulin in type 2 diabetes patients. *Indian Journal of Medical Research 126*, 471-474.

Aidoo, A.; Lyn-Cook, L. E.; Lensing, S. & Wamer, W. (1994). Ascorbic acid (vitamin C) modulates the mutagenic effects produced by an alkylating agent *in vivo. Environment and Molecular Mutagenesis, 24,* 220-228.

Alleva, R.; Di Donato, F.; Strafella, E.; Staffolani, S.; Nocchi, L.; Borghi, B.; Pignotti, E.; Santarelli, L. & Tomasetti, M. (2012). Effect of ascorbic acid-rich diet on *in vivo*-induced oxidative stress. *British Journal of Nutrition, 107,* 1645-1654.

Ames, B.N. (2001). DNA damage from micronutrient deficiencies is likely to be a major cause of cancer. *Mutation Research, 475*, 7-20.

Antunes, L. & Araujo, M. (2000) Mutagenicidade e antimutagenicidade dos principais corantes para alimentos. *Revista de Nutrição, 13(2),* 81-88. Campinas, Sao Paulo.

Arabi, M. (2004). Nicotine infertility: assessing DNA and plasma membrane integrity of human spermatozoa. *Andrologia, 36*, 305-310.

Argentin, G. & Cichetti, R. (2004) Genotoxic and antiapoptotic effect of nicotine on human gingival fibroblasts. *Toxicological Sciences*, 79, 75-81.

Argiles, J. M.; Carbo N.; Costelli, P. & Lopez-Soriano, F. J. (1998). Prevention of cancer and cardiovascular diseases: a common strategy? *Medicinal Research Reviews, 18,* 139-148.

Attia S.M. (2007). The genotoxic and cytotoxic effects of nicotine in the mouse bone marrow. *Mutation Research, 632,* 29-36.

Bartali, B.; Salvini, S.; Turrini, A.; Lauretani, F.; Russo, C. R.; Corsi, A. M.; Bandinelli, S.; D'Amicis, A.; Palli, D.; Guralnik, J. & Ferrucci, L. (2003). Age and disability affect dietary intake. *The Journal of Nutrition, 133*, 2868-2873.

Bartolomucci, A.; Cabassi, A.; Govoni, P.; Ceresini, G.; Cero, C.; Berra, D.; Dadomo, H.; Franceschini, P.; Dell'Omo, G.; Parmigiani, S. & Palanza, P. (2009). Metabolic consequences and vulnerability to diet-induced obesity in male mice under chronic social stress. *PLoS ONE, 4,* 1-12.

Benzie, I. F. (1996). Lipid peroxidation: a review of causes, consequences, measurement and dietary influences. *International Journal of Food Sciences and Nutrition, 47,* 233-261.

Benzie, I. F. (1999). Vitamin C: prospective functional markers for defining optimal nutritional status. *Proceedings of the Nutrition Society, 58,* 469-476.

Bingham, S. A.; Hughes, R. & Cross A. J. (2002). Effect of white versus red meat on endogenous: N-nitrosation in the human colon and further evidence of a dose response. *The Journal of Nutrition, 132,* 3522S-3525S.

Bishop, N. C. & Gleeson, M. (2009). Acute and chronic effects of exercise on markers of mucosal immunity. *Frontiers in Bioscience, 14,* 4444-4456.

Bjelakovic, G.; Nikolova, D.; Gluud, L. L.; Simonetti, R. G. & Gluud, C. (2007). Mortality in randomized trials of antioxidant supplements for primary and secondary prevention: systematic review and meta-analysis. *JAMA, 297,* 842-857.

Bjelakovic, G.; Nikolova, D.; Gluud, L. L.; Simonetti, R. G. & Gluud, C. Antioxidant supplements for prevention of mortality in healthy participants and patients with various diseases. Cochrane Database of Systematic Reviews. 2012. Available from: http://endosgine.com/core/pdfs/Antioxidant_supplements_for_prevention_of_mortality_i n_healthy_participants_and_patients_with_various_diseases.PDF.

Block, G. (1991). Vitamin C and cancer prevention: The epidemiologic evidence. *The American Journal of Clinical Nutrition, 53,* 270S-282S.

Boutelle, K. N.; Fulkerson, J. A.; Neumark-Sztainer, D.; Story, M. & French, S. A. (2007). Fast food for family meals: relationships with parents and adolescent food intake, home food availability and weight status. *Public Health Nutrition, 10,* 16-23.

Buettner G. R. & Jurkiewicz B. A. (1996). Catalytic metals, ascorbate and free radicals: combinations to avoid. *Radiation Research, 145,* 532-541.

Buettner, G. R. (1993). The pecking order of free radicals and antioxidants: Lipid peroxidation, alpha-tocopherol, and ascorbate. *Archives of Biochemistry and Biophysic, 300,* 535-543.

Carr, A. C. & Frei, B. (1999).Toward a new recommended dietary allowance for vitamin C based on antioxidant and health effects in humans. *The American Journal of Clinical Nutrition, 69,* 1086-1107.

Castro, M. A.; Angulo, C.; Brauchi, S.; Nualart, F. & Concha, I. (2008). Ascorbic acid participates in a general mechanism for concerted glucose transport inhibition and lactate transport stimulation. *Pflugers Archiv - European Journal of Physiology, 457(*2), 519-528.

Cerda, S. & Weitzman, S. (1997). Influence of oxygen radical injury on DNA methylation. *Mutation Research, 386,* 141-152.

Ceriello, A.; Kumar, S.; Piconi, L.; Esposito, K. & Giugliano, D. (2007). Simultaneous control of hyperglycemia and oxidative stress normalizes endothelial function in type 1 diabetes. *Diabetes Care, 30,* 649-54

Chinn, S. & Rona, R. J. (2001). Prevalence and trends in overweight and obesity in three cross sectional studies of British Children, 1974-1994. *British Medical Journal, 322,* 24–26.

Choi, S. W.; Benzie, I. F. F.; Lam, C. S. Y; Chat, S. W. S.; Lam, J.; Yiu, C. H.; Kwan, J. J.; Tang, Y. H.; Yeung, G. S. P.; Yeung, V. T. F.; Woo, G. C.; Hannigan, B. M. & Strain, J. J. (2005). Inter-relationships between DNA damage, ascorbic acid and glycaemic control in Type 2 diabetes mellitus. *Diabetic Medicine, 22,* 1347-1353.

Collins, B. H.; Horská, A.; Hotten, P. M.; Riddoch, C. & Collins, A. R. (2001). Kiwifruit protects against oxidative DNA damage in human cells and *in vivo*. *Nutrition and Cancer, 39,* 148-153.

Correa, P.; Malcom, G; Schmidt, B.; Fontham, E.; Ruiz, B.; Bravo, J. C.; Bravo, L. E.; Zarama, G. & Realpe, J. L. (1998). Antioxidant micronutrients and gastric cancer. *Alimentary Pharmacology & Therapeutics, 12,* 73-82.

Cooke, M. S.; Evans, M. D.; Podmore, I. D.; Herbert, K. E.; Mistry, N.; Mistry, P.; Hickenbotham, P. T.; Hussieni, A.; Griffiths, H. R. & Lunec, J. (1998). Novel repair action of vitamin C upon *in vivo* oxidative DNA damage. *FEBS Letters, 439,* 363-367.

Crott, J. W. & Fenech, M. (1999). Effect of vitamin C supplementation on chromosome damage, apoptosis and necrosis *ex vivo*. *Carcinogenesis 20,* 1035-1041.

Cosgrove, M. S. *(*2007*)*. Histone proteomics and the epigenetic regulation of nucleosome mobility. *Expert Review of Proteomics, 4,* 465–478.

Da Silva, F. R.; Erdtmann, B.; Dalpiaz, T.; Nunes, E.; Da Rosa, D. P.; Porawski, M.; Bona, S.; Simon, C. F.; Allgayer, M. C. & Da Silva, J. (2010). Effects of dermal exposure to *Nicotiana tabacum* (Jean Nicot, 1560) leaves in mouse evaluated by multiple methods and tissues. *Journal of Agricultural and Food Chemistry, 58,* 9868-9874.

Da Silva, F. R.; Da Silva, J.; Allgayer, M. C.; Simon, C. F.; Dias, J. F.; Santos, C. E. I.; Salvador, M.; Branco, C.; Schneider, N. B.; Kahl, V.; Rohr, P. & Kvitko, K. (2012a). Genotoxic biomonitoring of tobacco farmers: biomarkers of exposure, of early biological effects and of susceptibility. *Journal of Hazardous Materials,* 225-226.

Da Silva, F. R.; Da Silva, J.; Nunes, E.; Benedetti, D.; Kahl, V.; Rohr, P.; Abreu, M.B.; Thiesen, F. V. & Kvitko, K. (2012b). Application of the buccal micronuleus cytome assay and analysis of PON1Gln192Arg and CYP2A6*9(-48T>G) polymorphisms in tobacco farmers. *Environmental Molecular Mutagenesis, 53,* 525-534.

Dizdaroglu, M.; Jaruga, P.; Birincioglu, M. & Rodriguez, H. (2002). Free radical-induced damage to DNA: mechanisms and measurement. *Free Radic Biol Med.;32(11),* 1102-15.

Domitrovic, R. (2006). Vitamin C in disease prevention and therapy. *Biochemia Medica, 16,* 89–228.

Eikelis, N.; Schlaich, M.; Aggarwal, A.; Kaye, D. & Esler, M. (2003). Interactions between leptin and the human sympathetic nervous system. *Hypertension, 41,* 1072–1079.

Eichholzer, M.; Luthy, J.; Gutzwiller, F & Stahelin, H. (2001). The role of folate, antioxidant vitamins and other constituents in fruit and vegetables in the prevention of cardiovascular disease: the epidemiological evidence. *International Journal for Vitamin and Nutrition Research, 71,* 5-17.

Engler, M. M.; Engler, M. B.; Malloy, M. J.; Chiu, E. Y.; Scholoetter, M. C.; Paul, S. M.; Stuehlinger, M.; Lin, K.; Cooke, J.; Morrow, J.; Ridker, P.; Rifai, N.; Miller, E.; Witztum, J. & Mietus-Snyder, M. (2003). Antioxidant vitamins C and E improve endothelial function in children with hyperlipidemia: Endothelial Assessment of Risk from Lipids in Youth (EARLY) Trial. *Circulation, 108,* 1059-63.

Fadupin, G. T.; Akpoghor, A. U. & Okunade, K. A. (2007). A comparative study of serum ascorbic acid level in people with and without type 2 diabetes in Ibadan, Nigeria. *African Journal of Medicine and Medical Sciences, 36,* 335-339.

Fenech, M. & Ferguson, L. R. (2001). Vitamins/minerals and genomic stability in humans. *Mutation Research, 18,* 1-6.

Fenech, M. & Bonassi, S. (2011). The effect of age, gender, diet and lifestyle on DNA damage measured using micronucleus frequency in human peripheral blood lymphocytes. *Mutagenesis, 26,* 43-49.

Ferraz, C. M.; Steluti, J. & Marchioni, D. M. L. (2010). As vitaminas e minerais relacionados à estabilidade genômica e a proteção ao câncer. *Revista da Sociedade Brasileira de Alimentação e Nutrição, São Paulo, 35,* 181-199.

Fletcher, R. H. & Fairfield, K. M. (2002). Vitamins for chronic disease prevention in adults: clinical applications. *JAMA: The Journal of the American Medical Association, 287,* 3127-3129.

Flood, J. E.; Roe, L. S. & Rolls, B. J. (2006). The effect of increased beverage portion size on energy intake at a meal. *Journal of the American Dietetic Association, 106,* 1984–1990.

Franke, S. I. R.; Ckless, K.; Silveira, J. D.; Rubensam, G.; Brendel, M.; Erdtmann, B. & Henriques, J. A. P. (2004). Study of antioxidant and mutagenic activity of different orange juices. *Food Chemistry, 88,* 45-55.

Franke, S. I. R.; Pra, D.; da Silva, J.; Erdtmann, B. & Henriques, J. A. (2005a). Possible repair action of Vitamin C on DNA damage induced by methyl methanesulfonate, cyclophosphamide, FeSO4 and CuSO4 in mouse blood cells *in vivo. Mutation Research, 583,* 75-84.

Franke, S. I. R.; Pra, D.; Erdtmann, B.; Henriques, J. A. & da Silva, J. (2005b). Influence of orange juice over the genotoxicity induced by alkylating agents: an *in vivo* analysis. *Mutagenesis, 20,* 279-283.

Franke, S. I. R. (2006). *Suco de laranja e vitamina C: efeito sobre a estabilidade genômica.* Tese de doutorado. Programa de Pós-Graduação em Biologia Celular e Molecular, Universidade Federal do Rio Grande do Sul (UFRGS). Porto Alegre, RS: UFRGS.

Frei, B.; England, L. & Ames, B. N. (1989). Ascorbate is an outstanding antioxidant in human blood plasma. *Proceedings of the National Academy of Sciences of the United States of America, 86,* 6377–6381.

Gandini, S.; Merzenich, H.; Robertson, C. & Boyle, P. (2000). Meta-analysis of studies on breast cancer risk and diet: the role of fruit and vegetable consumption and intake of associated micronutrients. *European Journal of Cancer, 36,* 636-646.

Gardener, P. T.; White T. A. C.; McPhail, D. B. & Duthie, G. G. (2000). The relative contributions of vitamin C, carotenoids and phenolics to the antioxidant potential of fruit juices. *Food Chemistry, 68,* 471-474.

Ghaskadbi, S.; Rajmachikar, S.; Agate, C.; Kapadi, A. H. & Vaidya, VG. (1992). Modulation of cyclophosphamide mutagenicity by vitamin C in the in vivo rodent micronucleus assay. *Teratogenesis, Carcinogenesis, and Mutagenesis, 12,* 11-17.

Gey, K. F. (1995). Ten-year retrospective on the antioxidant hypothesis of arteriosclerosis: Threshold plasma levels of antioxidant micronutrients related to minimum cardiovascular risk. *The Journal of Nutritional Biochemistry, 6,* 206–236.

Goldman, R. & Shields, P. G. (2003). Food mutagens. *Journal of Nutrition,133,* 965S-973S.

Grinberg-Funes, R. A.; Singh, V. N.; Perera, F. P.; Bell, D. A.; Young, T. L.; Dickey, C.; Wang, L.W & Santella, R. M. (1994). Polycyclic aromatic hydrocarbon-DNA adducts in smvokers and their relationship to micronutrient levels and the glutathione- S-transferase M1 genotype, *Carcinogenesis, 15,* 2449-2454.

Guarnieri, S.; Loft, S.; Riso, P.; Porrini, M.; Risom, L.; Poulsen, H. E. & Dragsted, P. (2008). DNA repair phenotype and dietary antioxidant supplementation, *The British Journal of Nutrition, 99,* 1018–1024.

Gurbuz, N.; Ozkul, A. & Burgaz, S. (2009). Effects of vitamin C and N-acetylcysteine against cyclophosphamide-induced genotoxicity in exfoliated bladder cells of mice *in vivo. Journal of B.U.ON. : Official Journal of the Balkan Union of Oncology, 14,* 647-652.

Halliwell, B. (2001). Vitamin C and genomic stability. *Mutation Research, 475,* 29–35.

Halliwell, B. (1996). Antioxidants in human health and disease. *Annual Review of Nutrition, 16,* 33–50.

Halliwell, B. & Guterridge, J. M. C. (2000). *Free radicals in biology and medicine.* New York, NY: Oxford University Press.

Hara, S.; Mizukami, H.; Mukai, T.; Kurosaki, K.; Kuriiwa, F. & Endo, T. (2009). Involvement of extracellular ascorbate and iron in hydroxyl radical generation in rat striatum in carbon monoxide poisoning. *Toxicology, 264,* 69-73.

Harreus, U.; Baumeister, P.; Zieger, S. & Matthias, C. (2005). The influence of high doses of vitamin C and zinc on oxidative DNA damage. *Mutation Research, 681,* 51-67.

Hemilä, H. & Louhiala, P. Vitamin C for preventing and treating pneumonia. Cochrane Database of Systematic Reviews. 2007. Available from: http://dx.doi.org/10.1002/14651858.CD005532.pub2.

Hemilä, H. & Chalker, E. Vitamin C for preventing and treating the common cold. Cochrane Database of Systematic Reviews. 2007. Available from: http://onlinelibrary.wiley.com/doi/10.1002/14651858.CD000980.pub4.

Huang, H.Y.; Helzlsouer, J. & Appel, L. J. (2000). The Effects of Vitamin C and Vitamin E on Oxidative DNA Damage: Results from a Randomized Controlled Trial. *Cancer Epidemiology, Biomarkers & Prevention, 9,* 647-652.

Iannitti, T. & Palmieri, B. (2009). Antioxidant therapy effectiveness: an up to date. *European Review for Medical and Pharmacological Sciences, 13,* 245-278.

Imai, H. & Nakagawa, Y. (2003). Biological significance of phospholipid hydroperoxide glutathione peroxidase (PHGPx, GPx4) in mammalian cells. *Free Radical in Biology and Medicine, 34,* 145-169.

IOM (2000a). Institute of Medicine. *Dietary Reference Intakes for Vitamin C, Vitamin E, Selenium, and Carotenoids.* Food and Nutrition Board. Washington, DC: National Academy Press.

IOM (2000b). Institute of Medicine. *Dietary Reference Intakes: Applications in Dietary Assessment.* Food and Nutrition Board. Washington, DC: National Academy Press.

IOM (2003). Institute of Medicine. *Dietary Reference Intake: Applications in Dietary Planning.* Food and Nutritional Board. Washington, DC: National Academy Press.

Jacobson, J. S.; Begg, M. D.; Wang, L. W.; Wang, Q.; Agarwal, M.; Norkus, E.; Singh, V. N.; Young, E. L.; Yang, D. & Santella, R. M. (2000). Effects of a 6-month vitamin intervention on DNA damage in heavy smokers. *Cancer Epidemiology, Biomarkers & Prevention, 9,* 1303-1311.

Kagan, V. E.; Serbinova, E. A. & Packer, L. (1990). Generation and recycling of radicals from phenolic antioxidants. *Archiv Biochem. Biophys., 280(1)*, 33-39.

Kahl, V. F. S.; Reyes, J. M.; Sarmento, M. S. & da Silva, J. (2012). Mitigation by vitamin C of the genotoxic effects of nicotine in mice, assessed by the comet assay and micronucleus induction. *Mutation Research, 744*, 140-144.

Kliemann, M.; Prá, D.; Müller, L. L.; Hermes, L.; Horta, J. A.; Reckziegel, M. B.; Burgos, M. S.; Maluf S. W.; Franke, S. I. R. & Silva, J. D. (2012). DNA damage in children and adolescents with cardiovascular disease risk factors. *Anais da Academia Brasileira de Ciências, 84:*833-40.

Kloppel, G.; Lohr, M.; Habich, K.; Oberholzer, M. & Heitz P. U. (1985). Islet pathology and the pathogenesis of type 1 and type 2 diabetes mellitus revisited. *Survey and Synthesis of Pathology Research, 4*, 110-125.

Krone, C.A. & Ely, J. T .A. (2004). Ascorbic acid, glycation, glycohemoglobin an aging. *Medical Hypotheses, 62*, 275-279.

Ledikwe, J. H.; Blanck, H. M.; Khan, L. K.; Serdula, M. K.; Seymour, J. D.; Tohill, B. C. & Rolls, B. J. (2005). Dietary energy density determined by eight calculation methods in a nationally representative United States population. *Journal of Nutrition, 135*, 273–278.

Lee, K. W.; Lee, H. J.; Surh, Y. J. & Lee, C. Y. (2003). Vitamin C and cancer chemoprevention: reappraisal. *The American Journal of Clinical Nutrition, 78*, 1074-1078.

Leete, E. (1983). Biosynthesis and metabolism of the tobacco alkaloids. In S. W. Pelletier (Ed.), *Alkaloids Chemical and Biological Perspectives* (1st edition, 96-139). New York, NY: John Wiley and Sons.

Levine, M.; Conry-Cantilena, C.; Wang, Y.; Welch, R. W.; Washko, P. W.; Dhariwal, K. R.; Park, J. B.; Lazarev, A.; Graumlich, J. F.; King, J. & Cantilena, L. R. (1996). Vitamin C pharmacokinetics in healthy volunteers: evidence for a recommended dietary allowance. *Proceedings of the National Academy of Sciences of the United States of America, 93*, 3704-3709.

Linder, M. C. (2001). Copper and genomic stability in mammals. *Mutation Research, 475*, 141- 152.

Lloyd-Jones, D. M.; Larson, M. B.; & Levy, D. (1999). Lifetime risk of developing coronary heart disease. *Lancet, 353*, 89-92.

Loureiro, A. P.; Marques, S. A.; Garcia, C. M.; Di Mascio, P. & Medeiros, M. H. G. (2002). Development of an on-line liquid chromatography-electrospray tandem mass spectrometry assay to quantitatively determine 1,N2-etheno-2'-deoxyguanosine in DNA. *Chemical Research in Toxicology, 15*, 1302-1308.

Lunec, J.; Holloway, K. A.; Cooke, M. S.; Faux, S.; Griffiths, H. R. & Evans, M. D. (2002). Urinary 8-oxo-2-deoxyguanosine: redox regulation of DNA repair *in vivo. Free Radical Biology & Medicine, 33*, 875–885.

Machlin, L. J. (1995). Critical assessment of the epidemiological data concerning the impact of antioxidant nutrients on cancer and cardiovascular disease. *Critical reviews in food science and nutrition, 35*, 41-50.

Mahan, L. K.; Escott-Stump, S. & Raymond, J. L. (2011). *Krause's Food & the Nutrition Care Process*. Portland, Or: Elsevier Health Sciences.

Mahan, M. L. & Scott-Stump, S. E. (2005). *Alimentos, nutrição & dietoterapia* (11st ed.) São Paulo, SP: Roca.

Malo, C.; Wilson, J. X. (2000). Glucose modulates vitamin C transport in adult human small intestinal brush border membrane vesicles. *The Journal of Nutrition, 130,* 63-69.

Maxwell, S. R. & Lip, G. Y. (1997). Free radicals and antioxidants in cardiovascular disease. *British Journal of Clinical Pharmacology, 44,* 307-317.

Messner, B.; Frotsching, S.; Steinacher-Nigisch, A.; Winter, B.; Eichmair, E.; Gebetsberger, J.; Schwaiger, S.; Ploner, C.; Laufer, G. & Bernhard, D. Apoptosis and necrosis: two different outcomes of cigarette smoke condensate-induced endothelialcell death. 2012. Available from: http://www.ncbi.nlm.nih.gov/pmc/articles/PMC3542598/pdf/cddis2012162a.pdf.

Munzner, R. & Renner, H. W. (1989). Genotoxic investigations of tobacco protein using microbial and mammalian test systems. *Zeitschrift für Ernährungswissenschaft, 28,* 300-309.

Muralikrishnan, G.; Amalan Stanley, V. & Sadasivan Pillai, K. (2001). Dual role of vitamin C on lipid profile and combined application of cyclophosphamide, methotrexate and 5-fluorouracil treatment in fibrosarcoma-bearing rats. *Cancer Letters, 169,* 115-120.

Murphy, S. P. & Poos, M. I. (2002). Dietary Reference Intakes: summary of applications in dietary assessment. *Public Health Nutrition, 5,* 843-849.

Nakajima, M.; Yamamoto, T.; Nunoya, K.; Yokoi, T.; Nagashima, K.; Inoue, K.; Funae, Y.; Shimada, N.; Kamataki, T. & Kuroiwa Y. (1996). Role of human cytochrome P4502A6 in C-oxidation of nicotine. *Drug Metabolism and Disposition, 24,* 1212-1217.

Naska, A.; Orfanos, P.; Trichopoulou, A.; May, A. M.; Overvad, K.; Jakobsen, M. U.; Tjønneland, A.; Halkjær, J.; Fagherazzi, G.; Clavel-Chapelon, F.; Boutron-Ruault, M. C.; Rohrmann, S.; Hermann, S.; Steffen, A.; Haubrock, J.; Oikonomou, E.; Dilis, V.; Katsoulis, M.; Sacerdote, C.; Sieri, S.; Masala, G.; Tumino, R.; Mattiello, A.; Bueno-de-Mesquita, H. B.; Skeie, G.; Engeset, D.; Barricarte, A.; Rodríguez, L.; Dorronsoro, M.; Sánchez, M. J.; Chirlaque, M. D,.; Agudo, A.; Manjer, J.; Wirfält, E.; Hellström, V.; Shungin, D.; Khaw, K. T.; Wareham, N. J.; Spencer, E. A.; Freisling, H.; Slimani, N.; Vergnaud, A. C.; Mouw, T.; Romaguera, D.; Odysseos, A.; & Peeters, P. H. (2011). Eating out, weight and weight gain. A cross-sectional and prospective analysis in the context of the EPIC-PANACEA study. *International Journal of Obesity, 35,* 416–426.

Nelson, J. L.; Bernstein, P. S.; Schmidt, M. C.; Von Tress, M. S. & Askew, E. W. (2003). Dietary modification and moderate antioxidant supplementation differentially affect serum carotenoids, antioxidant levels and markers of oxidative stress in older humans. *Journal of Nutrition, 133,* 3117-3123.

Nunes, M. (2011). *Avaliação da Mutagenicidade de Pacientes em Tratamento com Anfepramona através do Teste de Micronúcleos em Mucosa Oral. Dissertação de Mestrado, PPGBioSaúde, ULBRA. Canoas, RS: ULBRA.*

Nunes, R. S.; Kahl, V. F. S.; Sarmento, M. S.; Richter, M. F.; Costa-Lotufo, L. V.; Rodrigues, F. A. R.; Abin-Carriquiry, J. A.; Martinez, M. M.; Ferronatto, S.; Ferraz, A. B. F. & Da Silva, J. (2011). Antigenotoxicity and antioxidant activity of acerola fruit (*Malpighia glabra* L.) at two stages of ripeness. *Plant Foods for Human Nutrition, 66,* 129-135.

Obrenovich, M.; Li, Y.; Parvathaneni K.; Yendluri, B.; Palacios, H.; Leszek, J & Aliev, G. (2011). Antioxidants in health, disease and aging. *CNS & Neurological Disorders Drug Targets, 10,* 192-207.

Ong, Z. Y.; Wanasuria, A. F.; Lin, M. Z.; Hiscock, J. & Muhlhausler, B. S. (2013). Chronic intake of a cafeteria diet and subsequent abstinence. Sex-specific effects on gene expression in the mesolimbic reward system. *Appetite, 65,* 189-199.

Padayatty, S. J. & Levine, M. (2001). New insights into the physiology and pharmacology of vitamin C. *CMAJ: Canadian Medical Association Journal, 164,* 353-355.

Padayatty, S. J.; Katz, A.; Wang, Y.; Eck, P.; Kwon, O.; Lee, J. H.; Chen, S.; Corpe, C.; Dutta, A.; Dutta, S. K. & Levine, M. (2003). Vitamin C as an antioxidant: evaluation of its role in disease prevention. *Journal of the American College of Nutrition, 22,* 18-35.

Pallàs, M.C. (2002). *Importancia de la nutrición en la persona de edad avanzada.* Barcelona: Novartis Consumer Health S.A.

Paoloni-Giacobino, A.; Grimble, R. & Pichard, C. (2003). Genomic interactions with disease and nutrition. *Clinical Nutrition, 6,* 507-14.

Paolisso, G.; D'Amore, A.; Galzerano, D.; Balbi, V.; Giugliano, D.; Varricchio, M. & D'Onofrio, F. (1993). Daily vitamin E supplements improve metabolic control but not insulin secretion in elderly type II diabetic patients. *Diabetes Care, 16,* 1433–1437.

Peluzio, M. C. G. & de Oliveira, V. P. (2008). Vitaminas. In: N. M. B. Costa & M. C. G. Peluzio (Eds.), *Nutrição e metabolismo* (1st edition, 209-262). Viçosa, MG: Editora UFV.

Da Silva, J.; Erdtmann, B.; Henriques, J. A. P.; Picada, J. N., Kern A. L.; Ramos, A. L. L. P. & Saffi, J. (2003). O estresse oxidativo e as defesas antioxidante. In: J. Da Silva; B. Erdtmann & J. A. Henriques (Eds.), *Genética Toxicológica* (1st edition, 251-264). Porto Alegre, RS: Alcance.

Planeta, C. S. & De Lucia, R. (1998). Involvement of dopamine receptors in diethylpropion-induced conditioning place preference. *Brazilian Journal of Medical and Biology Research, 31,* 561-564.

Poulsen, H. (2005). Oxidative DNA modifications. *Experimental and Toxicologic Pathology, 57,* 161-169.

Premkumar, K.; Min, K.; Alkan, Z.; Hawkes, W. C.; Ebeler, S. & Bowlus, C. L. (2007). The potentiating and protective effects of ascorbate on oxidative stress depend upon the concentration of dietary iron fed C3H mice. *The Journal of Nutritional Biochemistry, 18,* 272-278.

Quandt, S.A.; Arcury, T.A.; Preisser, J.S.; Norton, D. & Austin, C. (2000). Migrant farmworkers and green tobacco sickness: new issues for an understudied disease. *American Journal of Industrial Medicine, 37,* 307-315.

Rahman, K. (2007). Studies on free radicals, antioxidants, and co-factors. *Clinical Interventions and Aging, 2,* 219-36.

Riemersma, R. A. (1994). Epidemiology and the role of antioxidants in preventing coronary heart disease: a brief overview. *The Proceedings of the Nutrition Society, 53,* 59-65.

Riso, P.; Martini, D.; Moller, P.; Loft, S.; Bonacina, M.; Moro, M. & Porrini, M. (2010). DNA damage and repair activity after broccoli intake in young healthy smokers. *Mutagenesis, 25,* 595-602.

Risom, L.; Moller, P. & Loft, S. (2005). Oxidative stress-induced DNA damage by particulate air pollution. *Mutation Research, 592,* 119-137.

Rutkowski, M. & Grzegorczyk, K. (2012). Adverse effects of antioxidative vitamins. *International Journal of Occupational Medicine and Environmental Health, 25,* 105-121.

Saffi, J. & Henriques, J. A. P. (2003). Reparação de DNA em células eucarióticas. In: J. Da Silva; B. Erdtmann & J. A. Henriques (Eds.), *Genética Toxicológica* (1st edition, 183-205). Porto Alegre, RS: Alcance.

Samarin, R. & Garattini, S. (1993). Neurochemical mechanism of action of anoretic drugs. *Pharmacology & Toxicology, 73,* 63-68.

Samocha-Bonet, D.; Lichtenberg, D. & Pinchuk, I. (2005). Kinetic studies of copper-induced oxidation of urate, ascorbate and their mixtures. *Journal of Inorganic Biochemistry, 99,* 1963-1972.

Schneider, M.; Diemer, K.; Engelhart, K.; Zanki, H.; Trommer, W. E. & Biesalski, H. K. (2001). Protective effects of vitamins C and E on the number of micronuclei in lymphocytes in smokers and their role in ascorbate free radical formation in plasma. *Free Radical Research, 34,* 209–219.

Selvaraju, V.; Joshi, M.; Suresh, S.; Sanchez, J. A.; Maulik, N.; Maulik, G. (2012). Diabetes, oxidative stress, molecular mechanism, and cardiovascular disease--an overview. *Toxicology Mechanisms and Methods, 22,* 330-335.

Shen, J.; Gammon, M. D.; Terry, M. B.; Wang, Q.; Bradshaw, P.; Teitelbaum, S. L.; Neugut, A. I. & Santella, R. M. (2009). Telomere length, oxidative damage, antioxidants and breast cancer risk. *International Journal of Cancer, 124,* 1637-1643.

Sies, H. (1997). Oxidative stress: oxidants and antioxidants. *Experimental Physiology, 82,* 291–295.

Sies, H. (1993). Strategies of antioxidant defense. *European Journal of Biochemistry, 215,* 213-219.

Simon, J. (1992). Vitamin-C and Cardiovascular-Disease Review. *Journal of the American College of Nutrition, 11,* 107-125.

Slupphaug, G.; Kavli, B.; & Krokan, H. E. (2003). The interacting pathways for prevention and repair of oxidative DNA damage. *Mutation Research, 531,* 231-51.

Snyder, R. D. (2009). An update on the genotoxicity and carcinogenicity of marketed pharmaceuticals with reference to in silico predictivity. *Environmental and Molecular Mutagenesis, 50,* 435–450.

Snyder, R. D. (2010). Possible Structural and Functional Determinants Contributing to the Clastogenicity of Pharmaceuticals. *Environmental and Molecular Mutagenesis, 51,* 800-814.

Spada, P. D. S.; Souza, G. G. N.; Bortolini, G. V.; Henriques, J. A. P.; Salvador, M. (2008). Antioxidant, mutagenic, and antimutagenic activity of frozen fruits. *Journal of Medicinal Food, 11,* 144-151.

Sram, R. J.; Binkova, B.; Rossner Jr, P. (2012). Vitamin C for DNA damage prevention. *Mutation Research, 733,* 39-49.

Sweetman, S. F.; Strain, J. J. & McKelvey-Martin, V. J. (1997). Effect of antioxidant vitamin supplementation on DNA damage and repair in human lymphoblastoid cells. *Nutrition and Cancer, 27,* 122-130.

Thomas, P.; Hecker, J.; Faunt, J. & Fenech. M. (2007). Buccal micronucleus cytome biomarkers may be associated with Alzheimer's disease. *Mutagenesis, 22,* 371–379.

Tohamy, A. A.; Abdel Azeem, A. A.; Shafaa, M. W. & Mahmoud, W. S. (2012). Alleviation of genotoxic effects of cyclophosphamide using encapsulation into liposomes in the absence or presence of vitamin C. *General Physiology and Biophysics, 31,* 85-91.

Tomita, L. Y. (2006). Vitamina C. In: M. A. Cardoso (Ed.), *Nutrição e Metabolismo: Nutrição Humana* (1st edition, 198-215). Rio de Janeiro, RJ: Guanabara Koogan.

Tricker, A. R. (2003). Nicotine metabolism, human drug metabolism polymorphisms, and smoking behavior. *Toxicology, 183,* 151-173.

USDA. USDA National Nutrient Database for Standard Reference, Release 18: U.S. Department of Agriculture, Agricultural Research Service, Nutrient Data Laboratory. 2005. Available from: http://www.nal.usda.gov/fnic/foodcomp.

Valko, M.; Morris, H. & Cronin, M. T. (2005). Metals, toxicity and oxidative stress. *Current Medicine Chemistry, 12,* 1161–208.

Von Zglinick, T. (2002). Oxidative stress shortens telomeres. *Trends in Biochemical Sciences, 27,* 339-344.

Washi, S. A. & Ageib, M. B. (2010). Poor diet quality and food habits are related to impaired nutritional status in 13- to 18-year-old adolescents in Jeddah. *Nutrition Research, 30,* 527–534.

Wattanapitayakul, S. & Bauer, J. (2001). Oxidative pathways in cardiovascular disease: roles, mechanisms, and therapeutic implications. *Pharmacology & Therapeutics, 89,* 187-206.

Weber, C.; Wolfgang, E.; Weber, K. & Weber, P. C. (1996). Increased adhesiveness of isolated monocytes to endothelium is prevented by vitamin C intake in smokers. *Circulation, 93,* 1488–1492.

Willett, W.C. (2001). Diet and cancer: one view at the start of the millennium. *Cancer Epidemiology, Biomarkers & Prevention, 10,* 3-8.

Wild, S.; Roglic, G.; Green, A.; Sicree, R. & King, H. (2004). Global prevalence of diabetes: estimates for the year 2000 and projections for 2030. *Diabetes Care, 27,* 1047-1053.

Wilson, J. X. (2005). Regulation of vitamin C transport. *Annual Review of Nutrition, 25,* 105-125.

Wu, L. (1999). Review of risk factors for cardiovascular diseases. *Annals of Clinical Laboratory Science, 29,* 127-133.

Yin, J. J.; Fu, P. P.; Lutterodt, H.; Zhou, Y. T.; Antholine, W. E.; Wamer, W. (2012). Dual role of selected antioxidants found in dietary supplements: crossover between anti- and pro-oxidant activities in the presence of copper. *Journal of Agricultural and Food Chemistry, 60,* 2554-2561.

WHO.World Health Organization. *Guidelines on food fortification with micronutrients.* (2006). Available from: http://www.who.int/nutritionpublications/guide_food_ fortification_micronutrients.pdf.

Zhang, Z. W. & Farthing, M. J. (2005). The roles of vitamin C in *Helicobacter pylori* associated gastric carcinogenesis. *Chinese Journal of Digestive Diseases, 6,* 53-58.

In: Vitamin C
Editor: Raquel Guiné

ISBN: 978-1-62948-154-8
© 2013 Nova Science Publishers, Inc.

Chapter 2

AN OVERVIEW OF THE ANALYTICAL METHODS TO DETERMINE ASCORBIC ACID IN FOODSTUFFS

Julia López-Hernández[*] *and Ana Rodríguez-Bernaldo de Quirós*[†]

Department of Analytical Chemistry, Nutrition and Food Science,
University of Santiago de Compostela, Santiago de Compostela, Spain

ABSTRACT

Ascorbic acid is a natural antioxidant widely distributed in fruits and vegetables.

It is well known its participation in different biological processes such as, collagen formation, iron absorption and its involvement in neurotransmission and in immune responses. In addition is employed as additive to prevent food deterioration. Numerous analytical techniques have been developed for the determination of ascorbic acid in foods, including colorimetric, spectrophotometric, potentiometric, spectrofluorimetric, chromatographic and so on.

The present work intends to provide an updated review on the analytical methods for the analysis of ascorbic acid in foodstuffs. The analytical conditions, the advantages and the drawbacks and the method validation characteristics are commented on. Moreover, the extraction procedures of the antioxidant from the food matrix are reviewed.

1. INTRODUCTION

Ascorbic acid is a natural antioxidant widely distributed in vegetables and fruits, mainly citrus and tropical fruits. It is involved in different biochemical processes such as collagen formation, iron absorption and physiological functions including its involvement in neurotransmission and in immune responses (Spínola, et al. 2012; Martínez, 1998; Fenoll, et al. 2011; Pisoschi, et al. 2011). The ascorbic acid is not synthesized by the organism so it should be provided by the diet. The lack of the ascorbic acid can cause diseases such as scurvy. However, high levels of ascorbic acid in the human body could cause adverse effects.

---

[*], E-mail: julia.lopez.hernandez@usc.es.
[†] E-mail: ana.rodriguez.bernaldo@usc.es.

In addition, it is used as a food additive by the industry in different food items including, fruit juices, jams and dairy products among others, in order to avoid the oxidation (Adam, et al. 2012).

The study of the ascorbic acid has attracted the interest of the scientists in different fields; food science, pharmaceutical and clinical analysis. Therefore, sensitive and reliable methods to determine the antioxidant in different matrix are required. Several analytical techniques have been employed for its determination; including spectrophotometric, potentiometric, spectrofluorimetric, titrimetric, and chromatographic methods among others. The last ones are preferred because of their advantages of simplicity, short analysis time and sensitivity. Recently, ultra-high-performance liquid chromatography (UHPLC) has been successfully applied to determine the ascorbic acid as an excellent alternative to the conventional liquid chromatography. Regarding the detection systems; UV-Vis, fluorescence (FLD), electrochemical and mass spectrometry have been generally used. For fluorescence detection a derivatization step is necessary after treatment of the sample to obtain a fluorescent derivative of ascorbic acid. Mass spectrometry provides an excellent sensitivity and selectivity but its use become very expensive and it is not realistic for the routine analysis (Nováková et al. 2008).

The present chapter is focused on the methods of analysis of ascorbic acid particularly chromatography, although are also presented spectrophotometric, electrophoresis, voltametric and potentiometric.

2. Extraction Procedures of Ascorbic Acid From Foods

The extraction of ascorbic acid from foods generally involves a treatment with an aqueous acidic solution; followed by a homogenization or centrifugation. A derivation step is essential when fluorescence is used as a detection system. In Table 2.1 some of the commonly used extraction procedures of ascorbic acid from foods are summarized.

3. Analytical Techniques

3.1. High Performance Liquid Chromatography (HPLC)

Liquid chromatography coupled to different detection systems such as UV-Vis, electrochemical, fluorescence or mass spectrometry have been commonly employed to determine ascorbic acid. The separation of the vitamin was usually performed on a reversed stationary phase and employing a mobile phase at an acidic pH.

An isocratic and reversed-high-performance liquid chromatographic method to analyze ascorbic acid is reported by Janjarasskul et al. (2011). A C18 column, (25 cm x 4.6 mm i.d., 5 μm particles) (Supelco, Bellefonte, PA), with a C18 guard column (5 μm, Supelco) was employed as a stationary phase and an aqueous solution of phosphoric acid (pH 2.0) as the mobile phase. The flow rate was 1.0 mL/min. The wavelength was set at 245 nm.

Table 2.1. Extraction procedures of ascorbic acid from foods

Food matrix	Extraction solvent	Treatments	References
Fruits (passion fruits papayas, strawberries lemons) and vegetables (broccoli and green and red peppers).	3% metaphosphoric acid–8% acetic acid–1 mM ethylendiaminetetraacetic acid disodium salt (EDTA).	Homogenization and centrifugation (10,000 rpm, 10 min). Total ascorbic acid was determined after conversion of dehydroascorbic to L-ascorbic by using Tris buffer containing DL-1,4-dithiothreitol (DTT) at a concentration of 20mM; the reaction was stop by adding 0.4 M H_2SO_4.	Spinola et al. (2012).
Edible whey protein films.	Phosphoric acid solution (pH 2.0).	Homogenization and centrifugation (300 rpm for 1.5 min).	Janjarasskul et al. (2011).
Tomato paste.	2.5% m-phosphoric acid.	Vortex and centrifugation (4000 × g for 20 min). DL-1,4-Dithiothreital was used to convert dehydroascorbic to L-ascorbic.	Koh et al. (2012).
Honey.	Ultra pure water; NaOH 2M and 12.5mL of phosphate buffer 1M (pH = 5.5).	Homogenization and solubilization.	Ciulu et al. (2011).
Citrus fruits (Clementine mandarins and Meyer lemons).	Water and 3%meta phosphoric acid.	Homogenization and mixed.	Uckoo et al. (2011).
Different enriched food products.	2% (w/v) metaphosphoric acid solution.	Sonication and centrifugation (4100 g for 15 min).	Engel et al. (2010).
Biological matrices.	Aqueous solution of 10% meta-phosphoric acid (ascorbic acid). Aqueous solution of tris(2-carboxyethyl)phosphine solution in 0.05% trifluoroacetic acid.	Vortex-mixed and centrifugation (2500 g for 10 min).	Khan and Iqbal (2011).
Tomato, kiwi, and mango.	Methanol + a mixture of meta-phosphoric acid 3% and acetic acid 8%.	Homogenization.	Garrido Frenich et al. (2005).
Tropical fruits (banana, papaya, mango, and pineapple).	Two solvents extraction: -3% metaphosphoric acid- 8% acetic acid. -0.1% oxalic acid.	Homogenization and centrifugation (9000 g for 20 min).	Hernández et al. (2006).
Exotic fruits (mango, papaya, passion fruit, etc.).	10% (v/v) perchloric acid and 1% (w/v) metaphosphoric acid	Vortex (1min) and dilution.	Valente et al. (2011).
Strawberries, tomatoes and apples.	4.5% metaphosphoric solution.	Homogenization and centrifugation (22,100g for 15 min).	Odriozola-Serrano et al. (2007).
Pepper, tomato, orange and lemon.	0.05% (w/v) EDTA (Ethylendiami-netetraacetic acid disodium salt dehydrate).	Homogenization and centrifugation (10000g for 10 min).	Fenoll et al. (2011).

Table 2.1. (Continued)

Food matrix	Extraction solvent	Treatments	References
Green beans (*Phaseolus vulgaris* L.).	3% metaphosphoric acid with 8% acetic acid	Magnetic stirring. Ascorbic acid was oxidized to dehydroascorbic acid. Derivatization with o-phenylenediamine.	Sánchez-Mata et al. (2000).
Fruit juices, soft drinks and isotonic beverages.	No extraction only sample dilution when necessary.	Direct analysis.	Rodríguez-Bernaldo de Quirós et al. (2009).
Alpine food plant (*Phyteuma orbiculare* L.).	5% metaphosphoric acid.	Mixed in a mortar.	Abbet et al. (2013).
Sea urchin (*Paracentrotus lividus*, L.).	4.5% metaphosphoric acid.	Vortex (2 min) and centrifugation (5 min, 1100 rpm).	Rodríguez-Bernaldo de Quirós et al. (2001).
Orange juice, apple juice and orange drink concentrate.	Samples were diluted with double-distilled water.	Centrifugation (5 min, $10 \times 10^3 \times g$).	Tang and Wu (2005).
Beverages.	Sampled were diluted with water or with the running buffer.	Sonication (10 min).	Law et al. (2005).
Fruits (lemon, Sunkist, and pineapple) and spinach.	1 mM EDTA/0.2 M KH_2PO_4/0.474 M 27 mL H_3PO_4 (pH 2). 1 mM EDTA/3.0% methaphosphoric acid.	Homogenization and centrifugation (30 000 × g, 5 min).	Liao et al. (2001).
Food (Grapefruit juice, orange juice, apples, kiwi fruits, tomatoes, milk, endive, etc.)	1% (w/v) Methaphosphoric acid. Milk samples: 20% trichloroacetic acid.	Homogenization. Milk samples: centrifugation (4000 rpm, 10 min).	Burini (2007).
Wine samples.	Direct analysis.	Direct analysis.	Lopes et al. (2006).
Fruit juices (orange, pear, and mango), ground chestnuts.	Fruit juices: 6.25% m-phosphoric acid (MPA), 2.5 mM Tris(2-carboxyethyl) phosphine hydrochloride (TCEP), and 2.5 mM EDTA. Ground chestnuts: 5% MPA, 2 mM TCEP, and 2 mM EDTA.	Fruit juices: dilution. Ground chestnuts: centrifugation (3,000 × g, 5 min).	Barros et al. (2010).
Pharmaceutical preparation and energy drink.	Aqueous organic buffer containing 200 mg/L double-distilled water.	Dilution and sonication (10 min).	Karatapanis et al. (2009).

More recently, Koh et al. (2012) developed a method to determine ascorbic acid in tomato paste; in the analysis they used an Agilent Zorbax Eclipse XDBC18 column (4.6 × 250 mm, 5 μm) protected with a guard column (4.6 × 12.5 mm, 5 μm) of the same stationary phase and 0.05 mol L−1 KH2PO4 (pH 2.6) at a flow rate of 1.0 mL/ min as mobile phase. Chromatograms were recorded at a wavelength of 245 nm.

Ciuli et al. (2011) proposed a reversed-phase high-performance liquid chromatographic with UV-Vis detection method for the simultaneous determination of hidrosoluble vitamins including ascorbic acid in honey samples. A binary solvent gradient consisting of solvent (A) aqueous solution of trifluoroacetic acid (0.025%, v/v), and solvent (B) acetonitrile at a flow rate of 1.0 mL/min was employed. An Alltima C18 column (250 mm ×4.6 mm, 5μm particle size (Alltech, Sedriano, Italy) equipped with a guard cartridge of the same material was used for the separation of the water-soluble vitamins. With respect to performance characteristics, satisfactory limit of detection and quantification 0.10 mg/kg and 0.30 mg/kg, respectively, were achieved. Regarding the repeatability and reproducibility, appropriate values were obtained 7.3 and 3.3%, respectively (CV% exp, r.). Recovery values were around 104%.

Uckoo et al. (2011) proposed an isocratic method to determine amines and organic acids in citrus fruits. 3 mM phosphoric acid was used at a flow rate of 1.0 mL/min was used as a mobile phase. In the study they tested three stationary phases: Xbridge C18 (3.5 μm, 4.6 mm × 150 mm i.d.) from Waters ; Gemini C18 (5μm, 250 mm ×4.6 mm i.d.) from Phenomenex; and Luna C18 (5 μm, 250 mm × 4.6 mm i.d.) from Phenomenex. Ascorbic acid was detected at 254 nm. The limit of detection and quantification obtained were 5 and 9.8 ng, respectively. For ascorbic acid the recovery percentage ranged from 84.01 and 92.71%. depending on the sample spiked.

A gradient system consisted of (A) 0.1% (v/v %) formic acid in water (pH 2.55) and (B) 0.1% (v/v %) formic acid in methanol at a flow rate of 0.5 mL/min and a Restek Ultra Aqueous reverse phase C18 column (5 μm, 150 x 3.2 mm) equipped with a guard column was used to analyze free forms of B group vitamins and ascorbic acid in various fortified food products; detection was performed at wavelength of 266 nm (Engel et al. 2010). A limit of detection of 6 ng/mL for ascorbic acid was obtained.

Hernández et al. (2006) compared a titrimetic method and a reversed-phase high-performance liquid chromatographic method for the determination of ascorbic acid in tropical fruits. The chromatographic separation was performed on a Shodex RSpak KC- 811 column (250 x 4.6 mm i.d. 5 μm particle size) and using 0.2% orthophosphoric acid at a flow rate of 1.2 mL/min as mobile phase. The column temperature was set at 25 °C. Ascorbic acid was detected at 245 nm. Under these conditions the detection limit was 0.1 mg/L. The method presented a good linearity within the 0.5-50 mg/L range with a r2 of 0.999.

A reversed-phase high-performance liquid chromatography method with photodiode array detection to determine ascorbic acid in exotic fruits was proposed by Valente et al. (2011). The chromatographic conditions were as follows: the stationary was a Phenomenex, Synergi™Hydro-RP (150 × 4.6 mm i.d., 4.0 μm particle size) protected by a guard cartridge AQ C18 (40 × 2.0 mm i.d., 5 μm particle size), the column was thermostatted at 30 °C; a mobile phase composed by 20 mM ammonium dihydrogen phosphate, pH 3.5 (adjusted with orthophosphoric acid 85%), and containing 0.015% (w/v) of metaphosphoric acid was used. The flow rate and the injection volume were 0.6 mL/min and 20 μL, respectively. The detection was done at 254 nm. Appropriate limits of detection (0.035 µg/mL) and quantification (0.09 µg/mL) were achieved.

Two chromatographic methods with UV detection were compared in a study conducted by Odriozola-Serrano et al. (2007). In the first method a reverse phase C18 Spherisorb® ODS2 stainless steel column (250 x 4.6 mm, 5 µm) and an isocratic mobile phase consisting of a 0.01% solution of sulphuric acid adjusted to pH 2.6 were employed. In the second one the stationary phase was a NH2-Spherisorb S5 Column (250 x 4.6 mm, 5 µm) and 10 mM potassium dihydrogen phosphate buffer adjusted to pH 3.5 and acetonitrile (60:40 v/v) as the mobile phase were used. In both methods the flow rate was set at 1.0 mL/min. Chromatograms were monitored at 245 nm. Two reducing agents, DL-1,4-dithiotreitol and 2,3-dimercapto-1-propanol to convert dehydroascorbic to ascorbic acid were also compared. Both methods showed good sensibility with limits of detection and quantification ranging from 0.08 to 0.18 mg/100g and from 0.27 to 0.61 mg/100g, respectively. Recovery values were higher than 93.6% for both methods.

Rodríguez-Bernaldo de Quirós et al. (2009) proposed a simple and rapid method to determine ascorbic acid in fruit juices and soft drinks. The samples were analyzed directly without a previous treatment; dilution when necessary.

A novel stationary Teknokroma, Tr-010065 Mediterranea sea18 phase (15 x 0.4 cm, i.d., 3 µm) based on perfectly spherical particles of ultra-pure silica with a very low metal content were used to carried out the analysis; Milli-Q water (0.1% v/v formic acid) at a flow rate of 0.8 mL/min was employed as the mobile phase. Chromatograms were recorded at 245 nm. The method showed a extraordinary sensibility with a limit of detection of 0.01 mg/L. The within-day repeatability calculated as the relative standard deviation (R.S.D.) was lower than 2%.

Ferraces-Casais et al. (2012) in another study evaluated the ascorbic acid contents in fresh seaweed using a Kinetex C18 (150 × 4.6 mm, 2.6 µm; Phenomenex®, USA) column thermostatted at 30 ºC as stationary phase and a mobile phase consisting of acetic acid–Milli-Q water (0.1% v/v) at a flow rate of 0.7 mL/min. Detection was performed at λ 245 nm.

A gradient of two eluents, (A) water containing 1.03 g/L of n-hexane sodium sulfonic acid (pH adjusted to 2.6 with 40% H3PO4) and (B) and acetonitrile–water (8:2 v/v) was used for the determination of ascorbic acid in an Alpine food plant. The flow rate was 1 mL/min and the injection volume 10 µL. A EC Nucleosil C18 column (250 x 4.0 mm i.d., 100–5 µm) protected by a guard column (8.0 x 4.0 mm i.d.) packed with the same material was used as stationary phase and thermostatted at 25 ºC. The wavelength was set at 241 nm. The limits of detection and quantification obtained were 0.5 mg/100g and 2.0 mg/100g, respectively (Abbet et al., 2013).

A polymeric stationary phase PLRP-S 100Å (5 µm) column (150 mm×4.6 mm) was used to analyze ascorbic in wine samples. A gradient of two eluents (A) water-trifluoroacetic (99:1, v/v) and (B) acetonitrile-eluent A (80: 20 v/v) at a flow rate of 1 mL/min was used as mobile phase. The injection volume was 20 µL. Chromatograms were monitored at 243 nm. Under these analytical conditions detection and quantification limits were 1 and 5 mg/L, respectively; and recoveries were higher than 90% (Lopes et al. 2006).

Adam et al. (2012) determine ascorbic acid in beverages by using High-Performance-Liquid Chromatography-UV detection. The extraction of the vitamin from the drinks involves a microextraction by packed sorbent (MEPS). Concerning the chromatographic conditions, a

LiChrospher® 100 RP-18e (250 x 4 mm i.d., sorbent size 5 μm) protected by a guard column LiChrospher® 100 RP-18e (4 x 4 mm i.d., sorbent size 5 μm) was used as a stationary phase. The mobile phase consisted of water acidified with acetic acid pH 2.94 and methanol (B). The analysis was performed under isocratic conditions with 80% (A) and 20% (B) at a flow rate of 1mL/min. The wavelength used was 265 nm. The limits of detection and quantification of the method were 7.2 μg/mL and 24 μg/mL, respectively.

Two high-performance-liquid chromatographic methods with UV-Vis and fluorescence detection were compared for the determination of ascorbic acid in sea urchin samples. Direct determination of ascorbic acid at 245 nm was done with the UV-Vis detector; the HPLC-FLD method involves a oxidation of ascorbic acid to dehydroascorbic acid, followed by a derivatization with 1,2-phenylenediamine in order to obtain a fluorescence product (λem 430 nm λex 350 nm). The stationary phase was the same in both methods a Kromasil(25 x 0.4 cm),100, C18 5 μTeknokroma. The mobile phase was Milli-Q water adjusted to pH 2.2 with metaphosphoric acid, for the HPLC-UV method and methanol-0.1% metaphosphoric acid (7:3 v/v) for the HPLC-FLD method. The flow rate and injection volume were 1 mL/min and 20 μL, respectively. The authors found that the HPLC-FLD showed better sensitivity (LOD: 0.082 μg/mL) than the HPLC-UV (LOD: 0.19 μg/mL) (Rodríguez Bernaldo de Quirós, et al. 2001).

In a study carried out by Sánchez-Mata et al. (2000) a spectrofluorimetric assay and a chromatographic method were compared to determine ascorbic acid in green beans. The chromatographic method involves the use of Sphereclone ODS 2, 5 μm (Phenomenex) as a stationary phase and 1.8 mM H2SO4 in distilled water (pH 2.6) as the mobile phase. The flow rate was 0.9 mL/min and the injection volume was 20 μL. The detection was done with a UV-visible detector at 245 nm. Regarding the method validation parameters, a suitable sensibility (Detection Limit: 0.0097 mg/100 mL and Quantification Limit: 0.0323 mg/100 mL) were achieved. Coefficients of variation of repeatability were lower than 4.474% and coefficients of variation of reproducibility were 6.400% for ascorbic acid and 7.087% for Total Ascorbic Acid. The values of recovery ranged from 89.379% to 93.269%.

Liquid chromatography with fluorescence detection was used to determine total ascorbic acid in foods (Burini, 2007). The method involves the reaction of ascorbic acid with peroxyl radical generated in situ by thermal decomposition of an azo-compound, 2,2'- azobis(2-amidinopropane) dihydrochloride to produce dehydroasorbic followed by a derivatization to form a fluorescence derivative. The separation was performed on a Nova-Pak C18 (150mm×3.9mm i.d., 4μm particle size) column and using phosphate buffered solution (pH = 7.8) containing 16% MeOH (v/v) at a flow-rate of 0.8 mL/min as mobile phase. Detection was performed at λ_{ex} = 365 nm and λ_{em} = 425 nm. With regard to the sensibility, a limit of detection of 0.27 μg/mL was obtained.

A novel method for the determination of L-ascorbic acid, aminothiols, and methionine in biological matrices by ion-pairing reversed-phase high performance liquid-chromatography-electrochemical detection was reported by Khan and Iqbal (2011). The analyses were performed on a Supelco Discovery® HS C18 (250 mm x 4.6 mm, 5 μm; Bellefonte, USA) analytical column equipped with a

Perkin Elmer C18 (30 mm x 4.6 mm, 10 μm; Norwalk, USA) pre-column guard cartridge and using a isocratic mobile phase composed by methanol–aqueous solution of 0.05% trifluoroacetic acid (5:95, v/v), containing 0.1 mM 1-octane sulphonic acid as the ion-pairing agent. The flow rate was 1.5 mL/min. Regarding sensitivity, a limit of detection of 60 pg/mL was obtained for ascorbic acid.

High-performance liquid chromatography coupled to mass spectrometry (HPLC-MS) was used to determine simultaneously ascorbic acid, dehydroascorbic acid and 2,3-diketogulonic acid in a model juice system. In this study a gradient of two eluents, (A) water-acetonitrile-formic acid (95:5:0.95; v/v/v) adjusted to pH 1.8 and (B) acetonitrile at a flow rate of 1 mL/min was used. The separation was performed on a reverse phase/cation exchange column (Primesep-D, 4.6mm x150mm, particle size 5 μm) (Tikekar et al. 2011).

An isocratic method to determine ascorbic acid in vegetables and fruits by high-performance liquid chromatography coupled to mass spectrometry was developed by Garrido Frenich et al. (2005). Two coupled columns a Symmetry C18 (75 x 4.6 mm i.d. 3.5 μm) and then an Atlantis dC18 (150 x 2.0 mm i.d. 5 μm) were used to perform the analyses. The columns were thermostatted at 30 °C. The mobile phase consists of 70% methanol (0.005% acetic acid) and 30% acetic acid 0.05%. The injection volume was 10 μL. MS data were acquired in negative mode with electrospray ionization (ESI). The developed method was validated in terms of linearity, limits of detection and quantification, recovery and repeatability. The method showed an excellent sensitivity, with a limit of detection and quantification of 10 and 50 μg/L, respectively. The value obtained for the repeatability expressed as R.S.D.% was 8.7% and regarding the recovery a 85% was achieved.

Ascorbic and dehydroascorbic acids were determined in fruits and vegetables by LC-MS/MS using electrospray ionization (ESI) in the negative mode (Fenoll, et al. 2011). The analyses were performed on a Prontosil C18 analytical column (250 x 3 mm, 3 μm particle size). The column temperature was 20 °C. 0.2% (v/v) formic acid at a flow rate of 0.4 mL/min was used as mobile phase. The injection volume was 20 μL. The limits of detection were 13 and 11 ng/mL and the limits of quantification were 44 and 38 ng/mL for ascorbic and dehydroascorbic acids, respectively. Recoveries higher than 80% were obtained for both analytes.

Hydrophilic interaction chromatography (HILIC) has been used by Barros et al. (2010) to determine ascorbic and isoascorbic acids in different foods. The analyses were performed on a TSKgel Amide-80 (4.6 i.d. × 100 mm, 5 μm, Tosoh Bioscience, Japan) column thermostatted at 20 °C and using a gradient elution system consisted of (A) acetonitrile and (B) aqueous 0.1% trifluoroacetic acid (90:10, v/v) at a flow rate of 0.7 mL/min as mobile phase. The detection was done at 244 nm. A quantification limit of 1.5 mg/L was obtained for ascorbic acid.

Drivelos et al. (2010) tested several HILIC columns to analyze ascorbic and isoascorbic acids in fish tissue. APS-2 Hypersil (2.1 i.d.×50 mm, 3 μm, Thermo) was selected as the stationary phase and acetonitrile– ammonium acetate (90:10, v/v) at a flow rate of 0.4 mL/min as the mobile phase to carry out the analyses. The injection volume was 20μL and the optimum wavelength was 240 nm.

Karatapanis et al. (2009) used a HILIC-diol column to separate several water-soluble vitamins including ascorbic acid. The analytical conditions were as follows: HILIC Inertsil, diol column (150 mm x 4.6 mm, 5 μm particle size); the mobile phase was composed by ACN–H2O (90:10 v/v), containing ammonium acetate 10 mM, triethylamine 20 mM, pH 5.0; flow rate 0.8 mL/min and the ascorbic acid detection wavelength was 267 nm. Under these conditions a limit of detection of 0.3 μg/mL was obtained for ascorbic acid.

Hydrophilic interaction liquid chromatography coupled to a diode array detector (DAD) was employed to determine ascorbic acid (Nováková, 2008). The separation was carried out on a ZIC HILIC (150 x 2.1 mm, 3.5 μm) column; the mobile phase consisted of acetonitrile and 50 mM ammonium acetate buffer pH 6.8 (78:22 v/v); the flow rate was 0.30 mL/min and the injection volume 5 μL. The column temperature was 23 °C and the wavelength used 268 nm.

3.1.1. Ultrahigh-Performance Liquid Chromatographic (UPLC)

Lately, the ultrahigh-performance liquid chromatography has been used in the food analysis field due to its advantages in comparison with the conventional liquid chromatography, such as higher resolution and shorter analysis time, among others.

An UPLC-PAD method for the determination of L-ascorbic acid was reported by Spínola et al. (2012). The separation was performed on a Acquity HSS T3 analytical column (100 × 2.1 mm, 1.8 μm particle size) and using a mobile phase composed by an aqueous 0.1% (v/v) formic acid solution at a flow rate of 250 μL/min. The detection was done at 245 nm. Under these conditions the analysis was completed within 3 minutes. Regarding the method validation, an appropriate sensitivity (LOD: 22 ng/mL; LOQ: 67 ng/mL), good precision (R.S.D. < 4%) and satisfactory recoveries (96.6 ± 4.4% for L-ascorbic acid and 103.1 ± 4.8 % for total ascorbic acid) were achieved.

The method proposed by these authors is rapid, sensitive and environmental friendly when compared with conventional HPLC.

More recently, the same authors applied the UPLC-PAD method for the determination of ascorbic acid in different fruits and vegetables from Madeira. The chromatographic conditions employed were the same as previously reported (Spínola et al. 2013).

3.2. Gas Chromatography (GC)

In a study conducted by Silva (2005) a gas chromatographic method with flame ionization detector (FID) to determine total ascorbic acid in fresh squeezed orange juice was developed. The method involves the use of a Chrompack (Middelburg, Netherlands) (CP-Sil-5, 15 mm x 0.32 mm I.D., 0.25 μm film thickness) column as a stationary phase. Operating conditions were as follows: the injection port and detector temperatures were set at 300 °C, the ramp temperature was initially set at 150 °C for 1 min, then increased at 20 °C/min until 320 °C and held for 3 min. Injection was performed in the split mode with a split ratio of 100:1. A limit of detection of 4 mg/100 mL was obtained.

Vecci & Kaiser (1967) determined ascorbic acid by gas chromatography coupled to mass spectrometry as its trimethylsilylether derivative.

3.3. Capillary Electrophoresis

CE appears as an alternative to chromatographic methods for the determination of food components such as a vitamin's organic acids and so on. CE has been successfully applied for the determination of ascorbic acid in different food items (Cheung et al. 2007). This technique provides good sensitivity and high resolution.

Tang and Wu (2005) developed a simple and rapid capillary zone electrophoresis (CZE) method to determine ascorbic acid and sorbic acid in fruit juices. The analytes were separated under the follow conditions: 80 mmol/L boric acid–5 mmol/L borax (pH = 8.0) and a 75 μm-i.d., 360 μm-o.d. fused-silica capillary tube with a length of 55 cm. The detection was performed with a UV detector; the wavelength selected was 270 nm. For ascorbic acid the method showed a good linearity within 2.54–352.00 mg/L range. The limit of detection obtained was 1.70 mg/L.

Choi and Jo (1997) determined ascorbic acid in different foods including, ascorbic acid fortified biscuit, candy, chocolate and balanced nutrition biscuit, by capillary zone electrophoresis coupled to a diode array detector; the analysis was completed within two minutes. The wavelengths used were 245 and 265 nm. The separation was carried out on untreated fused-silica capillary of 27 cm of length x 57 μm I.D. and using a sodium borate buffer. Under these conditions the limits of detection and quantification achieved were 0.06 and 0.25 μg/mL, respectively. Recoveries higher than 95% were obtained.

A comparison of conventional capillary electrophoresis and microchip electrophoresis with capacitively coupled contactless conductivity detection for the determination of ascorbic acid in beverages is reported by Law et al. (2005). For the conventional capillary electrophoresis method a fused-silica

Capillaries (50 μm ID and 360 μm OD) with a length of 60 cm and buffer of 10mM histidine/ 0.135mM tartaric acid, 0.1mM CTAB, and 0.25% hydroxypropyl-β-CD (HP-β-CD) were used whereas for the microchip electrophoresis method PMMA microchips with dimensions of 90 x 16mm and histidine/tartrate buffer at pH 6.5, with 0.06% HP-β-CD and 0.25mM CTAB were employed. The limit of detection obtained with the conventional CE method was 3 mg/L and with the microchip 10 mg/L. But however, the analysis time was shorter with the microchip method.

Capillary zone electrophoresis has also been used by Liao et al. (2001) to quantify ascorbic acid in fruits and vegetables. The analyses were performed on an uncoated fused silica capillary tubing (57 cm length, 75 μm inner diameter) and using 0.2 M borate buffer (pH 9.0) as running buffer. The detection was done at wavelength of 265 nm. Recoveries ranged between 95% and 105%.

Three soluble vitamins including ascorbic acid were separated by means of poly(dimethylsiloxane) microchannel electrophoresis with electrochemical detection. 20 mM borate solution (pH 8.5) was used as a carrier buffer. The proposed method showed a good sensibility with a limit of detection of 1.0 μM, and appropriate recoveries ranging from 86.6 to 112.3% (Li et al. 2007).

3.4. Spectrophotometric and Spectrofluorimetric Methods

Spectrophotometric methods have been widely used to determine ascorbic acid in different matrices such as biological samples and pharmaceutical preparations among others. These methods are fast and simple (Arya et al. 1998).

Nejati-Yazdinejad (2007) developed a spectrophotometric method for the determination of ascorbic acid. Cu (II) was used as ascorbic acid oxidant, once the reaction was completed the excess of Cu (II) was determined by complexation with alizarin red s (ARS). The method showed a good sensibility with a limit of detection of 0.35 ppm and satisfactory recoveries (> 97%).

A spectrophotometric method that involves the use of iron (III), and p-carboxyphenylfluorone in a cationic surfactant micellar medium to analyze vitamin C in pharmaceutical preparations has been proposed by Fujita et al. (2001).

Spectrofluorimetry technique was applied to determine ascorbic acid, in green beans, after the oxidation to dehydroascorbic acid and derivatization with o-phenylenediamine. The wavelengths used were λex 350 nm and λem 430 nm, respectively. With regard to the method sensibility, a limit of quantification of 0.0998 mg/100 mL and a limit of detection of 0.0299 mg/100 mL, were obtained (Sánchez-Mata et al. 2000).

3.5. Other Methods

In this section other methods such as voltametric and potentiometric are commented on.

A voltametric determination of ascorbic acid in fruit juice samples has been reported by Romão Sartori and Fatibello-Filho (2012). The determination was performed using a glassy carbon electrode modified with functionalized multiwalled carbon nanotubes within a poly(allylaminehydrochloride) film.

Calibration curves were constructed within the 5.0 to 200.0 µM range and a limit of detection of 3.0 µM was obtained.

Differential pulse voltammetry and using a chitosan-graphene modified electrode was employed for the determination of ascorbic acid together with other analytes (Han et al. 2010). The linearity of the method was evaluated within a concentration range 50-1200 µM. The detection and quantification limits achieved were 50 and 166 µM, respectively.

Differential pulse voltammetry was also employed to determine ascorbic acid in fruit juices and wine samples in a method described by Pisoschi et al. (2011). The analyses were performed at Pt and carbon paste electrodes.

Baś et al. (2011) reported a method that involves a voltammetric determination of several vitamins including ascorbic acid, for that they used a silver liquid amalgam film–modified silver solid amalgam annular band electrode (AgLAF–AgSAE). The method showed a good linearity within the concentration range studied (0.05-12 mg/L) with a correlation coefficient of 0.9998, and an extraordinary sensitivity with a limit of detection of 0.02 mg/L.

A potentiometric sensor based on molecularly imprinted polypyrrole to determine ascorbic acid was developed by Tonelli et al. (2011). The sensor was successfully used to analyze ascorbic acid in food and pharmaceutical samples.

Llamas et al. (2011) used a flow injection spectrophotometric method (FIA) to determine ascorbic acid in fruit juices. The wavelength used to detect ascorbic acid was 300 nm. The method showed a good linearity within the concentration range (4.18-20.8 mg/L) studied (R2 0.9914). Detection and quantification limits were 2.26 and 7.5 mg/L, respectively. Appropriate recoveries were achieved (> 96%).

CONCLUSION

Different techniques including, spectrophotometry, spectrofluorometry, voltammetry, potentiometry, titrimetric methods, chromatography and electrophoresis among others have been applied to determine ascorbic acid in foods. Chromatographic techniques present several advantages such as simplicity, short analysis time and sensitivity. In this chapter an overview of the methods to determine ascorbic acid, particularly chromatography, is presented. The last trends in chromatographic techniques, such as ultra-high performance liquid chromatography (UPLC) are also included and commented on.

ACKNOWLEDGMENTS/REVISION

The present chapter has been reviewed by:

- Aida Moreira da Silva (PhD), Departamento de Ciência e Tecnología Alimentar, Escola Superior Agrária de Coimbra, Instituto Politécnico de Coimbra, Portugal.
- Ana I.R.N.A. Barros (PhD), Departamento de Química, Escola de Ciências da Vida e do Ambiente, Universidade de Tras-os-Montes e Alto Douro, Portugal.
- Mª José González Castro (PhD), Department of Analytical Chemistry, University of A Coruña, Spain.

REFERENCES

Abbet, C.; Slacanin, I.; Hamburger, M. & Potterat, O. (2013). Comprehensive analysis of Phyteuma orbiculare L., a wild Alpine food plant. *Food Chemistry*, 136, 595-603.

Adam, M.; Pavlíková, P.; Čížková, A.; Bajerová, P.& Ventura, K. (2012). Microextraction by packed sorbent (MEPS) as a suitable selective method for L-ascorbic acid determination in beverages. *Food Chemistry*, 135, 1613–1618.

Arya S. P.; Mahajan, M. & Jain. P. (1998). Photometric methods for the determination of vitamin C. *Analytical Sciences*, 14, 889-895.

Barros, A. I. R. N. A.; Silva, A. P.; Gonçalves, B. & Nunes, F. M. (2010). A fast, simple, and reliable hydrophilic interaction liquid chromatography method for the determination of ascorbic and isoascorbic acids. *Analytical and Bioanalytical Chemistry*, 396, 1863-1875.

Baś, B.; Jakubowska, M. & Górski, L. (2011). Application of renewable silver amalgam annular band electrode to voltammetric determination of vitamins C, B1 and B2. *Talanta*, 84, 1032-1037.

Burini, G. (2007). Development of a quantitative method for the analysis of total l-ascorbic acid in foods by high-performance liquid chromatography. *Journal of Chromatography A,* 1154, 97-102.

Cheung, R. H. F.; Marriott, P. J. & Small, D. M. (2007). CE methods applied to the analysis of micronutrients in foods. *Electrophoresis*, 28, 3390–3413.

Choi, O. K. & Jo, J. S. (1997). Determination of L-ascorbic acid in foods by capillary zone electrophoresis. *Journal of Chromatography A*, 781, 435-443.

Ciulu, M.; Solinas, S.; Floris, I.; Panzanelli, A.; Pilo, M. I.; Piu, P. C.; Spano, N. & Sanna, G. (2011). RP-HPLC determination of water-soluble vitamins in honey. *Talanta*, 83, 924-929.

Drivelos, S.; Dasenaki, M. E. & Thomaidis, N. S. (2010). Determination of isoascorbic acid in fish tissue by hydrophilic interaction liquid chromatography–ultraviolet detection. *Analytical and Bioanalytical Chemistry*, 397, 2199-2210.

Engel, R.; Stefanovits-Bányai, E. & Abranko, L. (2010). LC simultaneous determination of the free forms of B group vitamins and vitamin C in various fortified food products. *Chromatographia*,71, 1069-1074.

Fenoll, J.; Martínez, A.; Hellín, P. & Flores, P.(2011). Simultaneous determination of ascorbic and dehydroascorbic acids in vegetables and fruits by liquid chromatography with tandem-mass spectrometry. *Food Chemistry*, 127, 340-344.

Ferraces-Casais, P.; Lage-Yusty, M. A.; Rodríguez-Bernaldo de Quirós, A. & López-Hernández, J. (2012). Evaluation of Bioactive Compounds in Fresh Edible Seaweeds. *Food Analytical Methods*, 5, 828-834.

Fujita, Y.; Mori, I.; Yamaguchi, T.; Hoshino, M.; Shigemura, Y. & Shimano, M. (2001). Spectrophotometric determination of ascorbic acid with iron (III) and p-carboxyphenylfluorone in a cationic surfactant micellar medium. *Analytical Sciences*, 17, 853-857.

Garrido Frenich, A.; Hernández Torres, M. E.; Belmonte Vega, A.; Martínez Vidal, J. L. & Plaza Bolaños, P. (2005). Determination of ascorbic acid and carotenoids in food commodities by liquid chromatography with mass spectrometry detection. *Journal of Agricultural and Food Chemistry,* 53, 7371-7376.

Han, D.; Han, T.; Shan, C.; Ivaska, A. & Niu, L. (2010). Simultaneous Determination of ascorbic Acid, dopamine and uric acid with chitosan-graphene modified electrode. *Electroanalysis*, 22, 2001-2008.

Hernádez, Y.; Lobo, M.G. & González, M. (2006). Determination of vitamin C in tropical fruits: A comparative evaluation of methods. *Food Chemistry*, 96, 654-664.

Janjarasskul, T.; Min, S. C. & Krochta, J. M. (2011). Storage stability of ascorbic acid incorporated in edible whey protein films. *Journal of Agricultural and Food Chemistry,* 59, 12428-12432.

Karatapanis, A. E.; Fiamegos, Y. C. & Stalikas, C. D. (2009). HILIC separation and quantitation of water-soluble vitamins using diol column. *Journal of Separation Science,* 32, 909-917.

Khan, M. I. & Iqbal Z. (2011). Simultaneous determination of ascorbic acid, aminothiols, and methionine in biological matrices using ion-pairing RP-HPLC coupled with electrochemical detector. *Journal of Chromatography B*, 879, 2567– 2575.

Koh, E.; Charoenprasert, S. & Mitchell, A. E. (2012). Effects of industrial tomato paste processing on ascorbic acid, flavonoids and carotenoids and their stability over one-year storage. *Journal of the Science of Food and Agriculture*, 92, 23-28.

Law, W. S.; Kubáň, P.; Zhao, J. H.; Li, S. F. Y. & Hauser, P. C. (2005). Determination of vitamin C and preservatives in beverages by conventional capillary electrophoresis and microchip electrophoresis with capacitively coupled contactless conductivity detection. *Electrophoresis*, 26, 4648–4655.

Li, X. Y.; Zhang, Q. L.; Lian, H. Z.; Xu, J. J. & Chen, H. Y. (2007). Separation of three water-soluble vitamins by poly(dimethylsiloxane) microchannel electrophoresis with electrochemical detection. *Journal of Separation Science*, 30, 2320-2325.

Liao, T.; Jiang, C. M.; Wu, M. C.; Hwang, J. Y. & Chang, H. M. (2001). Quantification of L-ascorbic acid and total ascorbic acid in fruits and spinach bycapillaryzone electrophoresis. *Electrophoresis*, 22, 1484–1488.

Llamas, N. E.; Di Nezio, M. S.& Fernández Band, B. S. (2011). Flow-injection spectrophotometric method with on-line photodegradation for determination of ascorbic acid and total sugars in fruit juices. *Journal of Food Composition and Analysis*, 24, 127-130.

Lopes, P.; Drinkine, J.; Saucier, C. & Glories, Y. (2006). Determination of l-ascorbic acid in wines by direct injection liquid chromatography using a polymeric column. Analytica Chimica Acta, 555, 242–245.

Martínez, J. A. (1998). *Fundamentos teórico-prácticos de Nutrición y dietética*. España: McGraw-Hill, Interamericana.

Nejati-Yazdinejad, M. (2007). Indirect determination of ascorbic acid (vitamin C) by spectrophotometric method. *International Journal of Food Science and Technology*, 42, 1402–1407.

Nováková, L.; Solichová, D.; Pavlovičová, S. & Solich, P. (2008). Hydrophilic interaction liquid chromatography method for the determination of ascorbic acid. *Journal of Separation Science,* 31, 1634-1644.

Nováková, L.; Solich, P. & Solichová, D. (2008). HPLC methods for simultaneous determination of ascorbic and dehydroascorbic acids. *Trends in Analytical Chemistry*, 27, 942-958.

Odriozola-Serrano, I.; Hernádez-Jover, T. & Martín-Belloso, O. (2007). Comparative evaluation of UV-HPLC methods and reducing agents to determine vitamin C in fruits. *Food Chemistry*, 105, 1151-1158.

Pisoschi, A. M.; Pop, A.; Negulescu, G. P. & Pisoschi, A. (2011). Determination of ascorbic acid content of some fruit juices and wine by voltammetry performed at Pt and carbon paste electrodes. *Molecules*, 16, 1349-1365.

Rodríguez-Bernaldo de Quirós, A.; Lopez-Hernandez, J. & SirnaI-Lozano, J. (2001). Determination of Vitamin C in Sea Urchin: Comparison of Two HPLC Methods. *Chromatographia*, 53, Suppl, S246-S249.

Rodríguez-Bernaldo de Quirós, A.; Fernández-Arias, M. & López-Hernández, J. (2009). A screening method for the determination of ascorbic acid in fruit juices and soft drinks. *Food Chemistry*, 116, 509-512.

Romão Sartori, E. & Fatibello-Filho, O. (2012). Simultaneous voltammetric determination of ascorbic acid and sulfite in beverages employing a glassy carbon electrode modified with carbon nanotubes within a poly(allylamine hydrochloride) film. *Electroanalysis*, 24, 627-634.

Sánchez-Mata, M.; C.; Cámara-Hurtado, M.; Díez-Marqués, C. & Torija-Isasa, M. E. (2000). Comparison of high-performance liquid chromatography and spectrofluorimetry for vitamin C analysis of green beans (Phaseolus vulgaris L.). *European Food Research and Technology,* 210, 220-225.

Silva, F. O. (2005). Total ascorbic acid determination in fresh squeezed orange juice by gas chromatography. *Food Control*, 16, 55–58.

Spínola, V.; Mendes, B.; Câmara, J. S.;& Castilho, P. (2012). An improved and fast UHPLC-PDA methodology for determination of L-ascorbic and dehydroascorbic acids in fruits and vegetables. Evaluation of degradation rate during storage. *Analytical and Bioanalytical Chemistry*, 403, 1049-1058.

Spínola, V.; Mendes, B.; Câmara, J. S. & Castilho, P. C. (2013). Effect of time and temperature on vitamin C stability in horticultural extracts. UHPLC-PDA vs iodometric titration as analytical methods. *LWT - Food Science and Technology*, 50, 489-495.

Tang, Y. & Wu, M. (2005). A quick method for the simultaneous determination of ascorbic acid and sorbic acid in fruit juices by capillary zone electrophoresis. *Talanta*, 65, 794-798.

Tikekar, R. V.; Anantheswaran, R. C.; Elias, R. J. & LaBorde, L. F. (2011). Ultraviolet-Induced oxidation of ascorbic acid in a model juice system: identification of degradation products. *Journal of Agricultural and Food Chemistry*, 59, 8244-8248.

Tonelli, D.; Ballarin, B.; Guadagnini, L.; Mignani, A. & Scavetta, E. (2011). A novel potentiometric sensor for l-ascorbic acid based on molecularly imprinted polypyrrole. *Electrochimica Acta*, 56, 7149– 7154.

Uckoo, R. M.; Jayaprakasha, G. K.; Nelson, S.D. & Patil, B. S. (2011). Rapid simultaneous determination of amines and organic acids in citrus using high-performance liquid chromatography. *Talanta*, 83, 948-954.

Valente, A.; Gonçalves Albuquerque, T.; Sanches-Silva, A. & Costa, H. S. (2011). Ascorbic acid content in exotic fruits: A contribution to produce quality data for food composition databases. *Food Research International*, 44, 2237-2242.

Vecci, M. & Kaiser, K. (1967). Gas chromatographic determination of ascorbic acid in form of its trimethylsilyl ether derivative. *Journal of Chromatography*, 26, 22-29.

In: Vitamin C
Editor: Raquel Guiné

ISBN: 978-1-62948-154-8
© 2013 Nova Science Publishers, Inc.

Chapter 3

VITAMIN C DAILY SUPPLEMENTS AND ITS AMELIORATIVE EFFECTS

Said Said Elshama, Ayman EL-Meghawry EL-Kenawy and Hosam Eldin Osman*

[1]Department of Forensic Medicine and Clinical Toxicology - College of Medicine
Suez Canal University, Ismailia, Egypt
[2]Department of Molecular biology, Genetic Engineering and Biotechnology Inst.,
University of Menofia, Sadat city, Egypt
[3]Department of Anatomy, faculty of medicine, Al Azhar University,
Cairo, Egypt

ABSTRACT

Daily food supplementation rich by vitamin C is an important issue for our body. There is an individual difference of daily intake of dietary vitamin C depending on the age. Preventive and therapeutic doses of vitamin c range from 500 to 1000 mg per day. It is a recommended dose to prevent or treat many of disorders induced by vitamin C deficiency. It is used by the body to form cartilage, tendons, ligaments, skin and blood vessels. Vitamin c acts as an antioxidant by protecting the body against oxidative stress. It is a powerful reducing agent capable of rapidly scavenging a number of reactive oxygen species (ROS). The risk of developing some of diseases is reduced by recommended daily intake of dietary vitamin C according to recent studies. But taking vitamin C supplements will not prevent any of these conditions. Role of vitamin C for prevention or treatment of cancer is still controversial among different studies.

INTRODUCTION

Daily intake of vitamin C is an essential need for our body; it isn't stored in the body because it is a water-soluble vitamin. We should be depended on the daily food

---

* E-mail:saidelshama@yahoo.com, Temporary address: Saudi Arabia- Taif – College of Medicine -Taif University.

supplementation rich by vitamin c such as citrus fruits, broccoli, and tomatoes. Orange, spinach, red and green peppers, watermelon, papaya, grapefruit, cantaloupe, strawberries, kiwi, mango, Brussels sprouts, cauliflower, pineapple, potatoes and cabbage. Every person should eat these fruits and vegetables raw or lightly cooked because Vitamin C is sensitive to light, air and heat. Daily of dietary vitamin C intake should be calculated according to content of vitamin in every food such as one cup of Cantaloupe (59 mg) , one cup of Orange juice (97 mg), one cup of cooked Broccoli (74 mg) , one cup of Red cabbage(80 mg), one cup of Tomato juice (45 mg), one Kiwi (70 mg) and one cup of Green pepper (120 mg). Synthetic vitamin C is available in a variety of forms such as tablets, capsules, powdered crystalline, effervescent, liquid and chewable forms. The best way to take vitamin C supplements is 2 - 3 times per day, with meals, depending on the dosage, adults should take 250 - 500 mg twice per day as seen by Michaels & Frei (2012).

1. RECOMMENDED SUPPLEMENTATION

According to the National Academy of Sciences (NAS), daily intake of dietary vitamin C is different from person to another depending on his age. Newborn and infant up to 6 months should be taken 40 mg per day and raise to 50 mg per day until 12 months. Child of 1-3 years needs less daily intake around 15 mg and raise to 25 mg until 8 years and then 45 mg by end 13 years. Adolescent boys of 18 years need 75 mg per day but Adolescent girls of the same age need less daily intake around 65 mg. Pregnant women should be taken 80 – 85 mg per day but daily intake of Breastfeeding women ranges from 115- 120mg per day. Smoking depletes approximately 35 mg of vitamin C per day. The preventive and therapeutic dose of vitamin C ranges from 500 to 1000 mg per day. It is a recommended dose to prevent or treat many of disorders induced by vitamin C deficiency. Depending on antioxidants and health effects of vitamin C, recommended dietary allowance for vitamin C is 60 mg/day for healthy, non-smoking adults. It is determined by the rate of turnover and rate of depletion of an initial body pool of 1500 mg vitamin C and an assumed absorption of 85% of the vitamin at usual intakes. This amount provides an adequate margin of safety. Vitamin C is safe because our body gets rid of non-used vitamin C. But, high dose (more than 2000 mg per day) is limited for some persons because it causes diarrhea or git upset. Some patients of inherited diseases such as hemochromatosis should not take vitamin C supplements because it increases the amount of iron absorbed from foods as seen by McGregor & Biesalski (2006).

2. BASIS OF VITAMIN C ROLE

Collagen formation depends on the presence of vitamin C. It is used in the formation of cartilage, tendons, ligaments, skin and blood vessels and then Vitamin c plays an imperative role for healing wounds, repairing bones and teeth. Deficiency signs of vitamin C represent as gingivitis, bleeding gums, dry & scaly skin and defective healing wound but scurvy is the severe form of vitamin C deficiency. Oxidative stress means that free radicals (reactive oxygen species "ROS") in the body more than antioxidants. The oxidative process damages the important biological macromolecules such as DNA, proteins and lipids. The free radicals lead to aging process and development of some health conditions such as cancer, heart disease, and arthritis. Vitamin C acts as an antioxidant by protecting the body against oxidative stress. It is a powerful reducing agent capable of rapidly scavenging a number of reactive oxygen species (ROS). There are many controversial studies on role of vitamin C in the body. Is its role preventive or treatable for many diseases? Some studies conducted to conclusive answer that diet contained enough vitamin C lead to reduction the risk of developing some of diseases. But taking vitamin C supplements will not prevent any of these conditions as seen by Padayatty et al., (2003).

3. HEPATIC EFFECTS

The liver is the second largest organ in the human body and it is one of the five vital organs. The liver conducts several hundreds of functions; it metabolizes nutrients and substances. It also stores many vitamins and minerals. With liver diseases, Vitamin requirements increase for tissue repair and compensation of reduced storage capacity. The dietary intake of vitamin is often decreased because of git upset symptoms such as vomiting. It is known that vitamin C is involved in corticosteroid and cholesterol metabolism, electron transport processes and conversion of folic acid to folinic acid. This vitamin is considered the most potent antioxidant for liver because it protects hepatic cells from any chemical induced toxic effect. It antagonises the released free radicals of hepatic detoxification process. According to the above mentioned knowledge, some researchers searched about role for vitamin C in treatment of liver diseases. Ersöz et al. (2005) confirmed that Vitamin C with E is effective treatment option in patients with fatty liver disease in comparison with ursodeoxycholic acid as other therapeutic option for the same disease. Claudia et al. (2003) discovered that Vitamin C inhibits the development of experimental liver steatosis induced by choline-deficient diet in contrast to vitamin E which had not the same action for the same disease.

The University of Michigan, Medical School had many studies on relation of vitamin C and liver diseases especially alcoholic cirrhosis and fatty liver diseases. It was conducted that this vitamin can prevent or treat liver diseases depending on its dose ranging from 500 - 5000 mg/day according to type of hepatic disease and tolerance of the body to vitamin C. Ascorbic acid is considered as liver detox because it helps liver to detoxify any toxin and neutralizes any free radical release.

Acute viral hepatitis (hepatitis A), chronic hepatitis (hepatitis B) and non-A non-B hepatitis respond well to very large doses of vitamin C and B-complex vitamins. Myoglobinuria produce hepatic failure by oxidative reactions. It is induced by rhabdomyolysis (skeletal muscle injury). Sabzevarizadeh & Najafzadeh, (2012) discovered that myoglobinuric hepatic failure is modulated of by vitamin C administration is better than silymarin administration. Cisplatin is one of chemotherapy for cancer but it has a major side effect for liver because it reacts with hepatic vital compounds such as proteins or DNA. Liver degeneration and cell death is the end result of cisplatin use as therapeutic agent for cancer. Some researchers suggested that combination of spirulina and vitamin C can be given before and during chemotherapy cycles to reduce the risk of liver damage or renal failure with Cisplatin.

4. RENAL EFFECTS

The kidney is an excretory organ; it filters the blood except red blood cells and protein. Kidney maintains acid-base balance, recycles water and minerals and excretes waste products in the urine. Vitamin C is filtered and wasted through the kidneys, where vitamin C does not cause kidney problems but it prevents them from dysfunction as seen by (Sebastian et al. 2003). It stops the formation of oxalate stones and dissolves phosphate kidney stones. Ascorbic acid acidifies the urine and then dissolving phosphate stones and preventing their formation. Acidic urine dissolves also magnesium ammonium phosphate stones which require surgical removal. Both the urinary tract infections and stone are easily cured with large doses of vitamin C. Daily consumption of greater amounts than recommended of ascorbic acid prevent nearly 100% the urinary tract infections and stone. Ascorbate increases the body's production of oxalate but it does not increase oxalate stone formation. Vitamin C in the urine binds calcium and decreases its free form. This means less chance of occurrence of calcium oxalate stones formation. The diuretic effect of vitamin C reduces the static conditions which are necessary for stone formation. Dialysis is only and an important therapeutic option in cases of renal failure. Therefore, during dialysis, the water soluble vitamins such as B-complex and C are lost from the blood. Supplementation of these vitamins in these times is an essential issue. Deicher (2003) referred that 300 mg parenteral ascorbate is recommended for chronic kidney disease and hemodialysis patients because ascorbate represents one of the most prominent antioxidants both in plasma as well as intracellular, exerting beneficial effects by an inhibition of lipid peroxidation and reduction of endothelial dysfunction and then it decreases the accelerated atherosclerosis of chronic kidney disease patients. Reactive oxygen species is a fundamental issue in pathogenesis of chronic renal failure causing protein, lipid and DNA damage. Supplementation with antioxidants such as vitamin C prevents oxidative stress such as lipid peroxidation and then chronic renal failure and its complications as seen by (Ratna & Vasudha 2009). Rhabdomyolysis is one of the most important causes of acute renal failure. Free radicals have a vital role in pathogenesis of myoglobinuric acute renal failure. Thus Vitamin C has ability to prevent this disease because it is a major antioxidant. Ustundag et al. (2008) confirmed that 20 mg/kg of vitamin C may be beneficial for better functional and morphological recovery in rhabdomyolysis-induced acute renal failure.

5. CARDIOVASCULAR EFFECTS

There is an inverse relationship between blood ascorbate concentration and cardiovascular mortality in old age patients. It showed protective effects of vitamin C for cardiovascular diseases as seen by Cook et al. (2007). Vitamin C slows down the progression of atherosclerosis by prevention of plaques formation on arterial walls and keeps flexibility of arteries as seen by (Lonn, 2001; Langlois et al. 2001). Patients of low levels of vitamin C may be more likely to have a heart attack or peripheral artery disease such as atherosclerosis. Physicians recommended that foods rich in antioxidants such as vitamin C for patients of hypertension because it lowers risk of high blood pressure depending on population based studies. Oxidative stress and sympathetic activity are main issues for pathogenesis of essential hypertension. Reactive oxygen species can modulate sympathetic nerve activity. Vitamin C has a clear effect on sympathetic activity of muscle and sensitivity of baroreflex in hypertensive patients as seen by (Shinke et al. 2007).

6. RESPIRATORY EFFECTS

Ascorbic acid plays an important role for lung health especially if it suffers from serious effects of smoking. Clinical study confirmed that vitamin C may prevent symptoms of airway diseases such as cystic fibrosis and chronic obstructive lung diseases. Vitamin C maintains hydration of airway passages. So any shortage of vitamin C supplementation leads to dryness of airway passages and participation of respiratory infection. Other studies referred to importance of higher daily intake of vitamin C for good lung function. Recent studies showed that vitamin C reversed oxidative damage of proteins and lipids which were induced by cigarette smoke provided that discontinuation of cigarette smokes exposure as seen by Lykkesfeldt et al. (2000).

Relationship between lack of vitamin C and many respiratory disorders is well established by many studies in the last years. Enough daily intake of vitamin C for pregnant woman is essential for maturation of lung of premature baby. Number of recent studies indicated to importance of this vitamin for decreasing harmful effects of nicotine on fetal lung tissues as seen by Kompauer et al. (2006).

Some studies confirmed that vitamin C doesn't cure the common cold but regular daily intake of vitamin C leads to reduction of common cold duration. Until now, other studies still referred to the prevention role of vitamin C for common cold as seen by (Douglas et al. 2000; Braun et al. 2000; and Audera et al. 2001). Depending on population based studies, patients of bronchial asthma have low levels of vitamin C and then it reduces the risk of asthma especially exercise-induced asthma as seen by Ram et al. (2004).

7. ANTI-CANCER EFFECTS

According to some studies, antioxidants such as vitamin C reduce incidence of some cancers such as skin, breast and cervical cancer Rock et al. (2000) but there is one urgent question for this manner, is taking large doses of vitamin C by cancerous patient to help the cure from this disease? As seen by Padayatty & Levine (2000). Other studies have the answer for the previous question and confirmed that it is impossible that vitamin C has protection role against cancer and referred to large doses of antioxidants interfere with chemotherapy medications.

Furthermore, new studies referred that vitamin C enhances chemotherapy drugs action because of its ability to modulate the expression of transcription factor hypoxia inducible factor 1 (HIF-1) which is responsible for basic cell metabolism and controls cellular response to hypoxia. HIF-1 regulates many genes, enzymes and proteins coding involved in glycolysis and angiogenesis which is related to tumor growth. The above mentioned results support the use of intravenous administration of vitamin C as an adjuvant treatment for cancer as seen by (Heaney et al. 2008 & Gaziano et al. 2009).

8. OPHTHALMOLOGICAL EFFECTS

The leading cause of blindness in the United States is a macular degeneration. Combination of many antioxidants such as Vitamin C, zinc, beta-carotene and vitamin E protect the eyes against developing macular degeneration. Retinopathy of diabetes is one of common causes of blindness. Researchers showed that oxidative stress is responsible for pathogenesis of this condition. Lipid peroxidation and other biomarkers of oxidative stress such as malondialdehyde, superoxide dismutase and glutathione peroxidase are reduced by administration of antioxidants such as vitamin C and then severity and progression of this condition were reversed as seen by Taylor et al. (2002). Other population based studies observed that daily intake of vitamin C reduces incidence of cataract. These studies discovered that vitamin C supplementation for at least 10 years prevent occurrence of cataract as seen by (Head, 2001 & Mare-Perlman et al. 2000).

9. GYNAECOLOGICAL AND OBSTETRICAL EFFECTS

Some obstetricians suggested that vitamin C and vitamin E lowers occurrence of pre-eclampsia in high risk women. In contrast, some studies don't agree. There is a relationship between overdose of vitamin C and abortion, 12 gm per day regularly is effective to induce abortion. In the majority of cases the fetus dies within 5 days of taking Vitamin C. Ascorbic acid decreases the response of uterus to progesterone which is necessary for pregnancy as seen by (Sharma & Mittal 2004; Chappell et al. 2002).

Based on other studies, vitamin C is recommended for bacterial vaginosis of women in the first trimester of pregnancy because some topical antibiotics are contra-indicated. Vaginal vitamin C increases local acidification and decreases hydrogen peroxide which results from reduction of number of lactobacilli in vagina. Vitamin C reduces side effects of oral contraceptives by reduction of oxidative biomarkers and lipid peroxidation (potential cardiovascular risk factor) in receiving oral contraceptive pills as seen by Petersen et al. (2011).

10. TOXICOLOGICAL EFFECTS

This vitamin is one natural antidote and supplementation for many toxicological cases. Vitamin C enhances detoxification process and then reduces bio-accumulation of toxins and toxic minerals in body. It has essential role for modulation the toxicity of many agents and every day we discover a new use of vitamin C in the clinical toxicology field. Vitamin C modulates toxicity of some agents such as organophosphorous pesticides, aflatoxin induced liver cancer and monosodium glutamate induced hepatotoxicity as seen by EL-Meghawry et al. (2013). It abolishes chromosome damage resulted from the effect of toxic substances and help to protect the body against pollutants. Vitamin C reduces toxic effects of lindane poisoning on liver and brain because it overcomes oxidative stress induced by lindane. It has been demonstrated to be highly effective in neutralizing the toxic nature of mercury in all of its chemical forms. There are many medical reports about role of vitamin C as antidote of snake bite especially it is administrated by intravenous route. But its role as antivenin is still controversial until now. Food allergy can lead to anaphylactic shock for some persons according to degree of his sensitivity to this food. This condition is a life-threatening and requires urgent intervention. Vitamin C is a powerful antioxidant that can help to support immune system and kill free radicals that can lead to food sensitivities and produce symptoms similar to allergy reactions. Vitamin C should be given with antihistamines. Vitamin c supplements have capacity to relief mental and physical symptoms of some occupational diseases such as lead poisoning. It has a protective effect against arsenic, benzene and other chemicals, as well as such organic poisons as botulism, spider and scorpion bites.

Met hemoglobin is a type of hemoglobin that contains ferric iron and has a decreased ability to bind oxygen. Methemoglobinemia is abnormal condition characterized by the presence of a higher level of met hemoglobin in the blood. The ascorbic acid dosage is 200-500 mg/day can reduce cyanosis associated with chronic methemoglobinemia but long term oral therapy should be avoided because it can cause the formation of sodium oxalate stones as seen by Daniel & Nawarskas 2000; Bano & Bhatt 2010).

11. DERMATOLOGICAL EFFECTS

There is relationship between skin aging and low intake of vitamin C. A recent study including 4,025 women aged 40-74, found that higher vitamin C intake is associated with a lower incidence of a wrinkled appearance, dryness of the skin and a less skin-aging appearance. Vitamin C is responsible for collagen formation which makes skin elastic and reduces the risk of sunburn. It has an advantage for treatment of some dermatological disorders. Acne is one of these dermatological disorders which affect hair follicles and sebaceous glands. It is caused by the lack of collagen in the body. Vitamin C is the most important vitamin for treatment of acne because it is essential for collagen production. It also removes and prevents the toxins that damage skin cells. Vitamin C also reduces acne scars of severe cases and helps in their healing. Every day, there is a new fact about therapeutically benefits of vitamin C. New study revealed that vitamin C can relieve neurological pain and other dermatological symptoms of herpes zoster if it is administrated by intravenous route. It improves general fatigue and impaired concentration. It strengths the immunity and act as antiviral agent in the same time as seen by Masaki (2010).

12. ENDOCRINE EFFECTS

Vitamin C has many healthy effects which provide more viability for the body. It is involved in biosynthesis of hormone. It helps hormone to be potent action and decreases undesirable actions of hormone. Functions of neurotransmitter need vitamin C to induce more effective actions. Vitamin C has a relation for balance of some hormones in the body such as thyroxin hormone. The thyroid gland needs vitamin C to keep its healthy condition. Negative feedback of thyroxin level in the body causes the thyroid gland to secrete too much hormone to compensate this deficiency. There is an increase of thyroid stimulating hormone concentration, thyroid lipo-peroxidation and the thyroid gland weight. These changes of above mentioned parameters are modulated by pretreatment with vitamin C due to its antioxidant properties. Overactive thyroid needs extra vitamin C which is actually drained from the tissues of the body as seen by (Padayatty et al. 2007 & Suleiman et al. 2011).

Vitamin C is one of alternative medicine for obesity. It is a cofactor for burning of fat. Many researches confirmed that eating enough amount of food containing vitamin C which increases fat burn in the body during exercise by 25 % more than people with low blood levels of vitamin C.

It has anti- fatigue effect because it decreases heart rate, perception of fatigue and exertion during exercises. Other recent studies confirmed that obesity is associated with reduced growth hormone secretion and vitamin C levels are also reduced in obesity. Researchers discovered that dietary vitamin C intake has role for the regulation of growth hormone secretion and then the increasing vitamin C concentrations in obese will increase growth hormone secretion as seen by (Canoy et al. 2005; Furukawaet al 2004 & Flora, 2007).

13. PSYCHOLOGICAL EFFECTS

Stress lowers levels of vitamin C in the body because it is one of the nutrients sensitive to stress. It weakens immune system and enough daily intake of vitamin C improves condition of immune system. Some studies discovered that vitamin C decreases physical and psychological impact of stress. Patients of high levels of vitamin C have not any mental and physical signs of stress in acute psychological challenges. Vitamin C decreases secretion of cortisol in animals which is released by the adrenal glands in response to stress. Vitamin C is considered as an essential part of stress management by researchers (Levine et al., 2006).

14. NEUROPSYCHIATRIC EFFECTS

Psychiatric diseases such as vascular dementia, schizophrenia and Alzheimer have more benefit from using vitamin C as one of therapeutic option for these diseases because it is protective and improve cognitive function. Researchers observed that prevalence and incidence of Alzheimer are reduced among patients who received combination of vitamin C and E. According to recent experimental studies, vitamin C improves learning and memory in both sex but with different degree because of its antioxidants effects. Vitamin C may indirectly improve sleeping schedule and energy levels of daytime. According to the Mayo Clinic, it may improve iron absorption. Some people suffer from anemia due to poor iron absorption, which inhibits the ability to produce red blood cells and transport oxygen throughout the body. This can lead to feeling of fatigue and difficult sleep as seen by (David et al. 2010; Harrison, 2012).

So far, the relationship between vitamin c and brain function is not established although it's high concentration in the brain. Vitamin C improves cognition, alertness, language skills and increases IQ scores in normal and Down's. There are many studies about role of vitamin c for treatment of autism. We can use high doses of vitamin C for treatment of autism but by intravenous route to overcome its high dose side effects such as diarrhea. There is a link between autism in many children and vitamin C deficiency but this link is not well established because some autistic children have normal levels of vitamin C. It has a positive effect for change of behavior and improvement of autism symptoms such as oversensitivity to touch, light, or sound, aggression and difficulty with social interactions because it has a signaling effect on the brain, like a dopamine effect and then it is a cofactor for dopamine production. Some studies confirm that oxidative stress and free radicals play role for autism and then antioxidant property of vitamin c helps as alternative therapy line for autism. Vitamin C is not used as only one of autism treatment but it is added to vitamin mixtures. Autistic child with low level of vitamin C usually has a normal level after three months of oral supplementation with vitamin C as seen by (McGinnis, 2004 & Lisa, 2008).

Some studies suggest that vitamin C has high efficacy for treatment of some neurological disorders such as Parkinsonism. Tyrosine hydroxylase is responsible enzyme of dopamine biosynthesis. Vitamin C administration helps for regulation and increasing of this enzyme. Nurr1 gene is highly expressed in brain, midbrain dopaminergic cell development and survival. Vitamin C can increase Nurr1 protein expression. The progressive loss of dopaminergic neuron leads to motor function defect which is the cause of Parkinsonism. Status epilepticus is a neurologic disorder associated high mortality rate. It is characterized by alterations of normal brain function and cognitive state. Neurochemical and enzymatic activities studies suggest that status epilepticus can change free radical metabolism in brain. The oxidative stress has been associated with neuronal damage induced by seizures. The membrane lipid peroxidation can be produced by increase in free radicals levels and decrease in activities of antioxidant defense. The brain is a target for the peroxidative process because it has a high content of polyunsaturated fatty acids. Vitamin C is an exogenous antioxidant able to face the brain oxidative stress. According to experimental studies, vitamin C administration affects on latency of first seizures, percentage of seizures, mortality rate, lipid peroxidation levels and hippocampal catalase activity after seizures and status epilepticus as seen by Masaki et al. (2000).

15. ANTI-INFECTIVE AND IMMUNITY EFFECTS

Vitamin C is not an instant cure of whooping cough but it leads to significant decrease in cough severity because of neutralization of its toxin by this vitamin. Every breastfeeding mother should keep high levels of vitamin C in her body within 24 hours to relief whooping cough of her baby rapidly. Vitamin C is not antibacterial agent but it strengthens immune system by mobilization of neutrophils and phagocytes. There are other functions of vitamin C to keep the body against other toxins induced infectious diseases such as strengthening cellular and vascular collagen bonds, detoxifying the body and keeping mitochondria running properly. Clinical researches confirmed that large doses of vitamin C lead to therapeutic advantage for bums, injuries, surgical operations and infections. Phagocytosis and microbicidal activity of leukocytes are one of the major defense mechanisms of the host against infection. Vitamin C affects oxidative metabolism which causes an increase in hexose monophosphate shunt (HMS) activity. The process of phagocytosis by human polymorph nuclear leukocytes (PMN) is associated with changes of oxidative metabolism. HMS activity of leukocytes has an important role for the bactericidal activity of PMN. Although some recommends 2 grams or more of vitamin C for an adult as daily intake, but the use of vitamin C massive dose is still a controversial issue as seen by Azad et al. (2007).

A vaccination is a controversial issue because parents usually are unsatisfied about its side effects. Adverse effects and outcomes of vaccines result from allergic reactions depending on negative interaction with compromised immune systems. Any toxic effect or allergic reaction leads to oxidation of vital bio-molecules. Vitamin C is nonspecific antidote to any toxin or excess oxidative stress because its antioxidant effect. It should be included as part of any vaccination protocol for infants because of two reasons, the first it blocks the toxicity or side effects of vaccine and the second reason, it increases the antibody response of the immune system and then it improves efficacy of vaccine. Some studies demonstrated a protective role for vitamin C to decrease mortality rate of vaccinated infants if it is given before or after vaccinations as seen by (Amakye-Anim et al. 2000; Lauridsen& Jensen,2005; Cornford-Nairns 2012).

16. PHYSICAL PERFORMANCE EFFECTS

Vitamin C is useful for exercise metabolism and the health of exercising individuals because it is involved in some biochemical pathways. Some studies investigate requirement of vitamin C with exercise based on dietary vitamin C intakes. It assesses the response of body to supplementation of vitamin C and its changes of concentration in plasma, serum and leukocyte following both acute exercise and regular training. Exercise usually causes a transient increase in circulating ascorbic acid in the hours following exercise, but it declines below pre-exercise levels in the days after prolonged exercise. These changes are associated with increased exercise-induced oxidative stress. But it is still many questions so far on the role of regular exercise on increase metabolism of vitamin C. Some indicated that regular exercise does not increase the requirement of vitamin C in athletes. Others noticed a new finding such as attenuated levels of cortisol post-exercise after high doses of vitamin c. Athletes often take vitamin C supplements because severe muscular contractile activity results in oxidative stress. It is investigated by changes of glutathione concentrations in muscle and blood with increase in protein, DNA and lipid peroxidation. Oral administration of vitamin C decreases muscle mitochondrial biogenesis and training efficiency because it prevents some cellular adaptations to exercise. On the contrary other studies demonstrated that consuming 2 gram per day of vitamin C through five or more servings of fruit and vegetables may be sufficient to reduce oxidative stress and provide other health benefits without impairing training adaptations as indicated by Gandini et al. (2000).

17. VITAMIN C AND MINERALS

Vitamin C has a synergistic or parallel action with some minerals such as calcium. This action represents as alteration of cell permeability, decrease of nerve irritability, increase of blood coagulation, inhibition of allergic reactions, participation in tooth and bone growth, detoxification on heavy metals and arsenic. Vitamin C increases calcium absorption if it is taken with calcium supplements at the same time. Vitamin C and zinc have many health advantages such as potentiating of immunity; reducing the risk of age-related eye diseases and helping wounds heal. It helps the absorption of iron while zinc is required for the body to synthesize DNA and for cell division. The oral administration of the antioxidant vitamin C improves the performance of the iodine retention mechanism and treats defective cellular transport mechanism for iodine as seen by Morton et al. (2001); Maggini et al.(2012).

18. VITAMIN C AND STEM CELLS

In the last years, researchers discovered that Vitamin C is capable of generation of embryonic-like stem cells from adult cells by turning on set of genes. Adult cells are reprogrammed into cells with characteristics similar to embryonic stem cells. The reprogrammed cells (induced pluripotent stem cells "iPSCs") are potential for regeneration. Production of reactive oxygen species occurs during reprogramming. There is a potential link between high ROS and low reprogramming efficiency. Vitamin C is an essential antioxidant, so it enhances iPSC generation from both mouse and human cells. Vitamin C accelerated gene expression changes but other antioxidants do not have the same effect. Effect of Vitamin C on reprogramming is considered a reversal of the aging process at the cellular level. So it has anti-aging effects as seen by (Khaw et al. 2001 & Wei et al. 2012).

19. VITAMIN C AND LABORATORY INVESTIGATIONS

Vitamin C has an unwanted effect on laboratory investigations inducing false results and misdiagnosis. It reacts with chemical reagents of some tests and then it influences the results of tests. For example, Vitamin C blocks relevant chemical reactions, which may lead to false low blood glucose value. Two grams of vitamin C per day cause a positive result of urinary sugar test although glucose is not present, but it produces a negative result when glucose is present. Vitamin C affects other used tests such as enzymes activity assessment, uric acid and bilirubin. So physician should advise patient to stop taking the vitamins for two to three days prior to test. Vitamin C supplementation is recommended in haemodialysis patients because of diet limitations and losses with dialysis, (Luciak, 2004) but vitamin C effects on results of laboratory tests in haemodialysis patients. The lowest dose vitamin C leads to a false positive result whereas higher doses produce a false negative interference. Besides, there is a decrease in uric acid level with the high doses of vitamin C as seen by (Freemantle et al. 1994; Laight et al. 2000).

20. MISCELLANEOUS EFFECTS

Vitamin C has many ameliorative effects such as improving vision for uveitis, maintaining healthy gums, treating allergy conditions (eczema and allergic rhinitis) (Nurmatov et al. 2011), lowering of blood sugar in diabetic patients (Afkhami-Ardekani et al. 2007), strengthening of immune system and then high dose of vitamin C acts as antiviral agents. It exerts protective role against acute ultraviolet B-rays (Sunburn). Ascorbic acid has a prophylactic or therapeutic effect for some chronic diseases. Daily consumption of 1000 mg of vitamin C decreases blood glucose and lipids in patients of diabetes and thus reducing the risk of complications as seen by Tofler et al. (2000). Vitamin C is a new modern therapeutic line for fatty liver disease also. Increased vitamin C intake could prevent nephrotoxic effect. It assists in the prevention of blood clotting and bruising. It strengthens the walls of the capillaries. Vitamin C helps to reduce cholesterol levels and preventing atherosclerosis as seen by Kurowska et al. (2000). Vitamin C lowers risk of developing gout if it is taken regularly. It significantly lowered serum uric acid. According to results of previous studies, every 500 mg increase in vitamin C intake leads to decrease of risk for gout by 17 % as seen by (Choi et al., 2009).

Any joint consists of two covered bone with cartilage. Collagen is an essential part of cartilage. Vitamin C helps the body to form collagen. Destruction of this cartilage is called osteoarthritis. Some studies indicated to free radicals may be involved in destruction of cartilage. Incidence of this disease is reduced for persons who eat foods rich in vitamin C. Non-steroidal anti-inflammatory drugs are the first choice for treatment of osteoarthritis but it reduces levels of vitamin C. So taking of these drugs for osteoarthritis is associated with vitamin C supplement (Canter et al. 2007).

It protects susceptible cells from genotoxicity associated with antiestrogen metabolite-4-hydroxyl tamoxifen (4-OH tom) and inhibit DNA adduct induced by tamoxifen. Update study discovered that electromagnetic field of cell phone affects testes by increase of seminiferous tubules diameter with disorganization of sperm cycle. Effects of electromagnetic field were caused by oxidative stress. This study revealed that vitamin C can counter theses effects and restore the testes to normal condition.

CONCLUSION

Vitamin C (L-ascorbic acid) is an essential nutrient for humans. It scavenges reactive oxygen species and may, thereby, prevent oxidative damage to the important biological macromolecules, and could reduce aflatoxin induced liver cancer. Moreover, vitamin C abolishes chromosome damage resulting from the effect of toxic molecules, and help to protect the body against pollutants. Vitamin C is a biological reducing agent; it is also linked to the prevention of degenerative diseases such as cataracts, certain cancers and cardiovascular diseases. Increased vitamin C intake could possibly reduce and the prevent nephrotoxic effect. It assists in the prevention of blood clotting and bruising. It also strengthens the walls of the capillaries and in addition, it is well documented that vitamin C helps to reduce cholesterol levels, high blood pressure and prevent atherosclerosis. Vitamin C is absorbed by the intestine using a sodium-ion dependent channel, transported through the intestine via both glucose-sensitive and glucose-insensitive mechanisms. The presence of large quantities of sugar either in the intestines or in the blood can slow absorption. The richest natural sources are fruits, vegetables and some cuts of meat, especially liver. Plants are generally a good source of vitamin C, the amount in foods of plant origin depends on the precise variety of the plant, the soil condition, the climate in which it grew the length of time since it was picked, the storage conditions and the method of preparation. While in animals, vitamin C is most present in liver, muscle, mother's milk and in a lower amount in raw cow's milk, with pasteurized milk containing only trace amount. All excess vitamin C is disposed of through the urinary system. Moreover, during the cooking of food decomposes vitamin C chemically. The concentrations of various food substances decrease with time in proportion to the temperature they are stored at and cooking can reduce the vitamin C content of vegetables by around 60%.

REFERENCES

Afkhami-Ardekani M, Shojaoddiny-Ardekani A. Effect of vitamin C on blood glucose, serum lipids & serum insulin in type 2 diabetes patients (2007). *Indian J. Med. Res.*; 126(5):471-4.

Amakye-Anim, J., T. Lin, P. Hester, D. Thiagarajan, B. A. Watkins, and C. C. Wu. (2000). Ascorbic acid supplementation improved antibody response to infectious bursal disease vaccination in chickens. *Poultry Science* 79:680-688.

Audera C, Patulny RV, Sander BH, Douglas RM (2001). Mega-dose vitamin C in treatment of the common cold: a randomized controlled trial. *Med. J. Aust.*; 175(7):359-362.

Azad, I., J. Dayal, M. Poornima, and S. Ali. (2007). Supra dietary levels of vitamins C and E enhance antibody production and immune memory in juvenile milkfish, chanos (Forsskal) to formalin-killed Vibrio vulnificus. *Fish & Shellfish Immunology* 23:154-163.

Bano M, Bhatt DK. (2010). Ameliorative effect of a combination of vitamin E, vitamin C, alpha-lipoid acid and stilbene resveratrol on lindane induced toxicity in mice olfactory lobe and cerebrum. *Indian J. Exp. Biol.*; 48(2):150-8.

Braun BL, Fowles JB, Solberg L, Kind E, Healey M, Anderson R (2000). Patient beliefs about the characteristics, causes, and care of the common cold: an update. *J. Fam. Pract.*; 49(2):153-156.

Canoy D, Wareham N, Welch A, Bingham S, Luben R, Day N & Khaw KT. (2005). Plasma ascorbic acid concentrations and fat distribution in 19,068 British men and women in the European Prospective Investigation into Cancer and Nutrition Norfolk cohort study. *American Journal of Clinical Nutrition* 82; 1203–1209.

Canter PH, Wider B, Ernst E. (2007). The antioxidant vitamins A, C, E and selenium in the treatment of arthritis: a systematic review of randomized clinical trials. *Rheumatology*. 46(8):1223-33.

Chappell LC, Seed PT, Kelly FJ, Briley A, Hunt BJ, Charnock-Jones DS, et al. (2002).Vitamin C and E supplementation in women at risk of pre-eclampsia is associated with changes in indices of oxidative stress and placental function. *Am. J. Obstet. Gynecol;* 187(3):777–84.

Choi HK, Goa X, Curhan G. Vitamin C intake and the risk of gout in men. *Arch. Intern. Med* 2009; 169:502-7.

Claudia PMS Oliveira, Luiz Carlos da Costa Gayotto, Caroline Tatai, Bianca Ishimoto Della Nina, Emerson S Lima, Dulcinéia SP Abdulla, Fabio P Lopasso, Francisco RM Laurindo, and Deicher R, Hörl WH. (2003). Vitamin C in chronic kidney disease and hemodialysis patients. *Kidney Blood Press Res.*; 26(2):100-6.

Cornford-Nairns, R. (2012). "Construction and Preliminary Immunobiological Characterization of a Novel, Non-Reverting, Intranasal Live Attenuated Whooping Cough Vaccine Candidate." *J. Microbiol. Biotechnol.* 22(6), 856–865.

Cook NR, Albert CM, Gaziano JM, Zaharris E, MacFadyen J, Danielson E, Buring JE, Manson JE. (2007). a randomized factorial trial of vitamins C and E and beta carotene in the secondary prevention of cardiovascular events in women: results from the Women's Antioxidant Cardiovascular Study. *Arch. Intern. Med.*; 167(15):1610-8.

Daniel TA, Nawarskas JJ. (2000). Vitamin C in the prevention of nitrate tolerance. *Ann. Pharacother.;* 34(10):1193-1197.

David O. Kennedy, Rachel Veasey, Anthony Watson, Fiona Dodd, Emma Jones, Silvia Maggini, and Crystal F. Haskell. (2010). Effects of high-dose B vitamin complex with vitamin C and minerals on subjective mood and performance in healthy males. *Psychopharmacology (Berl).* 211(1): 55–68.

Douglas RM, Chalker EB, Treacy B. (2000). Vitamin C for preventing and treating the common cold. *Cochrane Database Syst. Rev.* (2):CD000980.

EL-Meghawry EL-Kenawy Ayman, Hosam Eldin Hussein Osman, Maha Hasan Daghestani (2013). The effect of vitamin C administration on monosodium glutamate induced liver injury. An experimental study. *Exp. Toxicol. Pathology*, in press.

Ersöz G, Günşar F, Karasu Z, Akay S, Batur Y, Akarca US. (2005). Management of fatty liver disease with vitamin E and C compared to ursodeoxycholic acid treatment, *Turk J. Gastroenterol.*, 16(3):124-8.

Flora SJ. (2007). Role of free radicals and antioxidants in health and disease. *Cellular and Molecular Biology* 53; 1–2.

Freemantle J, Freemantle MJ, Badrick T. (1994). Ascorbate interferences in common clinical assays performed on three analyzers. *Clin. Chem;* 40: 950–951.

Furukawa S, Fujita T, Shimabukuro M, Iwaki M, Yamada Y, Nakajima Y, Nakayama O, Makishima M, Matsuda M & Shimomura I. (2004). Increased oxidative stress in obesity and its impact on metabolic syndrome. *Journal of Clinical Investigation* 114; 1752–1761.

Gandini S, Merzenich H, Robertson C, Boyle P. (2000). Meta-analysis of studies on breast cancer risk and diet: the role of fruit and vegetable consumption and the intake of associated micronutrients. *Eur. J. Cancer.*; 36:636-646.

Gaziano JM, Glynn RJ, and Christen WG, et al. Vitamins E and C in the prevention of prostate total cancer in men: the physicians' health study II randomized controlled trial. *JAMA* 2009; 301:52-62.

Harrison FE. (2012). A critical review of vitamin C for the prevention of age-related cognitive decline and Alzheimer's disease. *J Alzheimer's Dis.* 29(4):711-26.

Head KA. (2001) Natural therapies for ocular disorders, part two: cataracts and glaucoma. *Altern Med Rev.*; 6(2):141-66.

Heaney ML, Gardner JR, Karasavvas N, et al. (2008).Vitamin C antagonizes the cytotoxic effects of antineoplastic drugs. *Cancer Res*; 68:8031-8.

Kompauer I, Heinrich J, Wolfram G, Linseisen J. (2006) Association of carotenoids, tocopherols, and vitamin C in plasma with allergic rhinitis and allergic sensitization in adults. *Public Health Nutr.* ; 9:472-9.

Khaw KT, Bingham S, Welch A, Luben R, Wareham N, Oakes S. & Day N. (2001). Relation between plasma ascorbic acid and mortality in men and women in EPIC-Norfolk prospective study: a prospective population study. European Prospective Investigation into Cancer and Nutrition. *Lancet*. 3; 357(9257):657-63.

Kurowska EM, Spence JD, Jordan J, Wetmore S, Freeman DJ, Piche LA, Serratore P. (2000). HDL-cholesterol-raising effect of orange juice in subjects with hypercholesterolemia. *Am J. Clin. Nutr.*72 (5):1095-1100.

Laight DW, Carrier MJ, Anggard EE. (2000). Antioxidants, diabetes and endothelial dysfunction. *Cardiovasc. Res.*; 47:457-464.

Langlois M, Duprez D, Delanghe J, De Buyzere M, Clement DL. (2001). Serum vitamin C concentration is low in peripheral arterial disease and is associated with inflammation and severity of atherosclerosis. *Circulation*, 103(14):1863-1868.

Lauridsen, C. & Jensen S. (2005). Influence of supplementation of all-rac-alpha-tocopheryl acetate pre weaning and vitamin C post weaning on alpha-tocopherol and immune responses in piglets. *Journal of Animal Science* 83:1274-1286.

Lisa A. Kurtz. (2008). "Understanding Controversial Therapies for Children with Autism, Attention Deficit Disorder, and Other Learning Disabilities: *A Guide to Complementary and Alternative Medicine*"; Jessica Kingsley Publishers.

Lon E. (2001). Do antioxidant vitamins protect against atherosclerosis? The proof is still lacking. *J. Am. Coll. Cardio.* ; 38:1795-8.

Luciak M (2004). Antioxidants in the treatment of patients with renal failure *Roczniki Akademii Medycznej w Bialymstoku* 49: 135- 260. Annales Academiae Medicae Bialostocensis.

Lykkesfeldt J, Christen S, Wallock LM, Chang HH, Jacob RA, Ames BN. (2000). Ascorbate is depleted by smoking and repleted by moderate supplementation: a study in male smokers and nonsmokers with matched dietary antioxidant intakes. *Am. J. Clin. Nutr.*, 71(2):530-536.

Maggini S, Beveridge S. & Suter M. (2012). A combination of high-dose vitamin C plus zinc for the common cold. *J Int Med Res.* 40(1):28-42.

Masaki H. (2010). Role of antioxidants in the skin: anti-aging effects. *J. Dermatol. Sci.* 2010; 58(2):85-90. Epub Mar 17.

Masaki KH, Losonczy KG, Izmirlian G. (2000). Association of vitamin E and C supplement use with cognitive function and dementia in elderly men. *Neurology*. 54:1265-1272.

Mares-Perlman JA, Lyle BJ, Klein R, et al. (2000). Vitamin supplements use and incident cataracts in a population-based study. *Arch. Ophthalmol.*118:1556-63.

Michaels A, Frei B. (2012). *"Vitamin C"*. In Caudill MA, Rogers M. Biochemical, Physiological, and Molecular Aspects of Human Nutrition (3 Ed.). Philadelphia: Saunders. pp. 627–654.

McGregor GP, Biesalski HK. (2006). "Rationale and impact of vitamin C in clinical nutrition". *Curr. Opin. Clin. Nutr. Metab. Care* 9 (6): 697–703.

McGinnis WR. (2004).Oxidative stress in autism. *Altern Ther Health Med*; 10(6):22-36; 37, 92. Morton DJ, Barrett-Connor EL. & Schneider DL. (2001). Vitamin C supplement use and bone mineral density in postmenopausal women. *J. Bone Miner. Res.*, 16(1):135-40.

Nurmatov U, Devereux G, Sheikh A. (2011). Nutrients and foods for the primary prevention of asthma and allergy: systematic review and meta-analysis. *J. Allergy Clin. Immunol;* 127(3):724-33.e1-30.

Padayatty SJ, Doppman JL, Chang R, Wang Y, Gill J, Papanicolaou DA, Levine M. (2007). Human adrenal glands secrete vitamin C in response to adrenocorticotrophic hormone. *Am. J. Clin. Nutr.*; 86(1):145-9.

Padayatty SJ, Katz A, Wang Y, Eck P, Kwon O, Lee JH, Chen S, Corpe C, Dutta A, Dutta SK, Levine M. (2003). "Vitamin C as an antioxidant: evaluation of its role in disease prevention". *J. Am. Coll. Nutr* 22 (1): 18–35.

Padayatty SJ, Levine M. (2000). Reevaluation of ascorbate in cancer treatment: emerging evidence, open minds and serendipity. *J. Am. Coll. Nutr.* 19(4):423-425.

Petersen EE, Genet M, Caserini M, Palmieri R. (2011). Efficacy of vitamin C vaginal tablets in the treatment of bacterial vaginosis: a randomized, double blind, placebo controlled clinical trial. *Arzneimittelforschung*, 61(4):260-5.

Ram FS, Rowe BH, Kaur B. (2004). Vitamin C supplementation for asthma. *Cochrane Database Syst Rev.* (3):CD000993.

Ratna Priya and Vasudha K. C. (2009). Antioxidant vitamins in chronic renal failure. *Biomedical Research* 2009; 20 (1): 67-70.

Rock CL, Michael CW, Reynolds RK, Ruffin MT. (2000). Prevention of cervix cancer. *Crit Rev. Oncol. Hematol.* 33(3):169-185.

Sabzevarizadeh M. & Najafzadeh H. (2012). Comparison Effect of Silymarin and Vitamin C on Liver Function in Myoglobinuric Status in Rats. *World Applied Sciences Journal* 17 (2): 228-232.

Sebastian J. Padayatty, Yaohui Wang, Oran Kwon (2003).Vitamin C as an Antioxidant: Evaluation of Its Role in Disease Prevention. *Journal of the American College of Nutrition*, 22, No. 1, 18–35.

Sharma JB, Mittal S. (2004). Oxidative stress and pre-eclampsia. *Obstet. Gynaecol. Today*; 9:551– 4.

Shinke T, Shite J, Takaoka H, Hata K, Inoue N, Yoshikawa R, Matsumoto H, Masai H, Watanabe S, Ozawa T, Otake H, Matsumoto D, Hirata K, Yokoyama M. (2007). Vitamin C restores the contractile response to dobutamine and improves myocardial efficiency in patients with HF. *Amer Heart* J.154 (4):645.1-8.

Suleiman F. Ambali, Chinedu Orieji, Woziri O. Abubakar, Muftau Shittu, and Mohammed U. Kawu. (2011).Ameliorative Effect of Vitamin C on Alterations in Thyroid Hormones Concentrations Induced by Sub chronic Co administration of Chlorpyrifos and Lead in Wistar Rats. *Journal of Thyroid Research*, 2; 1-6.

Taylor A, Jacques PF, Chylack LT Jr, et al. (2002). Long-term intake of vitamins and carotenoids and odds of early age-related cortical and posterior sub capsular lens opacities. *Am. J. Clin. Nutr.* 75(3):540-549.

Tofler GH, Stec JJ, Stubbe I, Beadle J, Feng D, Lipinska I, Taylor A. (2000).The effect of vitamin C supplementation on coagulability and lipid levels in healthy male subjects. *Thromb. Res.* 100(1):35-41.

Ustundag S, Yalcin O, Sen S, Cukur Z, Ciftci S, Demirkan B. (2008). Experimental myoglobinuric acute renal failure: the effect of vitamin C. *Ren. Fail.* ;30(7):727-35.

Wei F, Qu C, Song T, Ding G, Fan Z, Liu D, Liu Y, Zhang C, Shi S. & Wang S. (2012). Vitamin C treatment promotes mesenchymal stem cell sheet formation and tissue regeneration by elevating telomerase activity. *J. Cell. Physiol.*; 227(9):3216-24.

Reviewed by

El-kott A. F. (phD), Department of biology, Faculty of Science,
Damanhour University, Damanhour, Egypt

Metwally El-Sayed Metwally (PhD),
Forensic Medicine and clinical Toxicology Department, College of Medicine,
Suez Canal University, Ismailia, Egypt

In: Vitamin C
Editor: Raquel Guiné

ISBN: 978-1-62948-154-8
© 2013 Nova Science Publishers, Inc.

Chapter 4

IONIZING RADIATION EFFECTS ON VITAMIN C

Marcia N. C. Harder[1,], Valter Arthur[2,#], Suely S. H. Franco[2,†] and Paula B. Arthur[2,‡]*

[1]Department of Agroindustry,
Technology College of Piracicaba "Dep. Roque Trevisan",
FATEC Piracicaba, Santa Rosa, Piracicaba, Brazil
[2]Department of Radiobiology and Enviroment,
Center of Nuclear Energy in Agriculture, University of São Paulo,
CENA/USP, São Judas, Piracicaba, Brazil

ABSTRACT

The irradiation process has been the subject of increasing attention during the last decades because of the distinct advantages it offers over conventional methods of food processing: food can be processed after packaging; can be preserved in fresh state and perishable can be kept longer without quality loss. For fruits; fruit juices and vegetables are the most promising treatment is the combination of radiation and other treatments for sterilization. With irradiation alone, it may require higher doses of radiation and consequently promote enzyme's inactivation, wich are responsible for sensory changes during storage of these products. Food irradiation is not a new technology. The lethal effects of ionizing radiation on organisms are observed and reported since 1898 and techniques for using radiation in order to kill bacteria in food have been tested since 1916. The amounts of scientific data generated by various countries and international partnership programs during the past 50 years and together with research outweigh any other techniques for food processing. The percentage of vitaminis lost in food production will depend on: irradiation dose; food composition food temperature to be irradiated and the presence or absence of oxygen. Vitamins are more susceptible to irradiation in the presence of oxygen at temperatures above freezing. Generally the higher the radiation dose greatest is the loss of vitamins. Lost vitamins to food treated with irradiation below

[*] E-mail: marcia.harder@fatec.sp.gov.br.
[#] E-mail: arthur@cena.usp.br.
[†] E-mail: gilmita@uol.com.br.
[‡] E-mail: paula.arthur@hotmail.com.

1 kGy are minimum compatible with the loss in regards to heating foods treated and stored for long periods of time. Already doses above 10 kGy are likely to degrade these substances; however researchers indicated that these losses can be minimized by irradiation in oxygen-free packaging (cans or flexible packaging) or at cryogenic temperatures ranging from -20°C to -40°C. Aqueous solutions of vitamins are more vulnerable to destruction by irradiation than those in the matrix of dehydrated food or food. The objective of this study was to conduct a literature review pointing out studies that assessed changes in vitamin C caused by the action of ionizing radiation.

1. INTRODUCTION

The irradiation process has been the subject of increasing attention during the last decades due to the distinct advantages it offers over conventional methods of food processing: food can be processed after packaging; can be preserved in the fresh state; and perishable can be kept longer without quality loss.

For fruits; fruit juices and vegetables, the most promising treatment is the combination of radiation and other treatments because the sterilization with irradiation alone may require high doses of radiation and consequently promote enzyme inactivation responsible for sensory changes during storage of these products.

The fruits and vegetables treatment with ionizing radiation whose main purpose is to ensure its preservation, i.e., increase shelf life of food. This process may involve the inactivation of microorganisms (mainly fungi, bacteria and yeast); delay ripening and disinfestations among other mechanisms (Iemma et al, 1999).

Like other food processing techniques the irradiation can cause changes in the chemical composition and nutritional value. The nature and extent of these changes depends essentially of the type; variety and composition of the food; the radiation dose received and the environmental conditions during and after irradiation (Wiendl, 1984).

The ascorbic acid is known as a promoter of numerous chemical; biochemical and physiological characteristics, both in animals and in plants. It performs many functions in the body related to the immune system; collagen formation; iron absorption; inhibition of nitrosamines formation and antioxidant activity. Its contents can be influenced by soil type; cultivation; climatic conditions; agricultural procedures for harvesting and storage. Furthermore, the ascorbic acid in its pure form is very unstable and is easily destroyed by oxidation, particularly in high temperature; light; humidity; alkalinity; metal catalysts and physical damage (O'Keefe, 2001; Silva et al, 2004; Lima et al, 2009).

Studies have shown that among the water-soluble vitamins, the vitamin C is the most sensitive to radiation (Josephson, 1978). However, is necessary to remember that, the vitamin C as a relatively labile vitamin and similar results occur in its destruction treatments food by use of heat (Wiendl, 1984).

2. EFFECTS OF RADIATION ON FOOD

The food irradiation is not a new technology. The lethal effects of ionizing radiation on organisms are being observed and reported since 1898 and techniques for using radiation to kill bacteria in food have been tested since 1916. The amount of scientific data generated by various countries and international partnership programs during the past 50 years, the research outweighs any other technique for food processing (Mollins et al., 2001).

The Board of Experts on Food Irradiation Committee, formed by UN (United Nations) agencies (IAEA, WHO, among others) suggests that the process of food irradiation which is used gamma radiation from radionuclide originated Cobalto-60; Césio-137; and X-rays with energy up to 5MeV or electrons with energy up to 10MeV (Diehl, 1992; FAO/IAEA 1982). In general, the irradiation process at recommended doses causes little chemical changes in foods (Diehl et al., 1994, Al-Masri, 2003) however when inadequate doses are applied in food, they might have flavor or level components changed, making it unsuitable for consumption (ICGFI, 1999). According to Diehl (1992a, 1992b, 1995) at doses up to 1kGy the nutritional losses are considered insignificant and not known changes found in irradiated foods are harmful or dangerous being within the limits, normally found in foods (Satin, 1993; Delincee et al. 1998). For higher doses (over 10kGy) which are used for sterilization control and dangerous pathogens; nutritional losses are evaluated as lower or comparable with those arising from the cooking and cooling process (Grolinchova et al., 2004).

Radiation in proteins is able to induce changes in their configuration by the breaks through on the original connections as hydrogen bonds and SS bonds which stabilize their secondary and tertiary structures. With this change, its features can be compromised. It is important to note that these changes are related to pure chemicals compounds, when these elements are irradiated in complex mixtures (foods) there may be a variation in the sensitivity to the radiation (Grolinchova et al 2004). Fats are classified as one of the components most sensitive to ionizing radiation which can induce many hydrolytic reactions and auto-oxidant leading to undesirable organoleptic changes and loss of essential fatty acids. The range and nature of the changes caused by some radiation doses depend upon the material composition that is being irradiated; the type of fat and the unsaturated fatty acids content (Grolinchova et al 2004). Moreover, carbohydrates and minerals in foods are relatively radiation stable until 10kGy (Roberts & Weese, 2006).

The electromagnetic radiation absorption by biological tissues is the food, constitute is a function of the constituent molecules electron excitation. In the case of gamma radiation, the electronic excitation produced is sufficient to eject electrons from their respective orbitals resulting in the molecular ionization. One of the most important free radicals induced by radiation is the hydroxyl radical (HO-) formation that is involved in reactions of initiation and propagation of the chain reaction responsible for the effects of radiation (Riley, 1994).

The percentage of lost vitamins in food production will depend on: irradiation dose; food composition; food temperature to be irradiated; and presence or absence of oxygen. Vitamins are more susceptible to irradiation in the presence of oxygen at temperatures above freezing. Generally higher radiation dose causes higher losses of vitamins. A Committee formed by the FAO (Food and Agriculture Organization); WHO (World Health Organization) and IAEA (International Atomic Energy Agency) indicated that loss of vitamins to food treated with irradiation below 1kGy are minimum and are compatible losses in foods heating treated and stored for long periods of time (Roberts & Weese, 2006). Already doses above 10kGy can degrade these substances; however, researchers indicated that these losses can be minimized by irradiation in oxygen-free packaging (cans or flexible packaging) or at cryogenic temperatures ranging from -20°C to -40°C. Aqueous solutions of vitamins are more vulnerable to destruction by irradiation than those in the food matrix or the dehydrated food. Then the extrapolation of the nutritional losses of aqueous solutions is inappropriate for solid food (SCF, 2003).

Although there is a minimal vitamin losses associated to irradiation, especially some more sensitive as vitamins: B1; C and E, it is extremely unlikely that there are vitamins deficiencies due to consumption of irradiated foods (GAO, 2000). All other vitamins tend to be relatively stable to irradiation under 5kGy (Roberts & Weese, 2006).

In 1962 the WHO and the American Medical Association reported that irradiated food was produced according to good manufacturing practices (GMP) and should be considered safe and nutritionally adequate, because the radiation: a) does not induce a change in the composition of the food, which the toxicological point of view, that could lead to adverse effects on human health; b) does not induce changes in the food microflora, which could increase the microbiological risk to the consumer and; c) does not lead to nutrient losses, which could impose adverse effects to the individual or population state nutritional (Spolaore et al., 2003).

The Joint Expert Committee on Food Irradiation (JECFI), formed by FAO; WHO and IAEA in 1980 granted the 10kGy dose to irradiated foods as a safety condition: "any food irradiated to a dose of 10kGy did not caused toxicological problems, so toxicology tests with this kind of food are not necessary anymore". Moreover, the JECFI declared that food irradiation to a dose of 10kGy does not induce nutritional or microbiological problems. From these findings the Codex Alimentarius Commission, in association with the International Recommended Code of Practice for the Operation of Radiation Facilities used for the Treatment of Food presented in 1983 a General Standard for Irradiated Food. These codes were followed by many countries in the 80´s and 90´s thereafter initiated the procedures for this technology adoption for various irradiation applications. Currently 40 countries have radiating at least one or more products and 29 countries are already applying the irradiation process on a commercial basis (Kooij, [n/d]).

In 1997 the WHO together with FAO and IAEA held a meeting of experts to examine issues related to irradiation at doses above 10kGy and concluded that: "The food irradiated to any dose needs to have an appropriate dose to achieve the intended technological objective and both safe when to consume are nutritionally adequate" (GAO, 2000; Mollins et al., 2001). Irradiation doses above 10kGy are used for animal origin and very moist food; full meals for patients on immunotherapy; astronauts; military; and individuals in special activities outdoors and for decontamination of low moisture herbs and dried vegetables (SCF, 2003).

3. GAMMA IRRADIATION ON VITAMIN C

As any thermal treatment, loss of nutrients in foods from animal and plant sources occurs with irradiation, and nutrient loss increases with radiation´s dose. According to the World Health Organization, thiamin (vitamin B1), vitamin C, and the tocopherols (vitamin E) are extremely radiation sensitive. Much of the change in nutrient composition is a result of irradiation unexplainable-loss of certain nutrients is different for different foods. The most radiation-sensitive, fat-soluble vitamin is vitamin E, and then Carotene, vitamin A, vitamin D, and vitamin K follows in decreasing order of sensitivity. Vitamin B1 is the most radiation-sensitive, water-soluble vitamin, and then vitamin C, vitamin B6, vitamin B2, folate and niacin, and vitamin B12 follow in decreasing order of sensitivity (FAP/IAEA/WHO, 1999; Keller, 2013).

The organic and inorganic molecules and atoms, that contain one or more unpaired electrons, with independent existence, can be classified as free radicals (Halliwell, 1994). This configuration makes the free radicals highly unstable molecules with very short half-life and chemically very reactive (Bianchi & Antunes, 1999).

The continuous production of free radicals during the metabolic processes turns the development of many antioxidant defense mechanisms to limit the intracellular levels and prevent damage induction (Sies, 1993). Antioxidants are agents responsible for the inhibition and reduction of injuries caused by free radicals in cells (Bianchi & Antunes, 1999).

A broader definition of antioxidant is: "any substance that when present in low concentrations compared to oxidizable substrate delays or inhibits oxidation of the substrate effectively" (Stahl & Sies, 1997; Bianchi & Antunes, 1999).

These agents that protects cells against the effects of free radicals can be classified into antioxidants enzymatic or non-enzymatic (Sies, 1993). Vitamin C, for example, operates in the aqueous phase as an excellent antioxidant on free radicals, but it is not able to act on lipophilic compartments to inhibit the lipid peroxidation. Furthermore, in vitro studies showed that this vitamin in the presence of transition metals such as iron can act as a pro-oxidant molecule and generate OH and H2O2 radicals. Generally these metals are available in very limited quantities and the antioxidant properties of this vitamin predominates in vivo (Odin, 1997; Bianchi & Antunes, 1999).

The vitamin C (ascorbic acid) is usually consumed in large doses by humans, being added to many food products for inhibiting the formation of nitro carcinogenic metabolites. The vitamin C diet is absorbed quickly and efficiently by an energy-dependent process. Consumption of high doses can lead to increased concentration of this vitamin in the tissues and blood plasma (Bianchi & Antunes, 1999).

The benefits obtained in the vitamin C therapeutic use in biological assays with animals include a protective effect against damage caused by exposure to radiation and drugs (Amara-Mokrane et al., 1996). Epidemiological studies also attribute this vitamin as a possible protective role in the development of tumors in humans (Lupulescu, 1993; Duthie et al., 1996; Bianchi & Antunes, 1999).

However, the recommendation of this vitamin supplementation should be evaluated specifically for each case where there are many organic and inorganic components in cells that can modulate the activity of vitamin C, affecting their antioxidant activity (Bianchi & Antunes, 1999).

According to Graham & Stevenson (1997) the vitamin C content four varieties of strawberry and it was determined before and after treatment with ionizing radiation at doses of 1, 2 or 3 kGy and after storage for 5 and 10 days at 6°C, and also in potatoes which having been allowed a period of one month to recover from the effects of post-harvest stress, were irradiated at a sprout inhibition dose of 0•15 kGy, followed by storage and cooking. Total ascorbic acid (TAA), ascorbic acid (AA) and dehydroascorbic acid (DHAA) concentrations were measured using the technique of ion-exclusion high-performance liquid chromatography. Results from analysis of strawberry samples showed the DHAA content increased immediately following irradiation and must, therefore, be take into account when reporting vitamin C levels in irradiated produce. In addition, it was observed that whilst irradiation did affect the vitamin C concentration in all varieties of strawberry, the change was small in comparison with the large variations observed between varieties. With regard to potatoes results showed that, whilst irradiation, storage and cooking all had the effect of reducing vitamin C concentration, irradiated samples stored for 5 months had similar or marginally higher levels than their non-irradiated counterparts. Cooking did not markedly reduce TAA content of irradiated potatoes compared to non-irradiated potatoes and it was also noted that microwave cooking was more destructive than boiling in lightly salted water (Dionísio et al., 2009).

As seen, the ascorbic acid is one of the vitamins more sensitive font the irradiation. According to Proctor & Goldblith (1949), there are many fruits in which the level of ascorbic acid is not reduced significantly in a dose that fruit may tolerate (Maxie et al. 1964). These doses used to irradiate orange juice are above the tolerance level and the results showed a decrease in ascorbic acid with increasing radiation dose, reaching a lower value with the highest 7.5kGy dose (Spoto, 1988). These results are in agreement with those find by Munhoz-Burgos (1985) who observed a decrease in the vitamin C content with increasing radiation dose in orange juice; tangerine; tomato and passion fruit, being the orange and tangerine juices the most sensitive to radiation.

Wilska-Jeszka & Skorupinska (1975) also observed an ascorbic acid drastic decrease in tomato juices and blackcurrant and red syrups irradiated in relation to pasteurization by heating. This fact was also observed by Hussain & Maxie (1974) who observed losses of up to 70% of vitamin C in orange juice irradiated with doses of 2.5 to 10kGy.

Although there are some disagreement about the effects of radiation on the ascorbic acid content in citrus fruits, the results reported by the majority jobs shows unanimous in saying this lost in minimal when samples are irradiated with doses up to 1.0kGy. Exposure to doses higher than 1.0kGy can cause the destruction of this vitamin at a rate that increases proportionally with increasing doses of radiation to cite the work of: Romani et al., 1963; Ahmed et al., 1968; Ahmed, 1977; Guerrero et al., 1967; Dennison, 1968; Macfarlane and Roberts, 1968; Maxie et. al., 1964; Maxie et al., 1969; Kurosaki & Ogatta, 1971; Moshonas and Shaw 1984; Shaw and Moshonas, 1991.

Minimum ascorbic acid values found by Monseline & Khan (1966) arrived around 84% compared to controls and the differences were significant only in green fruit over ripe fruit. Josephson et al. (1978) observed that the retention of ascorbic acid in oranges; tangerines; tomatoes and papayas had a range of 73% to 100% when they were irradiated with doses from 0.4 to 3.0kGy. Spoto (1988) found a higher ascorbic acid loss when juices were heated at 50°C compared to 25°C irradiation temperature being lower than the variation between doses at that same temperature. Authors like Hussain & Maxie (1974); Dharkar (1964) reported that there is a higher ascorbic acid loss only by the irradiation than when compared to the combined treatment of irradiation and heating.

Munhoz-Burgos (1985) gave a better retention of acid ascorbic in tangerine juice irradiated, previously pasteurized as compared to only irradiated with a dose of 1.0kGy.

Much more pronounced than the effects of radiation dose and temperature of irradiation according to Spoto (1988) were the temperatures and storage periods which is consistent with the work of Wilska-Jeszka & Skorupinska (1975) that observed that the ascorbic acid losses percentage showed a variation of 15 to 23% in the juice irradiated with different doses of radiation over the pasteurized juice which was 76 to 80% during the storage period.

According to Dionísio et al. (2009):

- These are reports describing gradual loss of ascorbic acid in apples (Pyrus malus L.) irradiated with more than 2 kGy (Saito & Igarashi, 1970; Chunyao et al., 1993; Lastarria-Tapia & Sequeiros, 1985). However, after six months of storage at 0°C, no alterations in the ascorbic acid content of the fruits were observed (Saito & Igarashi, 1970). Destruction of vitamin C is a consequence of alteration of fruits metabolic oxidation pathways by radiation, which can convert vitamin C into dehydro-ascorbic acid, which can still be metabolized as vitamin C (Snauwart, 1973).
- Papaya and mango rot caused by fungi is a major problem during the storage and marketing. Gamma irradiation treatment was studied to determine its effect on the quality of papaya and mango irradiated at 0.5 to 0.95 kGy. The content of vitamin C was not significantly affected by the irradiation (Lacroix et al., 1990).
- Star fruit, mango, papaya, rambutan, and lichia were irradiated with 0.75 kGy and evaluated the vitamin C retention. Only star fruit presented significant vitamin C loss (Moy & Wong, 2002).
- Capsicums (green and red), cucumbers, custard apples, lemons, lychees, mandarins, mangoes, nectarines, papayas, peaches, persimmons, and zucchinis were irradiated at 0, 75, or 300 Gy. Commodities were analyzed shortly after the irradiation and again after 3 to 4 weeks of storage at 1-7°C for some parameters, such as vitamin C and dehydroascorbic acid. Significant ($p < 0.05$) small changes were recorded in some variables for some commodities. However, storage effects were higher than irradiation effects (Mitchell et al, 1992).
- Strawberries (Shasta variety, Fragaria sp.) presented minute, non-significant decrease in vitamin C levels when submitted to 1.0-2.0 kGy doses, during two and 11 days of storage at 5°C (Maxie et al., 1964). Similar observations were reported by Lopez et al. (1967). A study using higher radiation doses (3.0 and 4.0 kGy), resulted in 62 and 81% losses of ascorbic acid, respectively (Clark, 1959). However, 1.0-2.0 kGy doses are deemed enough to extend the shelf life of the fruits. Fruits irradiated with 2.0 kGy doses presented immediate increase in niacin contents, while thiamin was unaltered (Maxie & Sommer, 1968). A study with Selekta and Parafit varieties irradiated with 2 kGy doses, showed non-significant differences in riboflavin, thiamin and niacin contents, evaluated after 24 h. of exposure to the treatment (Beyers et al., 1979).
- In strawberry, vitamin C content was significantly affected by original content or the variety rather than treatments such as irradiation, heating or microwave. These results indicated that the losses of water-soluble vitamins, especially thiamin or vitamin C, were affected by the food temperature during the irradiation process (Chung & Yook, 2003).
- Irradiation can be an alternative for quarantining the papayas. Hot water treatment (immersion of fruits in water at 46 °C) can be used for the fruits smaller than 0.7 kg. However, it can harm fruit quality. It is not advisable to submit the mangos heavier

than 0.7 kg to hot water treatment because of lack of efficiency and intolerance of the product to the binomial time/temperature, which increases according to the fruit size (Hallman, 1999). Mangos and papayas irradiated with 2.0 kGy doses showed no loss of carotenoid; however, papayas stored at low temperatures without any kind of ionizing energy treatment showed large losses of these nutrients (Beyers & Thomas, 1979).

- Lycium, a popular fruit from China, was exposed to severe doses of gamma radiation (2-14 kGy), and decontaminating efficiency, changes in chemical composition and sensory characteristics were evaluated. Increasing the radiation dosage gradually decreased the fruits vitamin C concentration, but no alterations in β-carotene and riboflavin contents were registered (Wen et al., 2006). Reduction of vitamin C contents in irradiated Lycium is not a significant problem because this fruit is ordinarily used in traditional Chinese medicine for vision treatments, as an essential source of β-carotene and not vitamin C (Hsu et al., 1994).

- The importance of physiological state on vitamin loss was demonstrated with Early Park nº 7 tomato fruits irradiated with 4.0 kGy doses at the green-ripe stage. After ripening, tomatoes presented 8.6 % loss of ascorbic acid, while ripe fruits irradiated with 3.0 kGy showed 20.4% loss. However, because ripe fruits contained almost twice as much ascorbic acid, even after high destruction percentage of vitamin C by irradiation, still contained 5mg/100g more vitamin C than the control, harvested at green-ripe stage (Maxie & Sommer, 1968).

The loss of vitamin C of fresh-cutted lettuce irradiated with 1.0kGy was significantly (a = 0.05) lower than non-irradiated. The best treatment of maintaining quality of fresh-cutted lettuce appeared to be 1.0kGy irradiation (Zhang et al, 2006).

Adequate doses for insect disinfestations showed non-significant effects in vitamin C contents of citric fruits (Fan & Mattheis, 2001). Non significant losses of ascorbic acid were observed in the oranges irradiated and stored at 0ºC during 100 days. However, reduction of ascorbic acid content was observed in the lemons irradiated and stored at 15ºC during one month (Maxie et al., 1964).

Grapefruit Rio Red variety (Citrus paradisi Macf.) in different maturation stages, were irradiated to evaluate the influence of dose and storage period, showed the loss of some bioactive components and fruit quality. Fruit's response to irradiation depended on its maturation stage. Low irradiation doses (<0.2 kGy) applied to fruit harvested in the early season at 35 days of storage, promoted the formation of bioactive components, including β-caroten. Non-significant changes were recorded on vitamin C. High doses (0.4 and 0.7 kGy) affected the quality of fruit harvested in the early season. However, non-significant effects were observed in the fruits harvested in the late one (Patil et al., 2004).

Despite divergences regarding the effects of irradiation on ascorbic acid content of citric fruits, most research results demonstrated that the loss was minimun when doses up to 1.0 kGy were used. Exposure to higher doses can cause destruction of this vitamin in direct proportion to dose raise (Ahmed, 1977). Retention of ascorbic acid in oranges, tangerines, tomatoes and papayas varied from 100% to 72% with 0.4 to 3.0 kGy doses (Josephson et al., 1978).

Although most available data refer to irradiation-induced losses, especially of ascorbic acid in the reduced form, losses can actually be lower than reported, given that irradiation can convert ascorbic acid in reduced form into dehydroascorbic acid, biologically active form (Snauwart, 1973; Thomas, 1986).

The total of vitamin C in food is calculated by adding up ascorbic acid (AA) and dehydroascorbic acid (DHAA) activities. Almost all postharvest products contain only AA and many studies only determined the content of AA as vitamin C concentration measurement. However, the conversion of AA to DHAA during the storage and processing elicits significant concentration alterations. Therefore, some results reporting the effects of irradiation on vitamin C concentration seem conflicting because some studies only refer to AA concentrations, while others refer to the sum of both, AA and DHAA concentrations (Kilcast, 1994). Folates resistance to irradiation has not been widely studied yet (Diehl et al., 1991). Irradiation of spinach, green cabbage, and brussels sprouts reduced only 10% of the initial vitamins concentration of these produces. When dehydrated, the vitamin stability in these vegetables is higher than when they are fresh. In studies with fresh vegetables, the application of 10.0 kGy dose was only used to show that folate losses in analyzed foods depend on irradiation dosage (Müller & Diehl, 1996).

Ascorbic acid is one of the most sensitive vitamins to irradiation (Kilcast, 1994), but there are many fruit in which the level of ascorbic acid is not significantly reduced in tolerable doses (Maxie et al., 1964). Reduction of vitamin C contents with increasing irradiation doses were observed in orange, tangerine, tomato and passion fruit juices, with orange and tangerine being the most sensitive to irradiation (Munhoz-Burgos, 1985). Drastic reductions of ascorbic acid were observed in irradiated tomato juice and black and red currant syrups in comparison to losses resulting from pasteurization by heat (Wilska-Jeska & Skorupinska, 1975). For instance, 70.2 % vitamin C losses were registered for orange juice irradiated with 2.5 to 10 kGy (Hussain & Maxie, 1974). Studies showed that irradiation dose and temperature provoked only a slight reduction of ascorbic acid percentage in orange juice. This percentage was more drastically reduced because of temperature and storage period (Spoto, 1988).

Studies with carrot and kale juices evaluated the modifications in nutritional, microbiological and sensitive characteristics regarding irradiation. Results showed an increased reduction in the total ascorbic acid content with increasing irradiation dosage. However, total ascorbic acid concentration, including dehydro-ascorbic acid, remained stable with doses up to 3.0 kGy (Song et al., 2007).

With respect to irradiation in citrus Nagai & Moy (1985) observed that ascorbic acid losses in irradiated samples and compared with control treatment showed no significant differences during the storage period. The same result was also observed by Maxie et. al. (1964) irradiated on oranges and stored at 0°C for a period of 100 days. Lemons already irradiated and stored for 15°C for a month was had a reduction in the ascorbic acid content.

Most studies found in the literature are unanimous in stating that the losses of ascorbic acid induced by radiation occur mainly in ascorbic acid present mainly in reduced form. Probably this effective loss could be lower than that reported because the radiation can convert the ascorbic acid into the reduced form: dehydroascorbic acid which is biologically active (Thomas, 1986). In lemons variety Eureka irradiated at a dose of 4.0kGy the ascorbic acid losses was accompanied by an increase almost equivalent to dehydroascorbic acid (Romani et el. 1963). Similar findings were reported by Kurosaki & Ogatta (1971) in lemons and oranges of varieties Natsuma and Natsudaidai.

According to Oliveira (2011) the content of ascorbic acid was observed that decreased over the period of kiwifruit storage. On the 1st day the kiwifruits samples showed no significant difference between treatments. However, on the 7th and 14th day samples showed difference between them, the kiwifruits who received dose of 2kGy had lower ascorbic acid content when compared with the control sample. Considering that vitamin C is a water soluble vitamin and very sensitive to environmental factors such as temperature; light; presence of oxygen; humidity; pH; among other factors. The gamma radiation can also be a reducing agent that vitamin being observed during the storage period where it was found that there was degradation of vitamin C. Kim & Yook (2009) observed that the results for samples irradiated at doses kiwi 0 (control); 1 and 2kGy showed no significant difference, only the sample irradiated with 3kGy showed higher reduction in ascorbic acid content. However, in general, during the storage period kiwifruit irradiated showed low level of ascorbic acid over the control.

According to Franco et al. (2003), the losses that occur, specifically vitamins depend on the sensitivity of vitamins addition; the amount of energy that the food is exposed; and the nature and physical state of the medium in which it is present. The extent of this destruction is primarily a function of radiation dose and the medium temperature during irradiation. Some studies show that among the fat soluble vitamins and water soluble vitamins are more sensitive to ionizing radiation, and are the vitamins E and C. Samples containing 24 oranges of the variety pear juice were processed and divided into 7 lots of 100 ml each. Then, the lots containing 3 replicates were irradiated in an irradiator type Gammabeam 650 with doses of 0 (control); 1.0; 2.0; 3.0; 4.0; 5.0; and 6.0kGy. After irradiation was determined, the ascorbic acid contented the samples by titrimetric method. By the results obtained was concluded that the ascorbic acid content in orange juice gradually decreased with increasing radiation dose applied. At doses of 1.0 and 6.0kGy were decreases of 15.2 and 52.8% when compared with the control.

Oliveira et al. (2011) irradiated peaches with doses of 0 (control); 1.0 and 2.0kGy and between the treatments there was no significant difference in the content of vitamin C.

Harder & Arthur (2012) irradiated nectar of kiwi with doses 0 (control), 0,5; 1,0 and 2,0 kGy the results show that gamma radiation did not promote significant alterations in nectar of kiwi irradiated.

Bezerra, et al. (2012) irradiated lemon Thaiti, with doses of until 200 Gy, the results showed that the treatments there was no significant difference in the content of vitamin C.

According to Wyler et al. (2008) the increase of radiation dose and storage period in grapes cv. Niagara pink showed a tendency to decrease the total acidity; there was also dose versus time interaction regarding the pH; with the doses increasing and the storage period there was a downward trend, but there was no interaction between these two variables; with respect the color, the chroma (C *) also showed a change in relation to dose and storage time; there was no interaction between these variables. The other parameters (soluble solids, vitamin C, firmness of the berries and TSS/TS) had no significant changes. The grapes samples were irradiated with the following doses: 0 (control); 0.75; 1.0; 1.5kGy.

Perecin et al. (2009) showed that according to the results obtained in their work it was only the pH and soluble solids content (°Brix) showed significant difference over the period of storage and dose of radiation applied. However, no significant differences as to the parameters of texture, color, acidity and vitamin C content of minimally processed pineapple irradiated with doses of 0 (control); 1 and 2 kGy. The results related to the vitamin C content of pineapple spent through the statistical analysis showed that there was no significant difference during the entire period of study. However, the figures in the first day after irradiation, are higher than other results, therefore, it was found that the content of vitamin C is degraded with respect to applied dose and also over time. According to the authors Silva et al, (2008) the content of vitamin C decreased during the experiment with irradiated pineapples saying that this loss can be attributed to degradation or use of this acid in the first days after physiological maturity, may also be associated with stress the physical transportation, installation and implementation of treatment of the experiment.

CONCLUSION

Same as for other processing treatments, irradiation induces certains alterations that can modify the chemical composition and nutritive value of the foods. Vitamins presented different sensitivities regarding the treatment with ionizing energy. Vitamin C is one of the most sensitive to radiation and its degradation is proportional with an increase of dose of ionizing radiation. Neverthless, its sensitivity is also high in relation to several factors (exposure to oxygen, temperature elevation, pH modifications). In general, lower doses of irradiation treatment do not cause significant alterations in vitamins contents of foods. This method should be used because of its efficiency and low cost compared to other traditional methods.

ACKNOWLEDGMENTS/REVISION

The present chapter has been reviewed by:

- Liz Mary Bueno de Moraes (PhD), Research, University of Sao Paulo, Brazil.
- Hermas Amaral Germek (PhD), Director, Technology College of Piracicaba "Dep. Roque Trevisan", FATEC Piracicaba, Brazil.

REFERENCES

Ahmed, E. S. (1977). Biochemical responses of skim-coated citrus fruit irradiated for preservation. *Arabian Journal of Nuclear Science Appl.*, volume 10, 155-162.

Ahmed, E. S.; Dennison, R. S. & Merkley, M. S. (1968). Effects of low level irradiation upon preservation of foofd products. Report OKO-675, U.S. Atomic Energy Comission, Washington, D.C.

Al-Kahtani, H. A.; Abu-Tarboush, H. M.; Bajaber, A. S.; Atia, M.; Abou-Arab, A.A. & El-Mojaddidi, M. A. (1996). Chemical changes after irradiation and post-irradiation storage in tilapia and spanish mackerel. *Journal of Food Science*, volume 61, 729-733.

Al-Masri, M. R. (2003). Productive performance of broiler chicks fed diets containing irradiated meat-bone meal. *Bioresource Technology*, volume 90, 317-322.

Amara-Mokrane, Y. A.; Lehucher-Michel, M. P.; Balansard, G.; Duménil, G. & Botta, A. (1996). Protective effects of a-hederin, chlorophyllin and ascorbic acid towards the induction of micronuclei by doxorubicin in cultured human lymphocytes. *Mutagenesis*, volume 11, number 2, 161-167.

Beyers, M. & Thomas, A. C. (1979), Gamma irradiation of subtropical fruits.4. Changes in certain nutrients present in mangoes, papayas and litchis during canning, freezing and gamma irradiation. *Journal of Agriculture and Food Chemistry*, volume 27, 48-51.

Beyers, M.; Thomas, A. C.& Van Tonder, A. (1979). Gamma irradiation of subtropical fruits. Compositional tables of mango, papaya, strawberry, and litchi fruits at the edible-ripe stage. *Journal of Agriculture and Food Chemistry*, volume 27, 37-42.

Bezerra, D. N. F.; Silva, S. R.; Bassan, M. M.; Arthur, V. & Cantuarias-Avilés, T. (2012). Qualidade e conservação de frutos de lima ácida "Tahiti" submetidos a diferentes doses de radiação gama. XXII Congresso Brasileiro de Fruticultura, p. 4100-4103.

Bianchi, M. L. P. & Antunes, L. M. G. (1999). Free radicals and the main dietary antioxidants. *Revista de Nutrição*, volume 12, number 2, 123-130.

Chung, Y. J.; Yook, H-S. (2003). Effects of gamma irradiation and cooking methods on the content of thiamin in chicken breast and vitamin C in strawberry and mandarin orange. *Han'guk Sikp'um Yongyang Kwahak Hoechi*, volume 32, 864-869.

Chunyao, W; Mengyue, J.; Meixu, G.; Xiuye, M.; Shufen, Z & Shucheng, L. (1993). A study of the physiological changes and nutritional qualities of irradiated apples and the effect of irradiation on apples stored at room temperature. *Radiation, Physics and Chemistry*, volume 42, 347-350.

Clark, I. D. (1959). Possible applications of ionizing radiations in the fruit, vegetable and related industries. *International Jouranl Appl. Radiation Isotopes*, volume 6, 175-181.

Delincee, H.; Villavicencio, A. L. C. H. & Mancini-Filho, J. (1998). Protein quality of irradiated Brazilian beans. *Radiation, Physics and Chemistry*, v. 52, 1-6.

Dennison, R. S. (1968). Effects of low level irradiation upon the preservation of food products. *Progress Report in Agriculture Exp. STN*, Gainesville, 6-8.

Dharkar, S. E. (1964). Radiation of orange juice. *Indian Journal of Engenering and Technology*, volume 2, number 1, 24-30.

Diehel, J. F. & Josephson, E. S. (1994). Assessment of wholesomeness of irradiated food: a review. *Acta Alimentaria*, volume 23, number 2, 195-214.

Diehl, J. F. (1992). Food irradiation: is an alternative to chemical preservations. *Food Addition Contaminants*, volume 9, 409-416.

Diehl, J. F. (1992a). *Safety of irradiated foods*. 2th ed. New York: Marcel Dekker.

Diehl, J. F. (1992b), Nutritional effects of combining irradiation with other treatments. *Food. Control*, 2, 20-25.

Diehl, J. F. (1995). *Safety of Irradiated Foods*. 2. ed. revised and expanded. N.Y.: Marcel Dekker Inc.

Diehl, J. F., Hasselmann, C. & Kilcast, D. (1991). Regulation of food irradiation in the European Community: is nutrition an issue? *Food Control*, volume 2, 212-219.

Dionísio, A. P.; Gomes, R. T. & Oetterer, M. (2009). Ionizing radiation effects on food vitamins – A Review. *Brazilian Archives of Biology and Technology*, volume 52, number 5, 1267-1278.

Duthie, S. J.; Ma, A.; Ross, M. A. & Collins, A. R. (1996). Antioxidant supplementation decreases oxidative DNA damage in human lymphocytes. *Cancer Research*, volume 56, number 6, 1291-1295.

FAO/IAEA. (1982). *Training Manual on Food Irradiation Technology and Techniques.* 2. ed. FAO/IAEA.

FAP/IAEA/WHO. (1999). High-dose irradiation: wholesomeness of food irradiated with doses above 10 kGy. Report of a Joint FAP/IAEA/WHO Study Group. *World Health Organ. Tech. Rep. Ser.*; 890:i-vi, 1-197.

Franco, S. S. H.; Franco, J. G.; Franco, C. H.; Arthur, P. B. & Arthur, V. (2003). Efeitos da radiação gama sobre o conteúdo de acido ascórbico em suco de laranja. Reunião Anual do Instituto Biológico, RAIB, 157-157.

GAO (General Accounting Office of United States). (2000). Food Irradiation: Available Research indicates that benefits outweight risks – Report to Congressional Requesters.

Graham, W. D. & Stevenson, M. H. (1997). Effect of irradiation on vitamin C content of strawberries and potatoes in combination with storage and with further cooking in potatoes. *Journal of Science in Food and Agriculture*, volume 75, 371–377.

Grolinchova, M.; Dvorak, P. & Musilova, H. (2004). Employing ionizing radiation to enhance food safety – a review. *Acta Veterinaria Brno*, volume 73, 143-149.

Guerrero, F. P.; Maxie, E. C.; Johnson, C. F.; Eaks, I. L. & Sommer, N. F. Effect of post harvest gama irradiation on orange fruit. *Proc. American Society of Horticulture*, volume 90, 515-518.

Halliwell, B. (1994). Free radicals and antioxidants: a personal view. *Nutrition Reviews*, volume 52, number 8, 253-265.

Hallman, G. J. (1999). Ionising radiation quarantine treatments against tephritid. fruit flies. *Postharvest Biology and Technology*, volume 16, 93-106.

Harder, M. N. C. & Arthur, V. (2012). The effects of gamma radiation in nectar of kiwi (Actinidia deliciosa). In: *Gamma radiation*, 1. ed., p.305-320, Rijeka: InTech.

Hsu, H. Y.; Peacher, W. G. (eds). (1994). *Chinese Herb Medicine and Therapy*. Keats Publishing, New Canaan.

Hussain, A. & Maxie, E. C. (1974). Effect of gamma rays on shelf life and quality or orange juice. *International Biod. Bulletim*, volume 10, number 2, 81-86.

ICGFI (International Consultative Group on Food Irradiation). (1999). Fatos sobre irradiação de alimentos. Série de fichas descritivas do Grupo Consultivo Internacional sobre Irradiação de Alimentos. Centro de Desenvolvimento da Tecnologia Nuclear – CDTN.

Iemma, J.; Alcarde, A. R.; Domarco, R. E.; Spoto, M. H. F.; Blumer, L. & Matraia, C. Radiação gama na conservação do suco natural de laranja. *Scientia Agricola*, volume 56, number 4, 1193-1198.

Josephson, E. S. (1978). Nutritional aspects of food irradiation: an overview. *Journal of Food Processing and Preservation*, volume 2, 299-313.

Keller, J. L. Food Irradiation [online]. 2013 [2013/03/03]. Available from: http://www.healthyschoollunches.org/changes/irradiated.cfm.

Kilcast, D. (1994). Effect of irradiation on vitamins. *Food Chemistry*, volume 49, 157-164.

Kim, K. H. & Yook, H. S. (2009). Effect of gamma irradiation on quality of kiwifruit (Actinidia deliciosa var. deliciosa cv. Hayward). *Radiation, Physics and Chemistry*, volume 78, 414-421.

Kim, S. H.; Yook, H. S.; Byun, M. W. & Chung, Y. J. (2005). Effects of gamma irradiation on the content of riboflavin in egg powder and niacin in chicken breast. *Han'guk Sikp'um Yongyang Kwahak Hoechi*, volume 34, 1459-1463.

Kooij, J. [n/d]. Food irradiation makes progress. IAEA Bulletin, volume 26, number 2, 17-21.

Korasaki, T. & Ogatta, K. (1971). Effects of low doses gamma irradiation on the storage life of Satsuma oranges. *Engei Gakkaisassli*, volume 40, p. 85-89.

Lacroix, M.; Bernard, L.; Jobin, M.; Milot, S. & Gagnon, M. (1990). Effect of irradiation on the biochemical and organoleptic changes during the ripening of papaya and mango fruits. *International Journal of Radiation Applications and Instrumentation*. Part C. Radiation Physics and Chemistry, volume 35, 296-300.

Lastarria-Tapia, H. J. & Sequeiros, N. (1985). Efecto de la radiacion gamma em manzanas "delicias" almacenadas al médio ambiente y em refrigeracion. In: International Atomic Energy Agency. *Food Irradiation Processing*. Vienna, 55-60.

Lima, A. L. S.; Lima, K. S. C.; Coelho, M. J.; Silva, J. M.; Godoy, R. L. O. & Pacheco, S. (2009). Avaliação dos efeitos da radiação gama nos teores de carotenoides, ácido ascórbico e açúcares do fruto buriti do brejo (Maurita flexuosa L.). *Acta Amazonica*, volume 39, number 3, 649-654.

Lopez, G. M.; Rivas, G. A.; Ortin, S. N. & Val Cob, M. (1967). Preservation of food by irradiation. Preliminary investigation on strawberries. in Symp. *Application of Radioisotopes*, Madrid, 21-21.

Lupulescu, A. (1993). The role of vitamins A, b-carotene, E and C in cancer cell biology. *International Journal for Vitamin and Nutrition Research*, volume 63, number 3, 3-14.

Macfarlane, J. J. & Roberts, E. A. (1968). Some effects of gamma radiation on Washington Navel and Valencia oranges. *Australian Journal of Experimental Agriculture and Animal Husbandry*, volume 34, number 8, 625-629.

Maxie, E. C. & Sommer, N. F. (1968). Changes in some chemical constituints in irradiated fruits and vegetables. In: International Atomic Energy Agency. Preservation of fruit and vegetables by radiation. Vienna, 39-44.

Maxie, E. C.; Eaks, I. L. & Sommer, N. F. (1964). Some physiological effects of gamma irradiation on lemon fruit. *Radiation Botany*, volume 4, 405-411.

Maxie, E. C.; Sommer, N. F. & Eaks, I. L. (1969). Effect of gamma radiation on citrus fruits. In: International Citrus Symposium. *Proceedings*. Vienna IAEA, 1375-1387.

Mitchell, G. E.; McLauchlan, R. L.; Isaacs, A. R.; Williams, D. J. & Nottingham, S. M. (1992). Effect of low dose irradiation on composition of tropical fruits and vegetables. *Journal of Food Comp. Anal.*, volume 5, 291-311.

Mollins, R. A.; Motarjemi, Y. & Kaferstein, F. K. (2001). Irradiation: a critical control point in ensuring the microbiological safety of raw foods. *Food Control*, volume 12, 347-356.

Monseline, S. P. & Kahan, R. S. (1966). Changes in composition and enzymatic activities of flavour and juice of Shamonti oranges following gamma irradiation. *Radiation Botany*, volume 6, 265-274.

Moshonas, M. G. & Shaw, P. E. (1984). Effects of low dose y irradiation on grape-fruit productus. *Journal of Agriculture and Food Chemistry*, volume 32, 1098-1103.

Moy, J. H. & Wong, L. (2002). The efficacy and progress in using radiation as a quarantine treatment of tropical fruits - a case study in Hawaii. *Radiation, Physics and Chemistry*, volume 63, 397-401.

Müller, H. & Diehl, J. F. (1996). Effect of Ionizing Radiation on Folates in Food. *Lebens-Wiss. U.-Technol.*, volume 29, 187-199.

Munhoz-Burgos, R. A. (1985). Uso de La radiacion gama para extender el tiempo de conservation de jugos de algunas frutas exóticas. In: Seminario sobre irradiation de alimentos para paises da america latina, Vienna, IAEA,1-25.

Nagai, N. Y. & Moy, J. H. (1985). Quality of gamma irradiated California Valencia oranges. *Journal of Food Science*, volume 50, number 1, 215-219.

O'Keefe, T. (2001). Ascorbic Acid and Stable Ascorbate Esters as Sources of Vitamin C in Aquaculture Feeds. Singapore: American Soybean Association – United Soybean Board, *ASA Technical Bulletin*, volume AQ48-2001, 8-18.

Odin, A. P. (1997). Vitamins as antimutagens: advantages and some possible mechanisms of antimutagenic action. *Mutation Research*, v.386, n.1, 39-67.

Oliveira, A. C. S. (2011). Avaliação dos efeitos da radiação gama nas características físico-químicas de kiwi (Actinidia deliciosa) cv. Hayward minimante processado. MsC Thesis. IPEN/CNEN/University of São Paulo. São Paulo. Brazil.

Oliveira, A. C. S.; Silva, L. C. A. S.; Perecin, T. N.; Arthur, V.; Harder, M. N. C. & Canniatti-Brazaca, S. G. (2009). Conservação por radiação gama de pêssego Prunus pérsica minimamente processado: aspectos físico-químicos Biológico, volume 71, number 2, 157-157.

Patil, B. S.; Vanamala, J. & Hallman, G. (2004). Irradiation and storage influence on bioactive components and quality of early and late season "Rio Red" grapefruit (Citrus paradisi Macf.). *Postharvest Biology and Technoogy*, volume 34, 53-64.

Perecin, T. N.; Oliveira, A. C. S.; Silva, L. C. A. S.; Harder, M. N. C. & Arthur, V. Evaluation of the effects of gamma radiation on physical and chemical characteristics of pineapple (Annanas comosus) minimally processed. INAC Anal.

Proctor, B. E. & Goldblith, S. A. (1949). Effect of soft X-rays on vitamins (niacin, riboflavin and ascorbic acid). *Nucleonics*, volume 5, 56-62.

Riley, P. A. (1994). Free radicals in biology oxidative stress and the effects of ionizing radiation. *International Journal of Radiation and Biology*, volume 65, number 1, 27-33.

Roberts, T. & Weese, J. (1995). Food Irradiation. Alabama Cooperative Extension System. HE-727. Alabama A&M and Auburn University: Alabama.

Romani, R. J.; Kooy, J. V.; Lim, L. & Bowers. B. (1963). Radiation physiology of fruit-ascorbic, acid, sulphydryl and soluble nitrogen content or irradiated citrus. *Radiation Botany*, volume 3, 363-369.

Saito, Z. & Igarashi, Y. (1970). Effects of gamma irradation on changes in acidity, vitamin C, and nonprotein nitrogen in apples, *Hirosaki Daigaku Nogakubu Gakujutsu Hokoku*, volume 16, 1-9.

Satin, M. (1993). The case of food irradiation. International Conference of the Agricultural Research Institute, 93-110.

SCF (Scientific Committee on Food). (2003). Revision of the opinion the Scientific Committee on Food on the irradiation of food. European Commission – Health and Consumer Protection Directorate – General.

Shaw, P. E. & Moshonas, M. G. (1991). Ascorbic Acid Retention in Orange Juice Stored under Simulated Consumer Home Conditions. *Journal of Food Science*, volume 56, 867–868.

Sies, H. (1993). Strategies of antioxidant defence. Review. *European Journal of Biochemistry*, volume 215, number 2, 213-219.

Silva, J. M.; Silva, J. P. & Spoto, M. H. F. (2008). Características físico-químicas de abacaxi submetido à tecnologia de radiação ionizante como método de conservação pós-colheita. *Ciência e Tecnologia de Alimentos*, volume 28, number 1, 139-145.

Silva, M.R.; Silva, M.S. & Oliveira, J.S. (2004). Estabilidade de Ácido Ascórbico em Pseudofrutos de Caju-do-Cerrado Refrigerados e Congelados. *Pesquisa Agropecuária Tropical*, volume 34, number 1, 9-14.

Snauwart, F. (1973). Influence of gamma irradiation on the provitamin A (β-carotene) in solution. *Radiation Preservation of Food* (Proc. Symp. Bombay, 1972), IAEA, Vienna, 29.

Song, H. P.; Byun, M. W.; Jo, C.; Lee, C. H; Kim, K. S & Kim, D.H. (2007). Effects of gamma irradiation on the microbiological, nutritional, and sensory properties of fresh vegetable juice. *Food Control*, volume 18, 5-10.

Spolaore, A. J. G.; Germano, M. I. S. & Germano, P. M. L. (2003). Irradiação de alimentos. In: Germano, P. M. L.; Germano M. I. S. Higiene e Vigilância Sanitária de Alimentos – Qualidade das matérias primas, doenças transmitidas por alimentos, treinamento de recursos humanos. 2. ed. Varela.

Spoto, M. H. F. (1988) Radiação gama na conservação do suco concentrado de laranja. MsC Thesis. University of São Paulo. ESALQ/USP. Piracicaba, São Paulo. Brazil.

Stahl, W. & Sies, H. (1997). Antioxidant defence: vitamins E and C and carotenoids. *Diabetes*, volume 46, S14-S18.

Thomas, P. (1986). Radiation preservation of feed of plant origin III. Tropical fruits: bananas, mangoes and papayas. *CRC Crit. Rev. Food Science and Nutrition*, volume 23, 147-204.

Wen, H. W.; Chung, H. P.; Chou, F. I.; Lin, I. H. & Hsieh, P.C. (2006). Effect of gamma irradiation on microbial descontamination and chemical and sensory characteristic of lycium fruit. *Radiation, Physics and Chemistry*, volume 75, 596-603.

Wiendl, F. M. (1984). A salubridade dos alimentos irradiados. *Boletim SBCTA*, volume 18, 48-56.

Wilska-Jeska, J. & Skorupinska, A. (1975). Evalutaion of raduzired and pasteurized fruits juices during 12 months of storage. *Sesz. Nauk. Ploitech. Lodz. Chem. Spozywczea*, volume 23, 243-259.

Wyler, P.; Harder, M. N. C.; Arthur, V.; Silva, L. C. A..S. (2008). Efeito da radiação gama na conservação pós-colheita da uva cv. Niágara Rosada. SICUSP Anal.

Zhang, L.; Lu, Z.; Lu, F. & Bie, X. (2006). Effect of γ-irradiation on quality-maintaining of fresh-cut lettuce. *Food Control*, volume 17, 225-228.

Ziporin, Z. Z.; Kraybill, H. F. & Thach, H. J. (1957). Vitamin content of foods exposed to ionizing radiation. *Journal of Nutrient*, volume 63, 201-209.

In: Vitamin C   ISBN: 978-1-62948-154-8

Editor: Raquel Guiné   © 2013 Nova Science Publishers, Inc.

Chapter 5

VITAMIN C IN MARINE AND FRESHWATER TELEOSTS

Sungchul C. Bai, Kumar Katya† and Hyeonho Yun‡*

Department of Marine Bio-materials and Aquaculture,
Department of Fisheries Biology,
Feeds and Foods Nutrition Research Center (FFNRC),
Pukyong National University, Busan, Korea

ABSTRACT

This chapter reviews experiments conducted to evaluate vitamin C (ascorbic acid/AA) requirement, sources and deficiency symptoms in marine teleost, Korean rockfish, (*Sebastes schlegeli*), Olive flounder *(Paralicthys olivaceus)*, Parrot fish (*Oplegnathus fasciatus*) and in freshwater teleost, Japanese eel (*Anguilla japonica*).

In the 12 weeks of experiment with rockfish averaging 3.1 ± 0.02 g (mean $\pm$ SD) of initial body weight, results indicated that vitamin C requirement could be equal to or greater than 100 but less than 200 (mg AA kg^{-1} diet) in the form of L-ascorbyl-2-glucose (AA2G) as the dietary vitamin C source (average final body weight 15.3 ± 1.9 g). Based on findings from the 16 weeks of experiment with rockfish averaging 7.12 ± 0.02 g of initial body weight, it was concluded that dietary vitamin C level equal to or greater than 102 but less than 150 (mg AA kg^{-1} diet) for maximum growth and 1390 (mg AA kg^{-1}) in the form of dietary L-ascorbic acid could be required for the vitamin C saturation in various fish tissues (average final body weight 17.6 ± 3.2 g). From 8 weeks of experiment with rockfish averaging 12.6 ± 0.02 g of initial body weight, results indicated that vitamin C requirement could be equal to or greater than 39.7, but less than 144.6 (mg AA kg^{-1}) diet in the form of L-ascorbic acid for the maximum growth (average final body weight 52.6 ± 3.6 g). In the 12 weeks of experiment with juvenile olive flounder averaging 3 ± 0.06 g of initial body weight, the dietary vitamin C requirement could be equal to greater than 93 but less than 150 (mg AA kg^{-1} diet) in the form of L-ascorbyl-2-polyphosphate (average final body weight of 16.9 ± 3.1g). Findings from the 11 weeks of

---

* E-mail: scbai@pknu.ac.kr.

† E-mail: kumarkatya85@gmail.com.

‡ E-mail: yun841007@nate.com.

experiment with parrot fish averaging 3.9 ± 0.06 g of initial body weight, suggested that dietary vitamin C requirement could be equal to or greater than 118 ± 12 but less than 205 (mg AA kg^{-1}) diet in the form of L-ascorbyl-2-monophosphate (average final body weight of 14.3 ± 2.9 g). Results from the 12 weeks of experiment with Japanese eel averaging 15 ± 0.3 g of initial body weight, indicated that dietary vitamin C requirement could be equal to or greater than 41.1 but less than 52 (mg AA kg^{-1}) diet in the form of L-ascorbyl-2-monophosphate (average final body weight of 56.4 ± 8.79g).

1. INTRODUCTION

Most of the marine and freshwater teleosts are unable to synthesize vitamin C (ascorbic acid/AA) from D glucose due to the lack of enzyme, L-gulonolactone oxidase which is responsible for the synthesis of vitamin C *de novo* (Dabrowski, 1990; Fracalossi et al. 2001; Wilson, 1973). Although a few freshwater species such as sturgeon (*Acipenser fulvescens*) and marine crustaceans have been reported to have a limited ability to synthesize vitamin C but the findings are dubious and contradictory in many instances. Worth noting that title of this chapter covers "vitamin C in marine and freshawater teleost" while species of sturgeon and crustaceans are not teleost. In general, marine and freshwater teleosts fully depend upon the dietary supply for their ascorbic acid requirement. Many general physiological functions of L-ascorbic acid (AA) are well defined, the most important among them, being its capacity to act as a co-factor in the hydroxylation of proline to hydroxiproline, critical for helical structure of collagen. AA is also the most powerful reducing agent available to cells, losing two hydrogen atoms to become dehydroascorbic acid, and is of general importance as an antioxidant because of its high reducing potential (Bai, 2001). AA requirement in teleosts greatly varies with respect to differences in the biotic factors (species, age, physiological condition etc.) as well as various abiotic factors (rearing environmental condition). Consequently in the last three decades, AA requirement has been a highly debated and vast studied topic in aquaculture. Majority of economically important aquatic species have been the subject of AA requirement study and reports have been well documented. The updated reports in standard reference for aquatic species nutrition, *Nutrient Requirements of Fish and Shrimp* (NRC, 2011) evidenced the number of studies devoted to evaluate AA requirement. The previous edition (NRC, 1993) listed only a few economically important species in vitamin C section, while the current edition covers majority of commercially important species. A number of symptoms linked with vitamin C deficiency such as impaired collagen formation, spinal deformation, haemorrhaging, retarded growth and depressed immunity (Ai, Q. et al. 2006; Al-Amoudi et al. 1992; Gouillou-Coustans et al. 1998; Halver et al. 1969) used to be the common problems encountered at aquaculture farms. Aquaculture nutritionists' knowledge in vitamin C requirements has advanced significantly; as a result fish producers have got relief of severe economic loss linked with high and frequent incidence of malformed fish and subsequent mortality.

Whereas, a large discrepancy in quantitative requirements on vitamin C between and among the fish species has been acknowledged probably due to the differences in fish species, fish size as well as methodological approach and experimental condition (NRC, 1993). Dietary source of AA used in different experiments is one of the major and basic differences, which makes it complex to oversimplify the quantitative requirement of vitamin C in and among fish species. L-AA is the traditionally used vitamin C source in fish and shrimp feeds, but it is thermolabile, unstable and easily oxidized to an inactive form during feed processing and storage. Various derivatives of AA, including L-ascorbyl-2-sulfate (C2S), L-ascorbyl-2-monophosphate-Mg (C2MP-Mg), L-ascorbyl-2-monophosphate-Ca (C2MP-Ca), L-ascorbyl-2-polyphosphate (C2PP) and ascorbate-2-glucose (C2D), have been demonstrated more stable than the parent compound and have been shown to provide antiscorbutic activity in fish and shrimp. However, a strict comparison of the potency of each source of AA among different reports is noticed to be misleading because the experimental condition and purity of these derivatives also differ (NRC, 2011).

Apart from above mentioned biotic and abiotic factors affecting the level of AA requirement, the dietary level of various other nutrients has also been reported to alter the requirement and bioavailability of AA. The ability of AA to regenerate α-tocopherol by reducing tocopheroxyl radical, has been well characterized by *in vitro* studies in different species (Mukai et al. 1991; Packer et al. 1979; Tappl, 1968). On the other hand, bioflavonoids have been identified as having antiscorbutic (Regnault-Roger, 1988) and antioxidant (Pratt & Watts, 1964) properties as well as mutagenic activity (Brown, 1980). Rutin, one of the bioflavonoids, has been reported to produce vitamin C like effects as well as to spare vitamin C, even though it is not an indispensable food component equivalent to vitamins. The synergism between ascorbic acid and rutin has been established in guinea pigs (Crampton & Lloyd, 1950; Douglas & Kamp, 1959; Papageorge & Mitchell, 1949). However, in channel catfish limited synergetic effects of dietary rutin on vitamin C nutrition could be observed (Bai & Galtin, 1992). Lee & Dabrowski (2004) already stated that, do we need to reformulate the requirements of these micronutrients in fish based on their interaction, in comparison to the dietary requirement estimated for individual vitamins must be varified.

Korean rockfish (*Sebastes schlegeli*) (Hilgendorf) rank second in marine finfish aquaculture production in the Republic of Korea. It has been reported that in 2011, the total aquaculture production of Korean rockfish accounted for 17, 300 tons, contributing 23.89% of the total marine finfish aquaculture production in the country (KOSTAT, 2012). This species is having desirable characteristics for aquaculture such as high tolerance to wide range of temperatures, ease of seedling production due to viviparous reproductive style and the ability to withstand high stocking density. As a result, commercial fish culture of Korean rockfish has expanded rapidly in the last four decades. At present besides the indoor culture system (tank, recirculatory, flow through etc.), this species is also cultured at large scale in net, pen and cage aquaculture system. Korean rockfish of different age groups have been the subject of various macro and micronutrients requirement studies. Subsequently, nutrient requirement for this species have been well defined and established. Considering the complexity in evaluating the vitamin C requirement in fish, we initiated our research by developing the experimental model and semipurified diet design for Korean rockfish and other marine teleosts as well (Bai et al. 1996). Here, we summarize three experimental results, among a series of long and short term studies with different age group of Korean rockfish conducted to determine the vitamin C requirement.

Olive flounder (*Paralichthys olivaceus*) (Temminck & Schlegel) ranks first in the marine finfish aquaculture sector in Korea. In 2011, olive flounder production has been reported to be 40,800 ton, contributing 56.35% of total marine finfish aquaculture production (KOSTAT, 2012). The Republic of Korea has been the leading flatfish producer around the world. The establishment of seed production system and the favorable government policy could motivate farmers to expand the olive flounder aquaculture in the country. While the culture operation of this species has expanded rapidly, feeding practice is still dependent on moist pellets and trash fish. Approximately, 210, 403 tons of moist pellets have been reported to be consumed exclusively by olive flounder aquaculture in 2012. This feeding method causes many problems in aquaculture including disease, water pollution, high production cost and unbalanced nutrient supply. Thus, it is necessary to develop an economical and nutritionally complete diet in Korea to advance flounder aquaculture. Although Teshima et al. (1991) had done some vitamin C research in olive flounder, the data on juvenile olive flounder requirement are scarce. Therefore, we conducted an experiment to re-evaluate the vitamin C requirement in juvenile olive flounder using L-ascorbyl-2-polyphosphate (ASPP) as the vitamin C source.

Parrot fish is one of the emerging marine aquaculture species in Korea. Its high commercial value has attracted fish farmers and this species has been acknowledged as the promising aquaculture species in the future. However, there is no quantitative estimation of the dietary vitamin C requirement for this species (Ikeda et al., 1988; Ishibashi et al., 1992). Therefore, we conducted an experiment to determine the effects of different levels of dietary vitamin C on growth, tissue ascorbic acid and histolopathological changes in parrot fish.

In the Republic of Korea, freshwater aquaculture is dominated by Japanese eel (*Anguilla japonica*) production due to its overwhelming demand in domestic as well as overseas market. In 2011, Eel aquaculture production has been reported to be 7,250 tons by volume contributing 27.33% of the total finfish aquaculture production in the country (KOSTAT, 2012). Consequently, Japanese eel has been the subject of various macro and micro nutrient requirement studies. Although the dietary vitamin C requirement has been estimated in Japanese eel using L-ascorbic acid Ca as the source of vitamin C (Ren et al. 2005) this requirement could vary when other sources of vitamin C are used. Therefore, we conducted a study to re-evaluate the vitamin C requirement in juvenile eel, using L-ascorbyl-2-monophosphate as the vitamin C source.

Therefore, this chapter reviews our six experiments conducted to evaluate the vitamin C requirement in selected marine and freshwater teleosts.

2. VITAMIN C REQUIREMENT IN MARINE TELEOSTS

2.1. Materials and Methods

2.1.1. Experimental Semipurified Diets

Semipurified diet developed in our previous experiment (Bai et al. 1996) was little modified to match up with the nutrient and energy requirement of experimental fish (table 5.1). It was observed that the purified casein-gelatin based diet, low in fish meal (5%), was not readily accepted by experimental fish. Therefore, fish meal supplementation level was increased (10%) to enhance the diet palatability for the marine teleosts. Fish meal was extracted three times with a chloroform/methanol mixture (2:1, v/v) for one day and then air dried before incorporating into experimental diet (Lee et al. 1998). Vitamin C pre-mixture was added at different levels at the expense of cellulose.

Table 5.1. Composition of the basal diet (DM basis)

Ingredient	Percentage
Casein, vitamin free[1]	30.0
Gelatin[1]	10.0
White fish meal (defatted)[2]	10.0
Dextrin[1]	27.0
L-Arginine[3]	0.5
L-Lysine HCl[2]	0.5
DL-Methionine[2]	0.5
Pollack oil	5.0
Corn oil[4]	5.0
Carboxymethycellulose[1]	2.0
α-Cellulose[1]	2.5
Vitamin premix(Vit C free)[5]	3.0
Mineral premix[6]	4.0

[1] United States Biochemical, Cleveland, OH 44122, USA.

[2] Kum Sung Feed Co., Pusan, Korea.

[3] Yunsei Chemical Co., Japan.

[4] Corn oil 4.9% + DHA, EPA 0.1% (25% DHA + EPA mixture).

[5] Contains (as g per 100g premix): dl-calcium pantothenate, 0.5; choline bitartrate, 10; inositol, 0.5; menadion, 0.02; niacin, 0.5; pyridoxine HCl, 0.05; riboflavin, 0.1; thiamine mononitrate, 0.05; dl-α-tocopherylacetate, 0.2; retinyl acetate, 0.02; biotin, 0.005; folic acid, 0.018; B_{12}, 0.0002; colecalciferol, 0.008; α-cellulose, 87.06.

[6] H-440 premix No.5 (mineral) (NRC 1973).

Vitamin C concentrations in the experimental diets determined at the beginning and at the end of feeding trial by the modified procedure of Thenhen (1998) as described by Bai & Gatlin (1992). Less than 20% loss of AA activity was observed in the experimental diets during storage at -35°C for up to 4 months.

2.1.2. Experimental Diet, Fish and Feeding Trails

Experiment 1 (Korean Rockfish 3.1± 0.02 g)

Seven semipurified diets were prepared containing the equivalent of 0, 50, 100 or 200 mg L-AA kg^{-1} diet in the form of L-ascorbyl-2-glucose (AA2G) or L-ascorbyl-2-monphosphate Na/Ca (AMP-Na/Ca). The feeding trial was conducted in a flow-through system with 60-L aquaria receiving filtered seawater at a rate of 1 L min^{-1}. Supplemental aeration was provided to maintain dissolved oxygen level near saturation. Water temperature was maintained at 20 ± 1.5°C. Experimental fish averaging 3.1 ± 0.06g (mean ± SD) were randomly distributed into each group of 20 fish. Triplicate group of fish were fed with one of the seven experimental diets at 4-5% body weight/day for a period of 12 weeks.

Experiment 2 (Korean Rockfish 7.12 ± 0.02 g)

Six semipurified diets were formulated to contain 0, 25, 50, 75, 150, or 1500 mg AA kg^{-1} by adding the appropriate amounts of vitamin C pre-mixture (10 mg L-AA g^{-1} cellulose) at the expense of cellulose. The feeding trial was conducted in a flow-through system with 60-L aquaria receiving filtered seawater at a rate of 1L min^{-1}. Supplemental aeration was provided to maintain dissolved oxygen level near saturation. Water temperature was ranged from 18 ± 0.5°C at the begining to 13 ± 0.2°C (mean ± SD) at the end of the experiment because of the natural fluctuation in sea water temperature. Experimental fish averaging 7.12 ± 0.02 g (mean ± SD) were randomly distributed in each aquarium as a group of 25 fish. Triplicate group of fish were fed with one of the six experimental diets at approximately 3% body weight/day for 16 weeks. Fish were fed twice a day during the first 8 weeks and then once a day until the end of experiment.

Experiment 3 (Korean Rockfish 12.6 ± 0.02 g)

Six semipurified diets were formulated to contain 0, 25, 50, 75, 150 or 1500 mg AA kg^{-1} by adding appropriate amount of vitamin C pre-mixture (10 mg AA g^{-1} cellulose) at the expense of cellulose. The feeding trial was conducted in a flow-through system with 60-L aquaria receiving filtered seawater at a rate of 1L min^{-1}. Supplemental aeration was provided to maintain dissolved oxygen near saturation. Water temperature ranged from 15 ± 0.5°C at the beginning to 17 ± 0.5°C (mean ± SD) at the end of the experiment. Experimental fish, averaging 12.6 ± 0.02 g (mean ± SD), were randomly distributed in each aquarium in groups of 25 (total weight 316.3 ± 0.58 g). Experimental diets were fed at the rate of 2% of wet body weight per day for the experimental period of 8 weeks.

Experiment 4 (Olive Flounder 3± 0.06 g)

Semipurified diet developed for Rockfish experiment was little modified to match up with the protein (53%) and energy (17 kJ g^{-1}) requirement of olive flounder. Defated white fish meal (25%) and vitamin free casein (25%) was added as the dietary protein source. Six experimental diets were prepared containing equivalents of 0, 25, 50, 75, 150 or 1500 mg L-ascorbic acid (AA) kg^{-1} diet in the form of L- ascorbyl-2-polyphosphate (ASPP). Diets supplemented with an ascorbic acid source, an equivalent amount of cellulose was removed. The feeding trial was conducted in a recirculatory system with 54-L aquaria receiving filtered seawater at a rate of 1L min^{-1}. Supplemental aeration was provided to maintain dissolved oxygen level near saturation. Water temperature was maintained at 17 ± 1°C. Experimental fish averaging 3 ± 0.06g (mean ± SD) were randomly distributed into each group of 30 fish. Triplicate groups of fish were fed with one of the seven experimental diets at 2.5-4% body weight/day for a period of 12 weeks. The total fish weight in each aquarium was determined every 4 weeks, and the amount of diet fed was adjusted accordingly.

Experiment 5 (Parrot Fish 3.9 ± 0.06 g)

Semipurified diet developed in our previous experiment was little modified to match up with the protein (50%) and energy (21.7 kJg^{-1}) requirements of parrot fish. Defated fish meal (27.5%) and casein (27.5%) was added as the dietary protein source. Six diets were formulated to contain 0, 60, 120, 240, 480 and 2000 mg L-ascorbic acid (AA) per kg diet in the form of L-ascorbyl-2-monophosphate (AMP) on an AA equivalent basis, and two other diets were formulated to contain 60 and 240 mg L-ascorbic acid per kg diet. However, the analyzed AA levels were 0, 50, 100, 205, 426 and 1869 mg AA per kg diet in AMP-supplemented diets; 36 and 149 mg AA per kg diet in L-ascorbic acid supplemented diets. Thus, the diets were designated as AA-free, AMP$_{50}$, AMP$_{100}$, AMP$_{205}$, AMP$_{426}$, AMP$_{1869}$,

AA_{36} and AA_{149}. The feeding trial was conducted in a flow-through system with 60L aquaria receiving filtered seawater at a rate of 1.2 L/min. Supplemental aeration was provided to maintain dissolved oxygen level near saturation. Water temperature was $22^{\circ}C$ at the beginning of the feeding trial and was $17^{\circ}C$ at the end of the feeding trial according to the normal changes of natural water temperature. Fish averaging $3.9 \pm 0.06g$ (mean $\pm$ SD) were randomly distributed to each aquarium as groups of 20 fish and fed the experimental diets in triplicate at the rate of 4% to 5% of wet body weight per day for 11 weeks.

2.1.3. Sample Collection and Analyses

At the end of feeding trails, all fish were weighed and counted to calculate various biological parameters and morphological indices such as weight gain (WG), specific growth rate (SGR), feed efficiency (FE), protein efficiency ratio (PER), protein productive value (PPV), hepatosomatic index (HSI), condition factors (CF) and survival rate.

Weight gain (WG, %) = (final wt. - initial wt.) $\times$ 100 / initial wt

Specific growth rate (SGR, %) = ($\log_e$ final wt. - $\log_e$ initial wt.) $\times$ 100 / days

Feed efficiency (FE, %) = (wet weight gain / dry feed intake) $\times$ 100

Protein efficiency ratio (PER) = (wet weight gain / protein intake)

Protein productive value (PPV, %) = (body protein deposit/feed protein intake) $\times$ 100

Hepatosomatic index (HIS, %) = (liver weight/body weight) $\times$100

Condition factor (CF, %) = [fish wt (g)/fish length $(cm)^3$] $\times$100

Blood samples were collected from the caudal Vessel of experimental fish. Hematocrit (PCV) was determined by the microhematocrit method (Brown, 1980) and hemoglobin was measured in the same fish by cyanmethemoglobin procedure using Drabkin's solution. Hb standard prepared from human blood (Sigma Chemical, St. Louis, MO) was used. Tissue vitamin C concentrations of liver, muscle, gill and brain of fish were determined in triplicates. Each sample was prepared from five fish randomly selected per aquarium. In the experiment (1, 2, 3, and 4) Vitamin C was analyzed by the dinitrophenyldrazine (DNPH) spectrophotometric method (Schaffert et al. 1955) as described by Bai & Gatlin (1992). While in the experiment 5, Ascorbic acid concentrations in diets supplemented with L-ascorbic acid were determined directly by HPLC, and ascorbic acid concentrations in diets supplemented with AMP was calculated after analyzing the AMP contents in diets by HPLC (AMP was produced by Hoffman La Roche, containing 35% ascorbic acid activity). Ascorbic acid concentrations in gill, muscle, liver, and brain of pooled fish (five fish per aquarium) were determined by HPLC (Syknm, German) with a UV detector at 254 nm. The mobile phase was 0.1 M KH_2PO_4 at pH 2.8 and the flow rate was 0.4 ml/min. Preweighed samples were homogenized in 10% cold metaphosphoric acid. Homogenates were centrifuged at 10061g for 25 min and supernatants were analyzed on HPLC after filtered through a 0.45 mm pore-size syringe filter (Sartorius, Go¨ttingen, Germany). Whole body proximate composition including crude protein, moisture and ash were analyzed by AOAC methods (AOAC, 1995). Crude fat was determined by Soxtec system 1046 (Tecator AB, Swedan) after freeze drying the sample for 12 hours. All data were subjected to ANOVA using Statistix 3.1 (Analytical Software, St. Paul, MN). When a significant treatment was observed, a least significant difference test was used to compare means. Treatment effects were considered with the significant level at $P < 0.05$.

Table 5.2. Biological performances and morphological indices[1]

	Diets							Pooled SEM
	Vitamin C free	AMP-Na/Ca$_{50}$	AMP-Na/Ca$_{100}$	AMP-Na/Ca$_{200}$	AA2G$_{50}$	AA2G$_{100}$	AA2G$_{200}$	
WG (%)	285.1^c	362.8^{bc}	447.4^{ab}	475.8^a	386.9^{ab}	391.9^{ab}	411.1^{ab}	13.7
FER (%)	57.4^c	70.1^b	80.9^a	82.9^a	71.7^b	76.3^{ab}	78.1^a	2.0
HSI (%)	3.76^b	4.05^b	4.50^a	4.16^{ab}	3.86^b	4.05^b	4.10^{ab}	0.09
CF	1.47^b	1.59^{ab}	1.63^a	1.60^a	1.55^{ab}	1.57^{ab}	1.58^{ab}	0.02
Hb	5.67	5.80	5.84	5.92	5.74	5.87	5.86	0.07
PCV (%)	38.7^b	39.0^b	40.7^{ab}	44.8^a	39.2^b	39.7^b	40.3^b	0.87
SR (%)	88^b	96.7^a	98.3^a	98.3^a	96.7^a	100^a	98.3^a	1.05

[1] Values are means from triplicate groups of fish, and the means in each row with a different superscript are significantly different (P<0.05).

Table 5.3. Vitamin C concentration in different tissues[1]

	Diets							Pooled SEM
	Vit.C free	AMP-Na/Ca$_{50}$	AMP-Na/Ca$_{100}$	AMP-Na/Ca$_{200}$	AA2G$_{50}$	AA2G$_{100}$	AA2G$_{200}$	
Muscle	ND	6.7^b	12.5^{ab}	19.9^a	6.8^b	11.9^{ab}	20.1^a	2.5
Liver	ND	22.9^b	31.4^b	75.9^a	23.5^b	30.4^b	77.8^a	6.7

[1] Values are means from triplicate groups of fish, and the means in each row with a different superscript are significantly different (P<0.05).

2.2. Results

Experiment 1 (Korean Rockfish 3.1 ± 0.02 g)

The results of the biological performances and morphological indices are summarized in table 5.2. After 12 weeks of feeding, WG, FER and survival of fish fed vitamin C free diet were significantly lower than those of fish fed vitamin C supplemented diet in either form (AA2G or AMP-Na/Ca). WG, HSI, CF and survival of fish fed the vitamin C free diet were significantly lower than that of fish fed vitamin C supplemented diets, except those of fish fed the AMP-Na/Ca$_{50}$. There was no significant difference in Hb in fish fed any of the experimental diets. AA concentration in muscle and liver tissue could not be detected among the group fed vitamin C free diet. While, the AA concentrations in muscle and liver from fish fed diets containing 200 mg AA kg^{-1} diets were significantly higher than those from fish fed vitamin C free or 50 mg AA kg^{-1} diet with either of the dietary vitamin C sources (P < 0.05). However, no differences existed in muscle AA concentration between fish fed AMP-Na/Ca$_{50}$, AMP-Na/Ca$_{100}$, AA2G$_{50}$ and AA2G$_{100}$ diets (table 5.3). After the experimental period of nine weeks, fish fed vitamin C free diet began to show initial vitamin C deficiency signs such as anorexia and lethargy. At the end of 12 weeks, deficiency signs such as anorexia, scoliosis, exophthalmia and fin hemorrhages were pronounced. Overall performances indicated that optimum vitamin C requirement in Korean rockfish size 3.1 ± 0.02 g could be equal to or greater than 100 but less than 200 mg AA^{-1} diet in the form of L- ascorbyl-2-glucose (AA2G) as the dietary vitamin C source (average final body weight of 15.3 ± 1.9 g). WG, FE data and improved survival indicated that Korean rockfish can utilize AA2G effectively as a source of vitamin C as well as AMP-Na/Ca, which is extensively used in the aquatic feed industry.

Experiment 2 (Korean Rockfish 7.12 ± 0.02 g)

Results of biological performances and morphological indices are summarized in table 5.4 WG, SGR, PER, PPV and CF of fish fed vitamin C free diet were significantly lower than those of fish fed 150 mg AA^{-1} diet. While, there was no significant difference in these parameters among the group fed C_{25}-C_{1500} diets. Survival rate (SR) of fish fed vitamin C free diet was significantly lower than those of fish fed other diets. HSI of fish fed vitamin C free diet was lower than those of fish fed diets C_{50}-C_{1500} diets (P < 0.05). After 12 weeks of experimental period, fish fed vitamin C free diet exhibited a range of deficiency signs including scoliosis, shortened operculae, exophthalmia and fin hemorrhage. While, at the end of experiment, spinal deformity (5.3 ± 1.08%), shortened operculae, exopthalmia and fin hemorrhages were distinct among the group of fish fed vitamin C free diet. No significant difference existed in hematocrit, hemoglobin, whole body protein, whole body lipid and whole body moisture content among different groups (P < 0.05). However, ash contents of fish fed C_0 and C_{25} diets were higher than those of fish fed the other diets (P < 0.05). Muscle and liver AA concentration of fish fed C_0 diet were higher than those of fish fed C_{150} and C_{1500} diets (table 5.5). Broken line analysis of WG (figure 5.1) suggested the optimum dietary vitamin C level in Korean rockfish size 7.12 ± 0.02 g, could be equal to or greater than 102 but less than 150 mg AA kg^{-1} diet (average final body weight of 17.6 ± 3.2 g).

Table 5.4. Biological performances and morphological indices[1]

| | Diets | | | | | | Pooled SEM |
	C_0	C_{25}	C_{50}	C_{75}	C_{150}	C_{1500}	
Weight gain(%)	61^d	144^c	151^{b,c}	159^{b,c}	177^{a,b}	191^a	10.25
FCR	3.23^d	1.79^c	1.63^{b,c}	1.63^{b,c}	1.49^{a,b}	1.31^a	0.15
SGR(%)	0.44^d	0.85^c	0.89^b	0.90^{b,c}	0.99^{a,b}	1.08^a	0.05
PER	0.50^c	1.10^b	1.18^b	1.22^b	1.31^{a,b}	1.51^a	0.08
PPV(%)	8.8^c	17.3^b	19.1^b	19.6^b	21.2^{a,b}	24.9^a	1.23
HIS	2.73^c	3.14^{b,c}	3.65^{a,b}	3.88^{a,b}	4.04^a	4.33^a	0.15
CF	1.32^c	1.43^b	1.52^b	1.47^b	1.48^b	1.61^a	0.02
Haematocrit(%)	33.5	37.3	37.3	36.7	35.5	38.7	0.74
Haemoglobin(g/dl)	9.03	8.91	9.71	9.71	9.45	10.9	0.28
Survival	89^b	96^a	96^a	100^a	100^a	100^a	1.11

[1] Values are means from triplicate groups of fish, and the means in each row with a different superscript are significantly different (P<0.05).

Table 5.5. Vitamin C concentration in different tissues[1]

| | Diets | | | | | | Pooled SEM |
	C_0	C_{25}	C_{50}	C_{75}	C_{150}	C_{1500}	
Muscle	28.3^c	18.9^{b,c}	18.1^{b,c}	18.8^{b,c}	24.8^b	60.6^a	3.77
Liver	14.9^c	33.9^{b,c}	35.3^{b,c}	35.7^{b,c}	55.8^b	180.0^a	12.95
Gill	33.2^b	36.5^b	52.5^b	53.5^b	70.3^b	143.0^a	9.65
Brain	30.4^c	37.2^c	39.8^c	54.6^c	86.0^b	247.0^a	18.06

[1] Values are means from triplicate groups of fish, and the means in each row with a different superscript are significantly different (P<0.05).

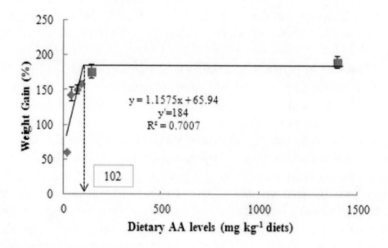

Figure 5.1. Broken line analysis based on weight gain.

Table 5.6. Biological performances and morphological indices[1]

	Diets					
	C_9	C_{25}	C_{50}	C_{74}	C_{150}	C_{1500}
Weight gain (%)	73.3^b	82.64^{ab}	81.85^{ab}	77.52^{ab}	84.35^a	87.09^a
	±1.87	±3.84	±0 .75	±2.76	±4.39	±1.59
FCR(%)	86.1^b	94.3^{ab}	90.2^{ab}	94.9^{ab}	100.4^a	103.8^a
	±2.1	±3.7	±2.8	±0.5	± 2.0	±2.8
Hematocrit(%)	34.7^b	41.3^a	42.0^{ab}	41.4^a	41.3^a	42.3^a
	±0.77	±1.79	±0.24	±0.92	±0.80	±0.65
Hemoglobin(g/dl)	8.00^a	8.34^a	8.01^a	8.08^a	8.28^a	8.23^a
	±0.23	±0.26	±0.31	±0.23	±0.17	±0.14
CF	1.79^a	1.84^a	1.80^a	1.80^a	1.81^a	1.81^a
	±0.02	±0.02	±0.03	±0.02	±0.03	±0.03

[1] Values are means from triplicate groups of fish, and the means in each row with a different superscript are significantly different (P<0.05).

Table 5.7. Vitamin C concentration in different tissues[1]

	Diets						Pooled
	C_0	C_{25}	C_{50}	C_{75}	C_{150}	C_{1500}	SEM
Muscle	4.84^c	10.70^{bc}	10.37^{bc}	12.36^{bc}	13.73^b	63.15^a	5.46
Liver	32.56^b	41.15^b	46.66^b	58.21^b	76.12^b	179.74^a	13.16
Gill	21.62^b	18.60^b	23.97^b	23.98^b	39.79^b	139.50^a	8.78
Brain	181.76^b	233.01^b	203.94^b	221.48^b	244.47^b	394.58^a	9.22

[1] Values are means from triplicate groups of fish, and the means in each row with a different superscript are significantly different (P<0.05).

Experiment 3 (Korean Rockfish 12.6 ± 0.02 g)

Results of biological performances and morphological indices are summarized in table 5.6. WG and FE of fish fed vitamin C free diet were significantly lower than those of fish fed diets C_{150} and C_{1500} (P < 0.05), while those of fish fed C_0, C_{150} or C_{1500} diet (P < 0.05). Average hematocrit (PCV) of fish fed C_0 was significantly lower than those of fish fed the other diets. No significant difference existed in survival rate, Hb, CF, whole body protein, whole-body lipid, whole body ash and whole body moisture content among the group fed six different level of vitamin C (P < 0.05). Muscle L-ascorbic acid (AA) concentrations of fish fed C_0 diet were lower than those of fish fed C_{150} and C_{1500} diets (P < 0.05), while there was no significant difference among fish fed diets C_0-C_{75} diet (P < 0.05). Liver, gill and brain AA concentrations of fish fed C_{1500} diet were significantly higher than those of fish fed diets C_0-C_{150} (P < 0.05), while these values were not significantly different among fish fed diets C_0-C_{150} (table 5.7). Overall results suggested the optimum dietary vitamin C level in Korean rockfish size 12.6 ± 0.02 g, could be equal to or greater than 39.7 mg AA, but less than 144.6 mg AA kg^{-1} diet in the form of L-ascorbic acid for the maximum growth (average final body weight of 52.6 ± 3.6 g)

Table 5.8. Biological performances and morphological indices[1]

| | Diets | | | | | | Pooled |
	C_0	C_{25}	C_{50}	C_{75}	C_{150}	C_{1500}	SEM
WG (%)	270.6^c	460.4^b	480.8^b	477.6^b	543.1^{ab}	557.9^a	22.0
FER (%)	41.3^a	65.8^b	74.6b^c	73.5^{bc}	76.3^{bc}	78.7^{bc}	3.37
PER	1.28^d	1.66^c	1.73b^c	1.73^{bc}	1.88^{ab}	1.95^a	0.06
HIS	2.01^b	1.98^b	2.26^{ab}	2.22^{ab}	2.69^a	2.52^{ab}	0.08
CF	0.85^b	0.88^{ab}	0.89^{ab}	0.91^{ab}	0.90^{ab}	0.93^a	0.10
SGR	1.56^c	2.05^b	2.11^b	2.07^b	2.14^{ab}	2.24^a	0.05
PCV (%)	20.4^{ab}	26.1^a	23.3^{ab}	19.7^b	22.7^{ab}	25.3^{ab}	0.89
Hb (g dL^{-1})	3.76^c	4.44^b	3.71^c	4.34^b	4.41^b	5.71^a	0.25
Survival	76.7	77.8	88.9	88.9	91.1	85.6	2.09

[1] Values are means from triplicate groups of fish, and the means in each row with a different superscript are significantly different (P<0.05).

Table 5.9. Vitamin C concentration in different tissues[1]

| | Diets | | | | | | Pooled |
	C0	C25	C50	C75	C150	C1500	SEM
Gill	36.1^e	40.1^{de}	51.3^{cd}	55.6^c	79.4^b	166.9^a	11.94
Kidney	24.5^e	36.2^d	45.0^d	67.1^c	97.6^b	254.9^a	20.90
Liver	27.7^e	37.0^d	39.1^{cd}	46.6^c	63.8^b	163.6^a	12.38
Muscle	16.6^e	21.6^d	29.5^{bc}	30.7^{bc}	36.6^b	56.2^a	3.37

[1] Values are means from triplicate groups of fish, and the means in each row with a different superscript are significantly different (P<0.05).

Experiment 4 (Olive Flounder 3 ± 0.06 g)

Results of bilological performances and morphological indices are summarized in table 5.8. WG and PER of fish fed the vitamin C free diet were significantly lower than those of fish fed the other diets (P < 0.05) and those of fish fed the C_{25}, C_{50}, C_{75} diets were significantly lower than those of fish fed the C_{1500} diet (P < 0.05). No significant difference existed in HSI, haematocrit, haemoglobin and survival among all the dietary treatments (P < 0.05). AA concentration in kidney, liver and muscle of fish fed vitamin C free diet were significantly lower than those of fish fed the C_{150} and C_{1500} diets (P < 0.05), while there was no significant difference among fish fed the C_0, C_{25} and C_{50} diets. However, AA concentration in kidney, liver and muscle from fish fed the C_{1500} diet were significantly higher than those of fish fed C_{150} diet (P < 0.05). Gill AA concentration of fish fed the C_{150} and C_{1500} diets were significantly higher than those of fish fed the C_0, C_{25}, C_{50}, and C_{75} diets (table 5.9). The initial symptoms of AA deficiency such as anorexia and lethargy were observed in fish fed the C_0 diet at the end of second week of the experimental period. Fish fed the vitamin C free diet exhibited scoliosis by the end of fourth week of the experimental period. Fin hemorrhage became apparent during the eleventh week in fish fed the vitamin C free diet. By the end of the tenth week, fish fed the C_{25} diet also exhibited initial deficiency symptoms exhibited by the fish fed the vitamin C free diet. While, no visible deficiency symptoms appeared in fish fed the C_{50}, C_{75}, C_{150} and C_{1500} diet during the 12 weeks of experimental period. Broken line model of WG suggested that optimum dietary level of AA in juvenile olive flounder size 3 ± 0.06 g, could be equal to greater than 93 mg but less than150 mg AA kg^{-1} diet in the form of L-ascorbyl-2-polyphosphate (average final body weight of 16.9 ± 3.1 g).

Table 5.10. Biological performances and morphological indices[1]

	Diets							
	AA-free	AMP_{50}	AMP_{100}	AMP_{205}	AMP_{426}	AMP_{1869}	AA_{36}	AA_{149}
WG (%)	47	180^c	271^b	291^b	306^{ab}	334^a	150^c	282^b
FE (%)		40.8^c	56.7^{bc}	62.5^b	65.1^b	74.9^a	37.6^c	68.2^b
HSI (%)		3.04	3.18	3.34	3.53	3.63	3.11	3.16
SR (%)		56.7^c	91.7^{ab}	91.7^{ab}	91.7^{ab}	98.3^a	36.7^d	83.3^b
PCV (%)		31.9	33.2	36.5	37.5	36.3	33.1	35.5
Hb (g/dl)		7.2	7.5	8.7	7.9	7.5	7.2	8.2

[1] Values are means from triplicate groups of fish, and the means in each row with a different superscript are significantly different (P<0.05).

Table 5.11. Vitamin C concentration in different tissues[1]

	Diets							
	AA-free	AMP_{50}	AMP_{100}	AMP_{205}	AMP_{426}	AMP_{1869}	AA_{36}	AA_{149}
Muscle	-	16.2^{bc}	19.9^{bc}	33.1^b	35.6^b	45.6^a	13.4^c	27.5^b
Liver	-	31.9^d	38.1^{cd}	48.4^b	55.0^b	109.6^a	37.7^{cd}	42.9^{bc}
Gill	-	33.1^d	72.4^c	90.5^{bc}	107.3^b	177.2^a	24.4^d	87.3^{bc}
Brain	31.5^f	89.6^e	131.7^d	289.9^c	368.1^b	467.0^a	79.9^e	253.6^c

[1] Values are means from triplicate groups of fish, and the means in each row with a different superscript are significantly different (P<0.05).

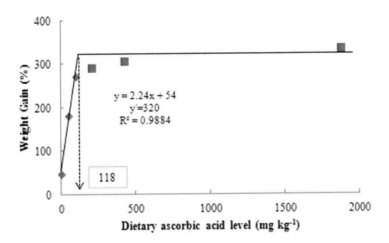

Figure 5.2. Broken line analysis based on weight gain.

Experiment 5 (Parrot Fish 3.9 ± 0.06 g)

Results of biological performances and morphological indices are summarized in table 5.10. WG of fish fed AMP_{50} and AA_{36} diets were significantly lower than that of the other groups, and fish fed AMP_{1869} showed a significant higher WG than did fish fed AMP_{50}, AMP_{100}, AMP_{205}, AA_{36} and AA_{149} diets ($P< 0.05$). However, there was no significant difference in WG between fish fed AMP_{426} and AMP_{1869} diets, and among fish fed AMP_{100}, AMP_{205}, AMP_{426} and AA_{149} diets. Fish fed the AA-free diet began to show vitamin C deficiency signs, such as retarded growth, darkening, anorexia, opercular deformity and high mortality, after 3 weeks of the feeding trial. By the end of the seventh week, all fish fed the AA-free diet were dead. There were no significant differences in HSI, hematocrit (PCV) and hemoglobin (Hb) among fish fed the various diets. Muscle, liver, gill and brain AA concentrations of fish fed AMP_{1869} diet were significantly higher than those from the other dietary groups (table 5.11). In general, there were no significant differences in tissue AA concentrations from fish fed AMP_{205}, AMP_{426}, and AA_{149} diets. Tissue AA concentration in fish fed AMP diets was higher than those from fish fed the AA diets at the same supplemented AA level. Broken line analysis of WG (figure 5.2) suggested that the optimum dietary vitamin C level in parrot fish size 3.9 ± 0.06 g could be equal to or greater than 118 ± 12 mg but less than 205 AA kg^{-1} diet in the form of L-ascorbyl-2-monophosphate (average final body weight of 14.3 ± 2.9 g).

2.3. Discussion

Prior to the start of each experiment, fish were fed the vitamin C free diet for 1- 4 weeks to adjust to the semi-purified diet and to reduce possible body reserves vitamin C. Furthermore, the anterior panels of the every aquaria were scrubbed once per week in addition to the daily siphoning of feaces to minimize algal and fungal growth, which could potentially provide vitamins C. Recorded WG in our few experiments could be lower than the reported value for the same species by other authors. The reason could be attributed differences in size of the fish, the experimental period, environmental condition and most importantly, the use of semipurified diets in these investigations. It was observed that the purified casein-gelatin based diet, low in fish meal (5%), was not readily accepted by experimental fish. Therefore, fish meal supplementation level was increased (10%) to enhance the diet palatability. Fish meal was extracted three times with a chloroform/methanol mixture (2:1, v/v) for one day and then air dried before incorporating into experimental diet (Lee et al. 1998).

The reduction in growth performance of fish fed the vitamin C free diet in these experiments may indicate that dietary AA has a specific effect on growth as suggested by Ram (1966). Similar results have been reported for tilapia (Shiau & Hsu, 1995) and channel catfish (Wilson et al. 1989). Fish species and age group responded differently to the different levels of dietary AA in terms of WG. Observation from the experiment 1, indicated that optimum vitamin C requirement in Korean rockfish size 3.1 ± 0.02 g could be equal to or greater than 100 but less than 200 mg AA $^{-1}$ diet in the form of L-ascorbyl-2-glucose. While, in the experiment 2, broken line model of WG indicated the optimum dietary vitamin C level could be equal to or greater than 102 mg AA^{-1} in the form of L-ascorbic acid for Korean rockfish size 7.12 ± 0.02 g. Results from the experiment 3, it is suggested that AA requirement is greater than 39.7 mg AA kg^{-1}, whereas 144.6 mg AA kg^{-1} in the form of L-ascorbic acid is adequate for the maximum growth of Korean rockfish size 12.6 ± 0.02 g. While, in the case of olive flounder (experiment 4), 93 mg AA kg^{-1} diet in the form of L-ascorbyl-2-polyphosphate was estimated to be required to support the reasonable growth in 3 ± 0.06 g size flounder. Teshima et al. (1991) could not detect significant differences among Japanese flounder fed 10-100 mg L-ascorbyl-2-phosphate-Mg (AMP) kg^{-1} diet fish meal based diets in flounder averaging 43 ± 5 g (mean $\pm$ SD) reared in a flow through system for 24 weeks. They concluded that 60-100 mg of AMP kg-^{1} diet was sufficient to support good growth and survival in Japanese flounder. Nevertheless, they did not observe any external signs of vitamin C deficiency in fish fed the control diet (without AMP supplementation) and diets containing AMP. They further postulated that a supplement of approximately 60 mg of AMP (equivalent to 28 mg of AA) kg^{-1} diet was sufficient to support the good growth and survival of the young Japanese flounder without external signs of vitamin C deficiency. The discrepancy from these two studies might demonstrate that the dietary requirement of AA might decrease with fish size, as has been shown in other studies (Hilton et al. 1978; Li & Lovell, 1985). The other reasons could be attributed such as differences in experimental condition as well as experimental diet. Furthermore, the native AA in the fish meal basal diet that Teshima et al. (1991) used might have also contributed some AA to the experimental diets and thus decreased apparent requirement level of supplemented AA in their diets. Broken line analysis of WG in parrot fish sized 3.9 ± 0.06 g suggested the dietary vitamin C requirement to be equal or greater than 118 ± 12 mg AA kg^{-1} diet in the form of L-ascorbyl-2-monophosphate. The value was higher than the dietary vitamin C requirement of catfish (Lim & Lovell, 1978), rainbow trout (Halver et al. 1969; Hilton et al. 1978), and Korean rockfish (Lee et al. 1998). It may indicate that parrot fish may have a higher vitamin C requirement than the other fish species. However, the vitamin C requirement value from the present study was much lower than 250 mg AAkg^{-1} diet reported in parrot fish from Ishibashi et al. (1992) using AA as the dietary vitamin C source. The main reason for the discrepancy among these two studies could be attributed the difference in source of vitamin C used for experimental diet.

Whereas various previous reports suggested that special attention must be given to vitamin C storage. Tissue levels of a given vitamin may be useful as an index of nutritional status of the animal with respect to that vitamin. In that case, they are complementary to growth studies in accessing the adequacy of the dietary concentration (Gouillou-Coustans & Kaushik, 2001). Liver AA concentration has been widely used as an index of AA status of fish (Hardie et al. 1991; Hilton et al. 1977; Murai et al. 1978; Skelbaek et al. 1990). Lim & Lovell (1978) and Murai et al. (1978) found a good correlation between the dietary and liver AA concentration in channel catfish. Hilton et al. (1977) and Skelbaek et al. (1990) also found significant correlation in rainbow trout. Whereas, Halver et al. (1975) preferred anterior kidney AA concentration although Lim & Lovell (1978) suggested that the kidney AA concentration of channel catfish did not reflect the differences among the AA concentartions of the diet. In our first experiment, the AA concentrations in the muscle and liver tissues from Rockfish fed diets containing 200 mg AA kg^{-1} diets were significantly higher than those from fish fed the vitamin C free or 50 mg AA kg^{-1} diets with either of the dietary vitamin C sources. Although, this experiment was confined by limited number of treatments but the observation is well supported by our previous long-term study. Juvenile Korean rockfish fed 1500 mg AA kg^{-1} diet for 28 weeks showed the liver AA concentration of 180.2μg AA g^{-1} tissue (Bai et al. 1996). A gradual increasing trend in the liver, muscle, gill and brain tissue AA concentration with a crosssponding increase in dietary vitamin C concentration clearly observed in our second and third experiment. In these experiments, the AA concentrations of these four tissues from fish fed the diet supplemented with 1500 mg AA kg^{-1} were 2-5 times higher than those of rockfish fed the diets supplemented with 25-150 mg AA kg^{-1}. In our investigation with olive flounder (experiment 4), liver AA concentrations showed the positive correlation ($r^2 = 0.98$) with dietary AA concentrations. The trend was similar in our experiment with parrot fish as well (experiment 5), muscle, liver, gill and brain AA concentrations of fish fed 1869 AMP kg^{-1} were significantly higher than those of group fed 50 - 426 AMP kg^{-1} diet. The results from the tissue vitamin C analyses indicated that the unit vitamin C concentration was highest in the brain and the lowest in muscle. Although the unit vitamin C concentration is lowest in muscle, the calculated total amounts of vitamin C in fish is the highest. This was well supported by the results from Al-Amoundi et al. (1992), Bai et al. (1996) and Bai & Lee (1996), Jauncey (1985), Soliman et al. (1986). Al-Amoudi et al. (1992) stated that AA in muscle may be in the consumable form which is readily available for physiological activities.

Overall observations in these experiments suggested a much higher dietary vitamin C requirement for the saturation of various tissues in fish body as compared to optimum dietary level estimated upon growth performance. Nevertheless, estimation of vitamin C requirement varies with the response criteria as well as methodological approach. We proposed the depletion-replition method to estimate a true quantitative requirement of a nutrient (Bai et al. 1991, 1998). Without having knowledge of nutritional history as well as the body reserved vitamin C concentration, true estimation could be missleading. Prior to the start of each experiment, fish were fed the vitamin C free diet for 1-4 weeks to deplete possible body reserves vitamin C. In our opinion, vitamin C requirement should be recommended at a level which could provide additional benefit beyond the basic requirement of fish. Taking into account the vitamin C saturation in various tissues, our results may suggest that requirement level could be greater than 1390mg AA kg^{-1} diet in the form of L- ascorbic acid for Korean rockfish, greater than 150 but less than 1500mg AA kg^{-1} diet in the form of L-ascorbyl-2-polyphosphate for juvenile olive flounder, while for parrot fish the level could be greater than 1869mg AA kg^{-1} in the form of L-ascorbyl-2-monophosphate.

The initial symptoms of AA deficiency were observed such as anorexia and lethargy just after an experimental period of 2-3 weeks in olive flounder and parrot fish experiments. While, Korean rockfish fed vitamin C free diet, exhibited these symptoms after an experimental period of 8-10 weeks, when the liver concentration amounted to <30μg AAg^{-1} tissue. Lim & Lovell (1978) observed deficiency symptoms in 2.3 g channel catfish after 8~12 weeks when liver AA concentrations was <30 μg AAg^{-1} tissue. Hilton et al. (1977) found that rainbow trout given an AA-free diet suffered from deficiency symptoms such as anorexia, lethargy and prostration when the liver concentration amounted to be <20 μg AAg^{-1} tissue after 12-14weeks. Hepatic atrophy symptoms were observed among the parrot fish fed vitamin C free diet after 3 weeks of feeding trail. In fact, parrot fish was found to be extremely sensitive to vitamin C deficiency, deficiency signs such as retarded growth, darkening, anorexia, opercular deformity as well as high mortality were pronounced just after an experimental period of 3 weeks. By the end of seventh weeks, all the parrot fish fed the AA free diet were dead. In all of our experiments deficiency symptoms were followed by deficiency signs such as scoliosis, shortened operculae, exopthalmia, and fin hemorrhage among the fish fed vitamin C free diet. Overall observation were identical with the signs and symptoms reported in various other fish species such as channel catfish (Andrew & Murai, 1975; Lim & Lovell, 1978; Murai et al. 1978; Wilson & Poe, 1973) coho salmon, *Oncorohynchus kisutch* (Walbaum), (Halver et al. 1969), rainbow trout (Hitlon et al, 1978; Sato et al, 1983; Tsujimura et al., 1978), carp, and yellow tail, *Seriola quinqueradiata* (Sakaguchi et al. 1969) fed vitamin C free or deficient diets. While, no such deficiency signs or symptoms were observed among fish fed vitamin C supplemented diet at different levels as reported in other studies.

L-AA is the traditionally used vitamin C source in fish and shrimp feeds, but it is thermolabile, unstable and easily oxidized to an inactive form during feed processing and storage. Derivatives of AA that are more stable than AA during diet processing and storage have antiscorbutic activity in many fish species (NRC, 1993). AA derivatives with sulfate and phosphate moitiies at the unstable carbon C-2 position in the lactone ring are highly resistant to oxidation (Shiau, 2001; Tolbert et al. 1979). Phosphate derivatives of AA have been shown to have antiscorbutic activity in channel catfish (El Naggar & Lovell, 1991), tilapia (Shiau & Hsu, 1995; Soliman et al. 1986), rainbow trout (Cho & Cowey, 1993; Dabrowski et al. 1996; Miyasaki et al. 1992), yellowtail (Kanazawa et al. 1992), Japanese flounder (Teshima et al. 1993) and marine shrimp (Shigueno & Itoh, 1988; Shiau & Hsu, 1994). Findings with 3.1 ± 0.02 g size rockfish (experiment 1) confirmed an equal efficiency of AA2G as the dietary vitamin C source compared to AMP-Na/Ca. L-Ascorbyl-2-glucose (AA2G), an AA derivative derived from Kimchi, a Korean traditional fermented vegetable food, is an α-glucose conjugate of AA at the C-2 position. AA2G is stable to ascorbate oxidase and heating, and it can be effectively hydrolysed *in vitro* by the rice seed enzyme α-glucosidase. AA2G was reported to have same vitamin C activity as AA on a molar basis for oral supplementation in guinea-pigs (Kumano et al. 1998; Wakamiya et al. 1992). However, it was the first experiment to measure the bioavailability of this derivative. Overall results suggested that for Rockfish dietary AA2G could be equally effective and practical derivative as a source of vitamin C like AMP-Na/Ca, which is extensively used in the aquatic feed industry. Matusiewicz & Dabrowski (1995) showed that phosphate derivatives of AA could be hydrolyzed by the action of rainbow trout intestinal alkaline phosphatase. While, taking into account the reason attributed before for the discrepancy between the reports of Teshima et al.

(1991) and our finding on vitamin C requirement for olive flounder. In our experiment with olive flounder (experiment 4), L-ascorby-2-polyphospahte (ASPP) as vitamin C source showed similar ascorbic activity as compared to other phosphate derivative of ascorbic acid. Moreover, obtained results with parrot fish reconfirmed that use of ascorbic monophosphate (AMP) as dietary vitamin C source can lead to significantly reduced loses and consequently lower the level of minimum requirement as described by Gouillou-Coustans & Kaushik (2001). As mentioned before the vitamin C requirement value from our study was much lower than 250 mg AA kg^{-1} diet reported in parrot fish from Ishibashi et al. (1992) using AA as the dietary vitamin C source. Observed results demonstrated a higher efficiency of phosphate derivative (AMP) in parrot fish as well.

Various derivatives of AA, including L-ascorbyl-2-sulfate (C2S), L-ascorbyl-2-monophosphate-Mg (C2MP-Mg), L-ascorbyl-2-monophosphate-Ca (C2MP-Ca), L-ascorbyl-2-polyphosphate (C2PP) and ascorbate-2-glucose (C2D), have been tested and encouraging results have been reported as compared to traditional source of vitamin C L-ascorbic acid. As mentioned in standard reference book NRC (2011), a strict comparison of the potency of each source of AA among different reports could be misleading because the experimental condition and purity of these derivatives may also differ.

3. VITAMIN C REQUIREMENT IN FRESHWATER TELEOSTS

3.1. Materials and Methods

3.1.1. Experimental Semipurified Diets

The experimental diets were formulated to contain 50% crude protein and 19.8 kJ gross energy g^{-1} diet (excluding indigestible gross energy). Fish meal was extracted four times by using 75-80°C hot ethanol (fish meal/ethanol = 1:2, W/V) before incorporation into the diet (Kosutarak et al. 1995). Vitamin-free casein and defatted fish meal were used as the main protein sources. Experimental diets were prepared by mixing the dry ingredients in an electric mixer, followed by the addition of oil and water. This mixture was formed into dough, and dry pellets were made by passing the dough through a screw-type pelleting machine and air drying the formed pellets for approximately 48 h. After drying, the pellets were broken up, sieved into the proper pellet size, sealed and stored at -20°C until use.

3.1.2. Experimental Diet, Fish and Feeding Trail

Five experimental diets were prepared to contain 0, 30, 60, 120 or 1,200 mg AMP kg^{-1} diet (dry matter basis, DM) in the form of L-ascorbyl-2-monophosphate (AMP) by adding appropriate amounts of AMP pre-mixture (10 mg AMP g^{-1} cellulose). The actual ascorbic acid concentrations of the experimental diets were determined by high-pressure liquid chromatography (HPLC) to be 0 (AMP$_0$), 24.1 (AMP$_{24}$), 52.3 (AMP$_{52}$), 107.9 (AMP$_{108}$) and 1,137 (AMP$_{1137}$) mg kg-1 diet. In diets supplemented with ascorbic acid, equivalent amounts of cellulose were removed. The feeding trail was conducted in a recirculatory system with a biofilter installed in a concrete water reservoir. All aquaria were equipped with the aeration system and water was heated by electric heaters in the concrete reservoir. Water temperature was maintained at 25 ± 1.0°C (mean ± SD) and water flow rate was 1 L min^{-1}. Experimental fish averaging 15±0.3g were randomly distributed to each of 15 aquaria (60 L capacity) as groups of 20 fish. Each diet was fed to triplicate groups of fish at a feeding rate of 3% of wet body weight for an experimental period of 12 weeks.

3.1.3. Sample Collection and Analyses

Weight gain (WG), specific growth rate (SRG), feed efficiency (FE), protein efficiency ratio (PER) and survival rate were measured and calculated after each weighing.

Weight gain (WG, %) = (final wt. - initial wt.) × 100 / initial wt
Specific growth rate (SGR, %) = ($\log_e$ final wt. - $\log_e$ initial wt.) × 100 / days
Feed efficiency (FE) = (wet weight gain / dry feed intake) × 100
Protein efficiency ratio (PER) = (wet weight gain / protein intake)

Samples of 20 fish at the beginning of the experiment and 6 fish per tank at the termination were collected and stored frozen at -20°C for determination of proximate carcass composition. Proximate composition analyses of experimental diets and fish bodies were performed by the standard methods of AOAC, (1995). Samples of diets and fish were dried to a constant weight at 105°C to determine moisture content. Ash was determined by incineration at 550°C, crude lipid by soxhlet extraction using the Soxtec system 1046 (Tecator AB, Hoganas, Sweden), and crude protein by the Kjeldahl method (N×6.25) after acid digestion. Vitamin C concentrations in experimental diets and carcasses of pooled fish (five fish per aquarium) were determined by high performance liquid chromatography (HPLC; Sykam, Eresing, German) with a UV detector at 254 nm.

Table 5.12. Composition of the basal diet (DM basis)

Ingredients	% of drymatter
Casein[1]	27.5
Defatted fishmeal[2]	27.5
Wheat flour[3]	11.3
Corn starch[3]	16.0
Fish oil[4]	3.1
Corn oil[5]	6.2
Vitamin premix (free vitamin C)[6]	3.0
Mineral premix[7]	3.0
Vitamin E premix[8]	0.0
Carboxymethylcellulose[1]	2.4

[1] United States Biochemical, Cleveland, Ohio, USA.
[2] Han Chang Fishmeal Co., Pusan, Korea.
[3] Young Nam Flour Mills Co., Pusan, Korea.
[4] E-Wha oil Co., Ltd., Pusan, Korea.
[5] Dong Suh Oil & Fats, Changwon, Korea.
[6] Vitamin premix (Wang et al., 2003a).
[7] Contains (as g kg-1 premix): NaCl, 43.3; MgSO4·7H2O, 136.6; NaH2PO4·2H2O, 86.9; KH2PO4, 239.0; Ca(H2PO4)2·H2O, 135.3; ZnSO4·7H2O, 21.9; Fe-citrate, 29.6; Ca-lactate, 303.89; AlCl3·6H2O, 0.15; KIO3, 0.15; Na2SeO3, 0.01; CuCl2, 0.2; MnSO4·H2O, 2.0; CoCl2·6H2O, 1.0.
[8] L-ascorbyl-2-monophosphate, Sigma, St. Louis, USA.

All the analyses were conducted according to standard methods (AOAC, 1995). All data were analyzed by one-way ANOVA to test for the effects of the dietary treatments. When a significant treatment effect was observed, a Least Significant Difference (LSD) test was used to compare means. Treatment effects were considered with the significance level at P <0.05. Broken-line analysis (Robbins et al. 1979) was used to estimate the optimum dietary level of vitamin C. All statistical analyses were carried out by SAS version 9.0 software (SAS Institute, Cary, NC, USA).

Table 5.13. Biological performances and morphological indices[1]

	WG (%)	SGR (% day^{-1})	FE (%)	PER	Survival(%)
Vitamin C (L-ascorbyl-2-monophosphate, AMP mg kg^{-1} diet)					
AMP$_0$	68.2±5.22^b	0.74±0.04^b	48.0±7.66^b	0.96±0.15^b	83.3±7.64^b
AMP$_{24}$	85.6±2.60^{ab}	0.88±0.02^{ab}	59.8±3.65^{ab}	1.20±0.07^{ab}	96.7±5.77^a
AMP$_{52}$	98.0±6.84^a	0.98±0.05^a	65.3±4.56^a	1.31±0.09^a	96.7±5.77^a
AMP$_{108}$	91.6±6.36^a	0.93±0.05^a	63.9±7.01^{ab}	1.28±0.14^{ab}	97.8±2.89^a
AMP$_{1137}$	89.1±4.84^{ab}	0.91±0.04^{ab}	62.2±7.56^{ab}	1.24±0.15^{ab}	98.3±2.89^a

[1] Values are means from triplicate groups of fish, and the means in each row with a different superscript are significantly different (P<0.05).

Table 5.14. Whole body proximate composition and vit C concentration[1]

	Moisture	Ash	Protein	Lipid	Vitamin C (μg g^{-1})
Vitamin C (L-ascorbyl-2-monophosphate, AMP mg kg^{-1} diet)					
AMP$_0$	61.0	3.2	17.1	44.5	ND
AMP$_{24}$	62.4	3.2	16.3	46.7	16.4^c
AMP$_{52}$	62.5	3.3	18.2	46.3	20.8^c
AMP$_{108}$	63.3	3.1	18.4	46.6	46.5^b
AMP$_{1137}$	62.8	3.4	18.4	46.6	78.3^a
Pooled SEM[2]	0.58	0.09	0.42	0.42	9.13

[1] Values are means from triplicate groups of fish, and the means in each row with a different superscript are significantly different (P<0.05).

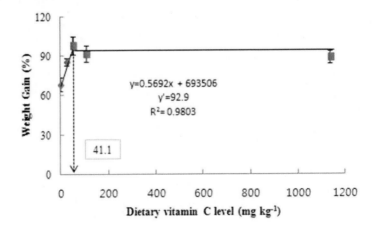

Figure 5.3. Broaken line abalysis based on weight gain.

3.2. Results

Biological performances of the experimental fish are summarized in table 5.13. WG and SGR for fish fed AMP_{52} and AMP_{108} were significantly higher than those of fish fed vitamin C free diet (P<0.05). However there were no significant difference among fish fed AMP_{24}, AMP_{52}, AMP_{108} and AMP_{1137} or among those fed AMP_0, AMP_{24} and AMP_{1137}. Similarly FE and PER of fish fed AMP_{52} were significantly higher than those of fish fed the diet without AMP supplementation (p<0.05). However, there were no significant differences in these parameters among fish fed AMP_{24}, AMP_{52}, AMP_{108} and AMP_{1137} or among those fish fed AMP_{24}, AMP_{52}, AMP_{108} and AMP_{1137} or among those fed AMP_0, AMP_{24}, AMP_{108} and AMP_{1137}. Survival of fish fed the AMP-supplemented diets was significantly higher than those of fish did not receive vitamin C supplementation. No vitamin C could be detected in whole body of fish fed AMP_0 diet. While the vitamin C level in fish fed AMP108 diet were significantly higher than those in fish fed AMP_{24} and AMP_{52}. Vitamin C level in fish fed AMP_{1137} diet were significantly higher than those in fish fed all other diets (table 5.14).

3.3. Discussion

Observed results indicated the essentiality of dietary vitamin C in juvenile eel. However, based on ANOVA test of growth parameters, there seemed to be no benefits of increasing vitamin C supplementation in diets beyond 24 mg AMP kg^{-1} diet, as fish fed any of the vitamin C supplemented diets had similar growth performance. Broken-line regression analysis on the basis of WG showed the dietary vitamin C requirement of juvenile eel could be equal to or greater than 41.1 mg kg^{-1} diet. The determined requirement based on broken-line analysis of WG is comparable to values obtained in common carp, *Cyprinus carpio* (45 mg AA kg^{-1} diet) (Gouillo-Coustan et al. 1998). Ren et al. (2005) reported the optimum dietary level of AA for the Japanese eel juvenile growth to be more than 27mg AA/kg without stating an upper limit. Although no significant differences were recorded above this minimum level, SGR continued to increase numerically up to the maximum supplementation level in their study. Ren et al. (2005) study was done using L-ascrobic acid Ca as the vitamin C source while L-ascorbyl-2-monophosphate was used in our study. Any differences could be attributed to the difference in the vitamin C source. But if broken line analysis had been done on the data in the previous study, the requirement might be similar, suggesting no differences in the availability of these vitamin C sources. Furthermore, no vitamin C deficiency signs such as anorexia, abnormal swimming, and hemorrhagic areas under the skin could be observed in our study in contrast to aforementioned study.

In our knowledge, number of studies devoted to investigate the vitamin C requirement in freshwater teleosts is less than the number of experiments conducted in marine teleost. For *O.mykiss* and *O. kisutch*, the minimum AA requirement based on WG and absence of deficiency signs has been reported to range between 20 - 100 mg kg A^{-1}. In the case of Atlantic salmon, *Salmo solar*, a dietary supplemental level of 50 AA mg kg^{-1} has been reported to be sufficient to support optimum growth (Lall et al. 1989). Sannes et al. (1992) concluded that the minimum dietray requirement for the optimal growth of Atlantic salmon could range between 10-20 mg AA kg^{-1} diet in the form of AMP.

However requirements recorded for Japanese eel experiments seem to be low when compared to the results obtained in marine teleosts mentioned in this article. Even though the value is lower than the reported value for vitamin C requirement in aquatic invertebrate, sea cucumber, *Apostichopus japonicas* (Okorie et al. 2008). Based upon a few existing reports, it would be misleading to conclude that freshwater teleost have a comparatively lower vitamin C requirement than the marine teleosts. Further studies are warranted to confirm the differences in efficiency of different AA derivatives in freshwater fish including eel.

4. GENERAL DISCUSSION AND SUMMARY

Aquaculture nutritionists' knowledge on vitamin C requirements has advanced significantly in the last three decades. Estimation of the true quantitative requirements of any nutrient is a critical issue. However, previously it was suggested that Salmonids differ from mammals with respect to vitamin C metabolism in being able to synthesize L-ascorbyl-2-sulphate (AS) and to use this compound as a storage form (Tucker & Halver, 1986). Also, Guerin (1986) found that AA concentrations were very low in tissues of channel catfish and these concentrations were postulated not to reflect dietary ascorbic acid levels. Thus, he concluded that AA was not an important storage form of vitamin C in channel catfish. While, in our experiment with channel catfish, ascorbic acid concentrations and thiobarbituric acid (TBA) values of fillet indicated that improved stability of channel catfish fllets may be achieved by enhancing tissue levels of vitamin C through dietary supplementation. Therefore, we proposed that Vitamin C can be stored in animal body (Bai & Galtin, 1992). The requirements of fat-soluble vitamins have been proposed by Shiau & Chen (2000) for vitamin A, by Shiau & Hwang (1994) for D, by Lee & Shiau (2004) for E and by Shiau & Liu (1994) for K.

Since vitamin C can be stored in the teleost body, body reserve and the nutritional history of experimental teleost must be taken into account prior to viamin C requirements study. Two approaches may be followed to determine the dietary requirement of an essential nutrient for growth. When turnover of the nutrient is rapid, or whole body has low reserves of that nutrient, normal growing animals can be fed diets containing graded levels of the nutrient and the requirement determined. However, for nutrients which require long time to deplete, animals may continue growing during early nutrient depletion by utilizing body reserves of the nutrient (Bai et al. 1989). In general, a requirement determined on repleted animals may result in an underestimation of the true requirement, because of the contribution of the body reserved vitamins. An alternate procedure to determine the requirement for a nutrient including vitamin C is to initially deplete animals by feeding a vitamin C deficient diet. Response criteria can be evaluated in animals repleted with graded of vitamin C. A requirement determined by the depletion - repletion method, unlike that determined on repleted animals, will tend to overestimate the true requirement, because some of the nutrient may be used to support compensatory growth or may be diverted to replenish body stores (Bai et al. 1991; 1998). In all the experiments experiments summarized in this chapter, the depletion- repletion procedure was adopted to estimate a true quantitative requirement of vitamin C.

Moreover, because of its reducing properties, vitamin C may influence the bioavailablity and thus the dietary requirement of other nutrients (Lovell, 2001). Rutin, one of the bioflavonoids, has been reported to produce vitamin C like effects as well as to spare vitamin C, eventhough it is not an indispensable food component equivalent to vitamin C. The synergism between ascorbic acid and rutin has been well established in guinea pigs (Crampton & Lloyd, 1950; Douglas & Kamp, 1959; Papageorge & Mitchell, 1949). While in our experiment with channel catfish dietary rutin was observed to have limited synergetic effect on vitamin C requirement. Duncan & Lovell (1994) reported a 10 times lower requirement for dietary folate in channel catfish when fish were fed at a marginal level of vitamin C excess 200 mg AA kg^{-1} diet. Among various other micronutrients, interaction effects of vitamn C and vitamin E has been well characterized. Packer et al. (1979) demonstrated that vitamin C spares vitamin E by regenerating it from tocopheroxyl radicals. Further studies investigated the interaction between AA and α -T *in vivo* in several animal species (Igarashi et al., 1991; Liu & Lee, 1998) and humans (Hamilton et al., 2000; Jacob et al., 1996;). The major concern as allready pointed out by Lee & Dabrowski (2004) remain unclear, do we need to reformulate the requirements of these micronutrients in fish based on their interaction, in comparison to the dietary requirement estimated for individual vitamins must be varified.

Based on findings under our experimental condition and methodological approach, the vitamin C requirement level for marine teleost Korean rockfish size 3.1 ± 0.02 g could be equal to or greater than 100 but less than 200 mg AA^{-1} diet in the form of either L-ascorbyl-2-glucose or L-ascorbyl-2-monophosphate. While, for Korean rockfish size 7.12 ± 0.02 g the requirement level could be equal to greater than 102 but less than 150 mg AA^{-1} diet while L-ascorbic acid used as the source of vitamin C. The requirement level is equal to greater than 39.7 mg AA kg^{-1}, whereas 144.6 mg AA kg^{-1} is for the maximum growth of Korean rockfish size 12.06 ± 0.02 g. While, in the case of olive flounder, equal to or greater than 93 but less than 150 mg AA kg^{-1} diet in the form of L-ascorbyl-2-polyphosphate was estimated to be required to support the reasonable growth in 3 ± 0.06 g size fish. In parrot fish sized 3.9 ± 0.06 g the dietary vitamin C requirement could be equal to greater than 118 ± 12 mg but less than 205 mg AA kg^{-1} diet in the form of L-ascorbyl-2-monophosphate. While, for freshwater teleost, Japanese eel the requirement level could be equal to or greater than 41.1 mg but less than 52 mg kg^{-1} diet when L-ascorbyl-2-monophosphate was used as the dietary vitamin C source. Taking into account the vitamin C saturation in different tissues to provide an additional benefit beyond the basic vitamin C requirement, the level could be greater than 1390 mg AA kg^{-1} diet in the form of L- ascorbic acid for Korean rockfish, greater than 150 but less than 1500 mg AA kg^{-1} diet in the form of L- ascorbyl-2-polyphosphate for juvenile olive flounder. While for parrot fish the level could be greater than 1869 mg AA kg^{-1} in the form of L-ascorbyl-2-monophosphate. For the vitamin C saturation in muscle of Japanese eel, the requirement level could be greater than 1137 mg AA kg^{-1} in the form of L-ascorbyl-2-monophosphate.

Furthermore, various derivatives of ascorbic acid could be more effective and practical source of vitamin C as compared to the traditional L- ascorbic acid. For rockfish an equal efficiency of L-Ascorbyl-2-glucose (AA2G) was observed as compared to AMP-Na/Ca. (AA2G), an AA derivative derived from Kimchi, a Korean traditional fermented vagetable food, is an α-glucose conjugate of AA at the C-2 position. In olive flounder, L-ascorbyl-2-polyphospahte (ASPP) as vitamin C source showed similar ascorbic activity as compared to other phosphate derivative of ascorbic acid. Moreover, obtained results with parrot fish reconfirmed that use of ascorbic monophosphate (AMP) as dietary vitamin C source could lead to significantly reduced loses and consequently lower the level of minimum requirement. However, in the case of freshwater teleost, Japanese eel no difference could be postulated between the bioavailability of L-ascrobic acid Ca and L-ascorbyl-2-monophosphate as the source of vitamin C source.

CONCLUSION

Observed results indicated the essentiality of dietary vitamin C in different species of marine and freshwater teleost. Overall observations from all these experiments demonstrated a specific vitamin C requirement in different species and size of marine and freshwater teleosts. Differences in AA requirements were noted based on the fish species, size, experimental period and the dietary vitamin C source as well. Variability in vitamin C requirements were also due to the differences in stability and bioavailability of different AA derivatives as dietary vitamin C sources. Phosphate derivatives of L- ascorbic acids demonstrated to be more stable and bioavailable than their parent compound. Findings were encouraging with AA2G, an AA derivative derived from Kimchi, a Korean traditional fermented vegetable food. Vitamin C deficiency symptoms such as scoliosis, shortened operculae, exophthalmia and fin hemorrhage exhibited among the group of fish fed vitamin C free diet. The deficiency symptoms were distinct in marine fish after an experimental period of 8 to 10 weeks. While, marine teleost parrot fish was found to be extremely sensitive, group of fish fed AA-free diet began to show deficiency signs just after 3 weeks. By the end of the seventh week, all the parrot fish fed the AA-free diet were dead. Adequate dietary supply of AA is obligatory to control the high incidences of malformed fish and subsequent mortality in practical fish farming. Although, deficiency signs and symptoms could not be observed in our experiment with freshwater teleost Japanese eel, growth parameters indicated dietary essentiality of vitamin C in freshwater teleost as well. In our knowledge, the number of vitamin C requirement studies devoted to freshwater teleosts is fewer than those of the marine teleost.

Based upon our earlier observation with channel catfish (*Ictalurus punctatus*), we proposed animal may store vitamin C in their muscle tissue (Bai & Galtin, 1992). A similar trend of gradual increase in fish muscle tissue vitamin C concentration with a corresponding increase in the dietary vitamin C level was observed in these experiments also. Dietary vitamin C requirement level must take in account the tissue vitamin C saturation also beside growth and disappearance of deficiency signs. Since, a large discrepancy on vitamin C requirement has been acknowledged in and among the different fish species, estimation of true quantitative requirement for vitamin C is a critical issue. Nutritional history of the fish as well as the knowledge of body reserved vitamin C are imperative prior to quantitative requirement study. Repletion-depletion method (Bai et al., 1991, 1998) should be followed to avoid the over estimation of true quantitative requirement. The interaction and synergetic effect of various nutrients altering the dietary vitamin C requirement level raises the concern as already pointed out by Lee & Dabrowski (2004), do we need to reformulate the requirements of these micronutrients in fish based on their interaction, in comparison to the dietary requirement estimated for individual vitamins must be varified. Vitamin C and E have long been known as strong antioxidant due to their protective role in scavenging free radical. Though considerable attention has been paid to study the antioxidant activity of vitamin E, vitamin C lags in enquiry. In a recent study conducted at our laboraotaory, dietary vitamin C at the concentration of 200 ppm demonstrated to have detoxification effects on induced inorganic mercury (Hg) toxicity in juvenile olive flounder (oral presentaion). Moreover, taking into account the ability of vitamin C to regenerate vitamin E from its tocopheroxyl radical, dietary combination of these two vitamins may have more protective effects on heavy metal toxicity in marine and freshwater teleosts. Furher studies are warranted to evaluate the detoxification effects of vitamin C individually as well as with the combination of other antioxidant micronutrients such as vitamin E and selenium (Se).

ACKNOWLEDGMENTS/REVISION

The present chapter has been reviewed by:

- K. Dinesh (PhD). Kerala University of Fisheries and Ocean Science (KUFOS), Puduveypu P. O. Kochi – 652-508, Kerala – India.
- Kyung Jun Lee (PhD). School of Marine Biomedical Science. College of Ocean Science, Jeju National University, Zip. 690-756. Jeju. Republic of Korea.

REFERENCES

AI, Q., Mai, K., Tan, B., Xu, W., Zhang, W., Ma, H. & Liufu, Z. (2006). Effects of dietary vitamin C on survival, growth and immunity of large yellow croaker, *Pseudosciaena crocea. Aquaculture, 242*: 489-500.

Al- Amoundi, A. A., El-Nakkadi, A. M. N. & El- Nouman, B. M. (1992). Evaluation of optimum dietary requirement of vitamin C for the growth of *Oreochromis sprilurus* fingerlings in water from the Red Sea. *Aquaculture, 105*; 165-173.

Andrew, J. W. & Murai T. (1975). Studies on the vitamin requirements of channel catfish (*Ictalurus punctatus*) *Journal of Nutrition* 105, 557-561.

AOAC. (1995). Official methods of analysis of 16th edn. Association of Official Analytical Chemists, Arlington, Virginia, USA.

Bai, S. C. & Gatlin D. M., III. (1992). Dietary rutin has limited synergetic effects on vitamin C nutrition of fingerlings channal catfish (*Ictalurus punctatus*). *Fish Physiology and Biochemistry* 10, 183-188.

Bai, S. C. & Lee, K. J. (1996). Long-term feeding effects of different dietary L-ascorbic acid levels on growth and tissue vitamin C concentrations in juvenile Korean rockfish. Journal of Korean rockfish, *Sebastes schlegeli. Journal of Korean Fisheries Society* 29, 643-650 (in Korean with English abstract).

Bai, S. C., David, A. Sampson, James G. Morris. & Quinton R. Rogers (1989). Vitamin B-6 requirement of growing Kittens. *American Institute of Nutrition*.

Bai, S. C., D. A Sampson, J. G. Morris & Q. R. Rogers. (1991). The level of dietary protein effects the vitamin B-6 requirements of cat. *Journal of nutrition* 121: 1054-1061.

Bai, S. C., Lee, K. J. & Jang, H. K. (1996). Development of an experimental model for vitamin C requirement study in Korean rockfish, *Sebastes schlegeli*. *Journal of Aquaculture* 9, 169-175. (In Korean with English abstract).

Bai, S. C. & Delbert, M. Gatlin III. (1992). Dietary rutin has limited synergetic effects on vitamin C nutrition of fingerlings channel catfish (*Ictalurus punctatus*). *Fish Physiology and Biochemistry* vol. 10 no. 3 pp 183-188.

Bai, S. C. (2001). Requirements of L-ascorbic acid in a viviparous marine teleost, Korean rockfish, *Sebastes schlegeli* (Hilgendorf). *Ascorbic acid in Aquatic organisms* 2001 by CRC press LLC. Chapter seven. pp. 69-85.

Bai, S. C., D. A. Sampson, J. G. Morris. & Q. R. Rogers. (1991). The level of dietary protein affects the vitamin B-6 requirement of Cats. *Journal of Nutrition* 121:1054-1061.

Bai, S. C., Q. R. Rogers, D. L. Wong, D. A. Sampson. & J. G. Morris. (1998). Vitamin B-6 deficiency and level of dietary protein affects hepatic tyrosine aminotransferase activity in cats. *Journal of Nutrition* 128:1995-2000.

Brown, J. P. (1980b). A review of the genetic effects of naturally occurring flavonoids, anthraquinones, and related compounds. *Mutat. Res.* 75: 243-277.

Coustans-Gouillo Marie F. & Kaushik J. Sadasivan. (2001). Ascorbic acid requirement in freshawater and marine fish: is there a difference? *Ascorbic acid in Aquatic organisms* 2001 by CRC press LLC. Chapter six. pp. 49-68.

Crampton, E. W. & Lloyd, L. E. (1950). A qualitative estimation of the effect of rutin on the biological potency of vitamin C. *Journal of Nutrition.* 41: 487-498.

Dabrowski, K. (1990). Absorption of ascorbic acid and ascorbic sulfate and ascorbic metabolism in common carp (*Cyprinus carpio L.*) *Journal of comparative physiology* B160, 549-561.

Douglas, C. D. & Kamp, G. H. (1959). The effect of orally administered rutin on the adrenal ascorbic acid level in guinea pigs. *Journal of Nutrition.* 67: 531-536.

El Naggar, G. O. & Lovell, R. T. (1991a). L-Ascorbyl-2-monophosphate has equal antiscorbutic activity as L-ascorbic acid but L-ascorbyl-2-sulfate is inferior to L-ascorbic acid for channel catfish. *Journal of Nutrition.* 121, 1622– 1626.

El Naggar, G. O. & Lovell, R. T. (1991b). Effect of source and dietary concentration of ascorbic acid on tissue concentrations of ascorbic acid in channel catfish. *Journal of World Aquaculture Society.* 22, 201– 206.

Fracalossi, D.M., Allen, M.E., Yuyama, L.K., & Oftedal, O.T. (2001). Ascorbic acid biosynthesis in Amazonian fishes. *Aquaculture* 192, 321–332.

Gouillou – Coustans, M. F., Bergot, P. & Kaushik, S. J., (1998). Dietary ascorbic acid needs of common carp (*Cyprinus carpio*). *Aquaculture*, 161: 453-461.

Guerin, M. (1986). Feeding elevated levels of ascorbic acid to channel catfish in ponds: Effects of tissue levels of ascorbic acids and ascorbate-2- sulfate on resistence to Edwardiella ictaluri. M. Sc. Thesis, Auburn University, U. S. A.

Halver J. E., Smith R. R., Tolbert B. M & Baker E. M. (1975). Utilization of ascorbic acid in fish. *Animals of the New York Academy of Science* 258, 81-102.

Halver, J. E., Ashley, L. M. & Smith, R. R. (1969). Ascorbic acid requirements of coho salmon and rainbow trout. *Trans. Am. Fish. Soc.* 98, 762–771.

Hardie, L. J., Fletcher T. C & Secombes C. J. (1991). The effect of dietary vitamin C on the immune response of the Atlantic salmon. *Aquaculture* 95, 201-214.

Hilton, J. W., Cho C. Y & Slinger S. J. (1978). effects of graded levels of supplemental ascorbic acid in practical diets fed to rainbow trout (*Salmon gairdneri*). *Journal of the Fisheries Research Board of Canada* 35, 431-436.

Hilton, J. W., cho C. Y. & Slinger S. J. (1977). Evaluation of ascorbic acid status of rainbow trout (*salmo gairdneri*). *Journal of the Fisheries Research Board of Canada* 34. 2207-2210.

Igarashi, O., Yonekawa, Y., & Fujiyama-Fujihara, Y., (1991). Synergistic action of vitamin E and vitamin C in vivo using a new mutant of Wistar-strain rats, ODS, unable to synthesize vitamin C. *J. Nutr. Sci. Vitaminol.* 37, 359– 369.

Ikeda, S., Ishibashi, Y., Murata, O., Nasu, T.& Harada, T. (1988). Qualitative requirements of the Japanese parrot fish for water-soluble vitamins. *Nippon Suisan Gakkaishi* 54, 2029–2035.

Ishibashi, Y., Ikeda, S., Murata, O., Nasu, T., & Harada, T. (1992). Optimal supplementary ascorbic acid level in the Japanese parrot fish diet. *Nippon Suisan Gakkaishi* 58, 267–270.

Jauncey, K., Soliman A. & Robert R. J. (1985). Ascorbic acid requirement in relation to wound healing in the cultured tilapia, *Oreochromis niloticus* (Trewavas). *Journal of Fisheries Management* 16, 139-149.

KOSTAT (2012), Statistics Korea.

Kumano Y., Sakamoto T., Egawa M., Iwai I.,Tanaka M. & Yamamoto I. (1998) In vitro and in vivo prolonged biological activities of novel vitamin C derivative,2-O-a-D glucopyranosyl- L-ascorbic acid (AA-2G), in cosmetic fields. *Journal of Nutritional Science and Vitaminology* 44,345-359.

Lee, K. J., Kim, K. W.& Bai, S. C. (1998). Effects of different dietary levels of L-ascorbic acid on growth and tissue vitamin C concentration in juvenile Korean rockfish, *Sebastes schlegeli* (Hilgendorf). *Aquaculture Research* 29, 237– 244.

Lee, M. H. & S. Y. Shiau. (2004). Vitamin E requirements of juvenile grass shrimp, *Penaeus monodon*, and effects on immune responses. *Fish and Shellfish Immunology* 16:475-485.

Li Y & Lovell R. T. (1985). Elevated levels of dietary ascorbic acid increase immune responses in channel catfish. *Ictalurus punctatus. Journal of Nutrition* 115, 123-131.

Lim C. & Lovell R. T. (1978). Pathology of vitamin C deficiency syndrome in channel catfish, *Ictalurus punctatus. Journal of Nutrition* 108, 1137-1146.

Miyasaki T. Sato M, Yoshinaka R., Yoshinaka R. & Sakaguchi M. (1992). Conversion of ascorbyl-2- polyphosphoate to asorbic acid in rainbow trout, *Nippon Suisan Gakkaishi* 58, 2101-2104.

Mukai, K., Nishimura, M. & Kikuchi, S. (1991). Stopped-flow investigation of the reaction of vitamin C with tocopheroxyl radical in aqueous Triton X-100 micellar solutions. The structure-activity relationship of the regeneration reaction of tocopherol by vitamin C. *J. Biol. Chem.* 266, 274– 278.

Murai T., Andreq J. W. & Bauernfeind J. C. (1978) Use of L-ascorbic acid, ethocel coated ascorbic acid and ascorbate-2-sulphate in diets for channel catfish (*Ictalurus punctatus*). *Journal of Nutrition* 108, 1761-1766.

NRC (National Research Council, 1993). *Nutrient requirements of Fish*. Washington, DC., National Academy Press.

NRC (National Research Council, 2011). *Nutrient requirements of Fish and Shrimp.* Washington, DC., National Academy Press.

Okorie, O. E., S. H. Ko, S. G. Go, S. H. Lee, J. Y. Bae, K. M. Han. & Bai. S. C. (2008). Preliminary study of the optimum dietary ascorbic acid level in sea cucumber, *Apostichopus japonicus* (Selenka). *Journal of World Aquaculture Society* 39(6):758-765.

Oral Presentaion. Protective effects of dietary vitamin C levels on mercury (Hg) toxicity in juvenile olive flounder, *Paralichthys olivaceus.* Presenter - Kumar Katya at World Aquaculture 2013, Nashville, U. S. A.

Packer, J. E., Slater, T. F. & Wilson, R. L. (1979). Direct observation of a free radical interaction between vitamin E and vitamin C. *Nature* 278, 737–738.

Papageorge, E. & Mitchell, G. L., Jr. (1949). The effect of oral administration of rutin on blood, liver and adrenal ascorbic acid and on liver and adrenal cholesterol in guinea pigs. *Journal of Nutrition* 37: 531-540.

Pratt, D. E. & Watts, B. M. (1964). Antioxidant activity of vegetable extracts. I. Flavone aglycons. *J. Food Sci.* 29: 27-33.

Ram M. M. (1966). Growth rate and protein utilization in vitamin C deficiency. *Indian Journal of Medical Research* 541, 946-970.

Regnault-Roger, C. (1988). The nutritional incidence of flavonoids: Some physiological and metabolic considerations. *Experientia* 44: 725-733.

Ren, T., S. Koshio, S. Teshima, M. Ishikawa, M. Alam, A. Panganiban, Y. Y. Moe, T. Kojima & H. Tokumitsu. (2005). Optimum dietary level of L-ascorbic acid for Japanese eel, *Anguilla japonica. Journal of World Aquaculture Society* 36(4):437-443.

Robbins, K. R., H. W. Norton & D. H. Baker. (1979). Estimation of nutrient requirements from growth data. *Journal of Nutrition* 109:1710-1714.

Sakaguchi H., Takeda F. & Tange K. (1969). Studies on vitamin requirements by yellowtail. 1. Vitamin B_6 and vitamin C deficiency symptoms. *Bulletin of Japanese Society of scientific Fisheries* 35, 1201-1206.

Sato M., Kondo T., Yoshinkae R. & Ikeda S. (1983). Effect of water temperetutre on the skeletol deformity in ascorbic acid defecient rainbow trout. *Bulletin of Japanese Socity of Scientific Fisheries* 49, 443-446.

Sato, P., Nishikimi, M. & Udenfriend, S. (1976). Is L-gulonolactone-oxidase the only enzyme missing in animals subject to scurvy? Biochem. *Biophys. Res. Commun.* 71, 293–299.

Shiau, S. Y. & J.Y. Hwang. (1994). The dietary requirement of juvenile grass shrimp, *Penaeus monodon*, for vitamin D. *Journal of Nutrition* 124:2445-2450.

Shiau, S. Y. & T. S. Hsu. (1994). Vitamin C requirement of grass shrimp, *Penaeus monodon*, as determined with L-ascorbyl-2- monophosphate. *Aquaculture* 122:347-357.

Shiau, S. Y. & Y. Chen. (2000). Estimation of the dietary vitamin A requirement of juvenile grass shrimp, *Penaeus monodon. Journal of Nutrition* 130:90-94.

Shiau, S. Y. & Hsu, T. S., (1995). L-Ascorbyl-2-sulfate has equal antiscorbutic activity as L-ascorbyl-2-monophosphate for tilapia, *Oreoochromis niloticus_O. aureus. Aquaculture* 133, 147–157.

Shiau, S. Y. & Hsu, T. S., (1994). Vitamin C requirement of grass shrimp Penaeus monodon, as determined with Lascorbyl- 2-monophosphate. *Aquaculture* 122, 347– 357.

Shigueno, K., Itoh, S., (1988). Use of Mg– L-ascorbyl-2-phosphate as a vitamin C source in shrimp diets. *Journal of World Aquaculture Society* 19, 168–174.

Skelbaek, T., Andersen N. G., Winning M. & Westergaard S. (1990). Stability in fish feed and bioavilability too rainbow trout of two ascorbic acid forms. *Aquaculture* 84, 335-343.

Soliman, A. K., Jauncey K. & Roberts R. J. (1986). The effect of varying forms of dietary ascorbic acid on the nutrition of juvenile tilapias (*Orechromis niloticus*). *Aquaculture* 52, 1-10.

Tappl, A. L. (1968). Will antioxidant nutrients slow aging processes? Geriatrics 23, 97–105.

Teshima, S. L., Kanazawa A., Koshio S. & Itoh S. (1991). L-ascorbyl-2-phosphate-Mg as vitamin C source for the Japanese flounder (*Paralichthys olivaceus*) In: *Fish Nutrition in Practice*, (ed by S. J. Kaushik & P. Luquet) pp. 157-166. Biarritz. France.

Thenen, S. W. (1989). Megadose effects of vitamin C on vitamin B-12 status in the rat. *Journal of Nutrition* 119, 1107-1114.

Tolbert, B. M. (1979). Ascorbic acid metabolism and physiological function. *Int. J. Vitam. Nutr. Res., Suppl.* 19, 127– 142.

Tsujimura, M., Yoshikawa H., Hasagawa T., Suzuki T, Kaisai T., Suwa T. & Suwa T. & Kitamura S. (1978). Studies on the vitamin C activity of ascorbic acid 2- sulafate on the feeding test of newborn rainbow trout. *Vitamins* (Japan) 52, 35-44.

Tucker, B. W. & Halver, J. E.. (1986). Utilization of ascorbate 2- sulfate in fish. *Fish Physiol. Biochem.* 2: 151-160.

Wakamiya, H., Suzuki E.,Yamamoto I., Akiba M., Otsuka M. & Arakawa N. (1992). Vitamin C activity of 2-O-a-D-glucopyranosyl- L-ascorbic acid in guinea pigs. *Journal of Nutritional Science and Vitaminology* 38, 235-245.

Wilson, R. P. & Poe W. E. (1973). Absence of ascorbic acid synthesis in channel catfish (*Ictalurus punctatus*) and blue catfish (*Ictalurus furcatus*). *Comp. Biochem. Physiol.,* B 46, 635–638.

Wilson, R. P. & Poe, W. E., Robinson, E. H. (1989). Evaluation of L-ascorbyl-2-polyphosphate (C2PP) as a dietary ascorbic acid source for channel catfish. *Aquaculture* 81, 129– 136.

In: Vitamin C
Editor: Raquel Guiné

ISBN: 978-1-62948-154-8
© 2013 Nova Science Publishers, Inc.

Chapter 6

EFFECTS OF ASCORBIC ACID ON IMMUNITY AND LOW GRADE SYSTEMIC INFLAMMATION

Edite Teixeira de Lemos [1,2*], *Luís Pedro Teixeira de Lemos* [3†] *and Maria João Reis Lima* [1,4‡]

[1]Department of Food Industry, Polythecnic Institute of Viseu, Portugal
[2]Institute for Biomedical Imaging and Life Sciences (IBILI), Faculty of Medicine, University of Coimbra, Portugal
[3]Faculty of Medicine, University of Coimbra, Portugal
[4]Educational Technologies and Health Study Center
Quinta da Alagoa, Estrada de Nelas, Viseu, Portugal

ABSTRACT

Vitamin C or ascorbic acid, has long been known to have an important role in the synthesis of collagen in connective tissue. In fact, its name reflects its relation with scurvy, the disease caused by Vitamin C deficiency. Therefore, it's only natural that its recommended dietary allowance has traditionally been based on the prevention of this disease. However, higher intakes of vitamin C may exert additional health benefits.

For the past few decades vitamin C has been the subject of many investigations in order to have a better understanding of the biological mechanisms in which it is involved and its possible effects on the primary prevention of chronic low grade systemic inflammation. It has been found that vitamin C supplementation ameliorates atherosclerosis, diabetes, cancer and aging. As an antioxidant, vitamin C influences various metabolic processes that are directly associated with inflammation and immune functions.

Therefore, the objective of the present chapter is to clarify the interactions between the immune system and micronutrients, with a focus on the immunobiologically relevant functions of vitamin C. Its ability to decrease low grade systemic inflammation, thus preventing and improving chronic diseases, is another main point of this chapter.

---

[*] Edite Teixeira de Lemos: E-mail: etlemos2@gmail.com.
[†] Luís Pedro Teixeira de Lemos: E-mail: lupelemos@gmail.com.
[‡] Maria João Reis Lima: E-mail: mjoaolima@esav.ipv.pt.

Finally, a concentration-function approach will be taken in order to review vitamin C's recently discovered physiological and pharmacological effects.

1. INTRODUCTION

Ascorbic acid is a simple six carbon compound whose IUPAC nomenclature is (2R)-2-[(1S)-1,2-dihydroxyethyl]-4,5-dihydroxyfuran-3-one. From a chemical point of view, it is a sugar acid well soluble in water and poorly penetrating into lipid fraction. Ascorbic acid salts (sodium, calcium and potassium) and acid esters are frequently used as food additive.

In the body, L-Ascorbic acid (L-Ascorbic acid, AA, 2, 3-endiol-L-gulonic acid-g-lactone) (Figure 6.1) acts as Vitamin C. Its discovery, that in 2013 celebrates its 85th anniversary, was considered an important landmark due to the fact that vitamin C malnutrition has a serious impact on human health. The name ascorbic acid is an acronym of the two Latin words: *scorbutus* referring to scurvy and prefix "*a*" indicating that there is no scurvy during the adequate compound intake. Scurvy is then a disease caused by a lack of ascorbic acid intake and was well recognized for thousands of years typically affecting sailors whose diet is scanty in fresh fruits and vegetables. While cutaneous manifestations, bleeding and gum symptoms are the most striking symptoms of scurvy, the disease also leads to psychical alterations (Verrax and Calderon, 2008). Though scurvy is not a typical disease in population with an adequate access to food, the disease is still diagnosed.

The Recommended Dietary Allowances (RDA) are about 75 mg/day and 90 mg/day, established for adult women and men, respectively; and 45 mg/day for children 9–12 years old (Food and Nutrition Board, Institute of Medicine, 2000). There are practically no toxicity problems related to ascorbic acid, since its excess is rapidly excreted in urine due to it being water-soluble, as seen by Korolkovas and Burckhalter (2008).

The water-soluble vitamin C influences biochemical reactions that involve oxidation and acts as an antioxidant in aqueous environments of cellular components (Institute of Medicine, 2000). Vitamin C has been shown to play an important role in immune system function when supplied at dietary levels higher than standard doses, namely in several fish groups (Blazer, 1992).

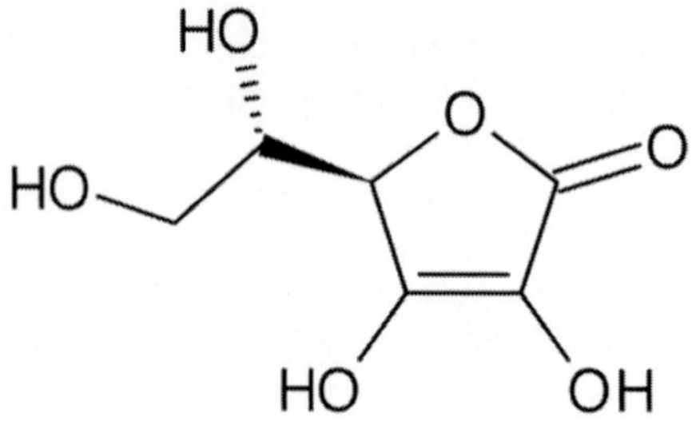

Figure 6.1. L-Ascorbic Acid.

Vitamin C is mainly found in fruits and vegetables. Fruit sources rich in vitamin C include cantaloupe, grapefruit, honeydew, kiwi, mango orange, papaya, strawberries, tangelo, tangerine and watermelon. Fruit juices containing vitamin C in abundance include grapefruit and orange juices, while several others, such as the apple, cranberry and grape juices, are fortified with vitamin C. Rich vegetable sources of vitamin C include asparagus, broccoli, brussels sprouts, cabbage, cauliflower, kale, mustard greens, pepper (red or green), plantains, potatoes, snow peas, sweet potatoes and tomatoes. Variables that affect vitamin C content of fruits and vegetables are harvesting season, duration of transport to the marketplace, period of storage and cooking practices (Wanden-Berghe and Martín-Rodero, 2012).

Although most mammals are capable of synthesizing ascorbate endogenously, during evolution humans lost the capacity to produce this vitamin as seen by Aguirre and May (2008). Ascorbic acid (AA) is a cofactor in numerous physiological reactions, including the post-translational hydroxylation of proline and lysine residues in collagen and other connective tissue proteins, collagen gene expression, synthesis of norepinephrine and adrenal hormones, activation of many peptide hormones and synthesis of carnitine (Johnston et al., 2007). Ascorbic acid also participates in numerous cellular processes such as phenylalanine and tyrosine oxidation. The recommendations for human intake of vitamin C should take into account ascorbate absorption and excretion, which are governed by the following: (i) bioavailability and absorption in the gastrointestinal tract; (ii) concentrations in circulation; (iii) tissue distribution; (iv) excretion and (v) metabolism, as seen by Rumsey and Levine (1998). Despite the fact that ascorbic acid was discovered long time ago and that its role in the body is relatively understood, an extensive research focusing on both benefits of the compound and the role of its depletion during deterioration processes in the organism is still ongoing. In recent years, endogenous as well as exogenous ascorbic acid have been investigated as an antioxidant with treatment potential in low grade systemic inflammatory diseases. The present chapter aims to summarize the immunobiologically relevant functions of vitamin C. Its ability to decrease low grade systemic inflammation, thus preventing and improving chronic diseases and conditions, such as atherosclerosis, diabetes, cancer and aging, is another of the main points of this chapter. Finally, a concentration-function approach will be taken in order to review vitamin C's recently discovered physiological and pharmacological effects and its potential therapeutic usages.

2. General Aspects of the Inflammatory Process and the Role of Vitamin C

Inflammation is a physiological response to infection and tissue injury; it initiates pathogen killing as well as tissue repair processes and helps to restore homeostasis at infected or damaged sites. According to the different mechanisms activated in response to injury, inflammation may be classified into four types:

i   inflammation caused by innate and acquired immunity against infectious agents, in which cells are activated and mediators released to prevent or combat infection and remove foreign material;

ii   inflammation caused by different inhaled agents ('irritants');

iii   allergic inflammation, in which specific IgE antibodies bound to mast cells upon cross-linking by an allergen cause the immediate release of a number of inflammatory mediators and activation of inflammatory cells;

iv   neurogenic inflammation, mediated by the nervous system.

All these different forms of inflammation have in common a first moment where the presence of an unfamiliar substance is sensed by different kinds of cells and a second moment where the intruder is eliminated by the inflammatory response.

The acute response to inflammation involves:

i   An increased blood supply to the site of inflammation.

ii   An increased capillary permeability (caused by retraction of endothelial cells). These allow larger molecules to traverse the endothelium and thus deliver soluble mediators to the site of inflammation.

iii   Leucocyte migration from the capillaries into the surrounding tissue. This is promoted by the release of chemoattractants from the site of inflammation (in a process called chemotaxis) and by the upregulation of adhesion molecules on the endothelium. Once in the tissue the leucocytes move to the site of inflammation.

iv   The release of mediators from leucocytes at the site of inflammation.

Depending on the cell type involved, the nature of the inflammatory stimuli, the anatomical site involved and the stage of the inflammatory response, the released mediators may include lipid mediators (e.g. prostaglandins (PG), leukotrienes), peptide mediators (e.g. cytokines), reactive oxygen species (ROS, e.g. superoxide), amino acid derivatives (e.g. histamine) and enzymes (e.g. matrix proteases).

All these mediators normally play a role in host defense, but when produced inappropriately or in an unregulated fashion, they can lead to disease. Several of these mediators may amplify the inflammatory process acting, for example, as chemoattractants. These inflammatory mediators can also exert systemic effects if they escape into circulation. For example, the cytokine interleukine-6 (IL-6) induces hepatic synthesis of the acute phase C-reactive protein (CRP), while the cytokine tumor necrosis factor-α (TNF-α) elicits metabolic effects within skeletal muscle, adipose tissue and bone.

Acute inflammatory reactions are usually self-limiting and resolve rapidly, due to the involvement of negative feedback mechanisms.

However, inflammatory responses that fail to regulate themselves can become chronic and contribute to the perpetuation and progression of disease. Therefore, regulated inflammatory responses are essential to remain healthy and maintain homeostasis.

In the following sections the effects of vitamin C in the acute response to inflammation (innate immune system) will firstly be discussed; followed by the connection between acute and chronic inflammation and the putative effects of vitamin C not only in the mechanisms of chronic low inflammation but also the effects on several non-transmissible chronic diseases, including atherosclerosis, diabetes, cancer and aging.

2.1. Actions of Vitamin C in the Innate Immune System

The immune system is an intricate network of specialized tissues organs, cells and substances, protecting the host from infectious agents and other noxious insults. Although defense mechanisms of both innate and adaptive immunity are very complex, they can be described as being organized in three main clusters: physical barriers (e.g. skin, mucosa, mucus secretions), immune cells and antibodies. Inter-individual variations in many immune functions exist within the normal healthy population and are due to genetics, age, gender, smoking habits, habitual levels of exercise, alcohol consumption, diet, stage in the female menstrual cycle and stress, as seen by Calder and Kew (2002). Nutrient status is an important factor contributing to immunocompetence and the profound interactions between nutrition, infection and health have been recognized by Calder and Jackson (2000). In the recent decade, substantial research has focused on the role of nutrition and especially on the contribution of the role of micronutrients to an optimum functioning of the immune system.

A number of studies (Padayatty and Levine, 2001; Kaelin, 2005; Mandl et al., 2009; Siddiq et al., 2008) focus on the role of ascorbate in various hydroxylation reactions and in the redox homeostasis of subcellular compartments including mitochondria and the endoplasmic reticulum. Of particular importance is its role in hydroxylation reactions catalyzed by mono- and dioxygenases, which include, among others:

i   the cotranslational hydroxylation of residual proline and lysine in procollagen;
ii   the hydroxylation of tryptophan in serotonin biosynthesis;
ii   the synthesis of catecholamines;
iv   the α-amidation in the biosynthesis of numerous peptide hormones such as gastrin, cholecystokinin, calcitonin, vasopressin and oxytocin;
v   the hydroxylation of β-hydroxy-ε-N-trimethyllysine and ɤ-butyrobetaine in endogenous carnitine synthesis.

Other physiological activities of ascorbic acid include:

i   a role in iron transfer from the iron transporting protein transferrin to the iron storage protein ferritin,
ii   detoxification of numerous substances in the liver by stimulating the synthesis of cytochrome P450,
iii   promotion of intestinal iron absorption by reducing non-absorbable Fe^{3+} to more easily absorbable Fe^{2+} and by inhibiting the production of insoluble iron-tannin and iron-phytate complexes.
iv   the participation in the antioxidant defense localized in the hydrophilic compartment of cells.

The immunological function of vitamin C is indicated by the fact that the concentration of vitamin C in immunocompetent cells (lymphocytes, neutrophils and monocytes) is 10 to 100 fold higher than its concentration in plasma (Wintergerst et al., 2006; Vissers and Wilkie, 2007).

In adults, the association between vitamin C dose intake and immune cell concentration underlines the specific function of vitamin C in cellular immune response.

Indeed, experimentally-induced vitamin C deficiency impairs cellular but not humoral immune defense (Levine et al., 2001; Vissers and Hampton, 2004). Webb and Villamor (2007) reviewed the impact of vitamin C supplementation on parameters of innate and adaptive immunity and mentioned the association between high circulating levels of serum vitamin C and enhanced antibody response, neutrophil function and mitogenic response. The functional significance of vitamin C in infection resistance in humans and other species has also been proven. Vitamin C deficiency reduces resistance to various microbial agents, such as *Mycobacterium tuberculosis* and *Rickettsia,* as well as fungal infections such as *Candida albicans* (Ströhle and Hahn, 2009). An improved vitamin C supply increases the antibody reaction and the activity of neutrophils as well as resistance to infections (White et al., 1986; Cathcart, 1984; Hovi et al., 1995; Harakeh, et al., 1995; Hemilä and Douglas, 1999).

Based on the biochemical functions of vitamin C the immunomodulating effects of this micronutrient probably result from its antioxidant potential as seen by Wintergerst et al. (2006); its role in the *de-novo* synthesis of carnitine (Rebouche, 1991; Carr et al., 2013); its relevance to the synthesis of tetrahydrobiopterin (Huang et al., 2000; Nakai et al. 2003) and its iron metabolism modulating effects (Hallberg and Hulthén, 2000; Hurrell and Egli 2010).

2.1.1. Immunobiological Relevance of the Antioxidant Capacity of Vitamin C

Wintergerst et al. (2006) have observed that during infections, the concentration of vitamin C in the plasma and leukocytes rapidly decline during infections and stress because ascorbate is oxidized due to augmented production of ROS and the fact that the endogenous enzymatic reduction have reached their functional limit.

It is well known that reactive oxygen species (ROS), generated by activated immune cells during the process of phagocytosis, can be scavenged by non-enzymatic antioxidants, such as vitamin C or by enzyme action. While ROS play essential roles in intracellular killing of bacteria and other invading organisms, the immune system and other molecules may also be vulnerable to oxidative attack. If ROS are produced in high concentrations, they can cause oxidative stress, leading to an impaired immune response, loss of cell membrane integrity, altered membrane fluidity and alteration of cell-cell communication, as seen by Maggini et al. (2007). These alterations can contribute to degenerative disorders such as cancer and cardiovascular disease. Therefore, vitamin C plays a pivotal role in the integrity of phagocytes because it acts as an effective water-soluble antioxidant, trapping excess oxygen radicals and thus protecting immune cells against damage (Dagher and Pick, 2007). Biophysically, this can be explained by the ability of the organism to efficiently regenerate the oxidized form of ascorbic acid, which ensures that sufficient amounts of biologically active vitamin C are available (Murphy and DeCoursey, 2006; Mizrahi et al., 2006; Kunes et al., 2009; Loyd and Lynch, 2011).

2.1.2. Immunobiological Relevance of Vitamin C by Its Involvement in the Carnitine Synthesis

The hydroxycarbonic acid carnitine (3-hydroxy-4-N-trimethylaminobutyric acid) metabolite is essential for the transport of long-chain fatty acids from the cytosol into the mitochondrial matrix and is an important player in energy production via β-oxidation.

Therefore, carnitine depletion causes a failure of ATP production and an accumulation of triglycerides in tissues, such as the liver, skeletal muscle and heart (Ramsay et al., 2001).

Carnitine is endogenously synthesized from the aminoacids lysine and methionine in a multi-stage process. Vitamin C is required for its synthesis serving as a cofactor for two enzymes involved in the process: β-hydroxy-N-trimethyl lysine hydroxylase (EC 1.14.11.8) and butyrobetaine hydroxylase (EC 1.14.11.1). The first enzyme catalyzes the mitochondrial hydroxylation of ε-N-trimethyl lysine, which is released by cellular proteins, whereas the second enzyme promotes the hydroxylation of butyrobetaine localized in the cytosol (Ramsay et al., 2001; Famularo et al., 2004).

In addition to its function as a carrier of long-chain fatty acids, several authors suggest carnitine has important immunological effects, such as the stimulation of phagocytosis and chemotaxis in granulocytes and macrophages (Izgüt-Uysal et al., 2003, 2004), the stimulation of immunoglobulin synthesis (IgG) (Mast et al., 2000) and the stimulation of the acute phase response (Buyse et al., 2007).

2.1.3. Influence on the Synthesis of Tetrahydrobiopterin and Nitric Oxide

Tetrahydrobiopterin (BH$_4$) acts as a single-electron donor and is a cofactor of inducible nitric oxide (NO) synthase that oxidizes arginine *via* multiple steps, generating citrulline and NO. BH$_4$ easily reacts with ROS and RNS, especially peroxynitrite (Patel et al., 2002). Being oxidized to a trihydrobiopterin radical in this process, BH$_4$ is inactivated and thus removed from NO synthesis (Patel et al., 2002; Schmidt and Alp, 2007). Ascorbate increases NO synthesis by reducing trihydrobiopterin radicals to active tetrahydrobiopterin (BH$_4$) and/or protecting BH$_4$ against oxidation (Gorren and Mayer, 2002; Wu and Meininger, 2002). Therefore, vitamin C plays an important role for the NO supply of the cell. The immunological relevance of this fact becomes clear when the role of NO as a key substance for cellular immunity is considered. Cytokine-activated macrophages produce increasing amounts of NO (Korhonen et al., 2005; Coleman, 2001; Hibbs, 2002), which exhibit microbicidal effects (Hibbs, 2002; Nagy et al., 2007), modulate the function of T lymphocytes (Nagy et al.; 2007; Nagy et al., 2008) and induce the transformation of Th1 to Th2 helper cells (Korhonen et al., 2005).

2.2. Chronic Inflammation

As mentioned above, inflammation is defined as a wide variety of adaptive physiological and pathological processes to avoid infection and repair damage, restoring the organism to the usual state of homeostasis; inflammation is usually triggered by harmful stimuli and agents like infection and tissue injury.

The organism may have different forms of adaptation and maintenance of tissue/cell homeostasis in relation to inflammation. If conditions waver in between homeostasis and infection, such as mild/slowly progressive stress or modest malfunction, the tissue/cells tend to finely adapt to the slightly changed conditions and restore tissue/cell functionality by inducing para-inflammation, sub-inflammation, low-level inflammation, sterile inflammation, physiological inflammation or "inflammaging", as Franceschi proposed (Franceschi and Bonafe, 2003; Giunta, 2006). A significant body of evidence highlights the key role of abnormal innate immune responses and chronic low-grade inflammation.

However, if the response is not properly phased and the process lasts for a long period of time, chronic low-grade inflammation sets and may predispose the host to various illnesses, as well as forming the underlying basis for several body systems and tissues, including the circulatory (atherosclerosis, heart failure), endocrine (insulin resistance, metabolic syndrome, type 1 and type 2 diabetes, obesity), skeletal (sarcopenia, arthritis, osteoporosis), pulmonary (chronic obstructive pulmonary disease) and neurological (dementia, depression) systems; in addition, some data strongly suggests that chronic inflammation aging-related disability and Alzheimer's disease are connected (Niklas and Brinkley, 2009).

Emerging evidence suggests that during inflammation, mast cells and leukocytes are recruited to the site of damage, leading to a respiratory "burst" due to an increased uptake of oxygen and consequently to an increased release and accumulation of reactive oxygen (ROS) and nitrogen species (RNS) at the site of damage (Zhou et al., 2009). The excessive release of pro-inflammatory cytokines and chemokines that takes place during chronic inflammation can result in dysregulation of processes such as glucose and lipid metabolism and vascular function, via the effects of cytokines on adipocytes, muscle tissue, the liver and blood vessels (Garcia-Bailo et al., 2011; Fernandez-Real and Pickup, 2007).

In addition, chronic inflammation is closely associated with oxidative stress, which is characterized by an elevated presence of highly reactive, potentially harmful molecular compounds, such as reactive oxygen and nitrogen species and free radicals (Abd et al., 2011; Da et al., 2012).

These reactive molecules contribute to further oxidative damage and inflammation through their ability to generate pathways leading to the activation of transcriptor factors of nuclear factor-κB family as well as other molecules such as signal transducer and activator of transcription 3 (STAT3), hypoxia-inducible factor-1 α (HIF1-α), activator protein-1 (AP-1), nuclear factor of activated T cells (NFAT) and NF-E2 related factor-2 (Nrf2), which mediate immediate cellular stress responses. Induction of cyclooxygenase-2 (COX-2), inducible nitric oxide synthase (iNOS), aberrant expression of inflammatory cytokines (TNF-α, interleukin-1 (IL-1), IL-6, interleukin-8 (IL-8); chemokine receptor 4 (CXCR4)) as well as alterations in the expression of specific microRNAs have also been reported to play a role in oxidative stress-induced inflammation (Oeckinghaus et al., 2011; Wan and Lenardo, 2010).

Thus we may consider that the potential forces that drive low grade systemic inflammation are pro-inflammatory cytokines and substances as listed in Table 6.1. CRP and fibrinogen, the major clinical markers of inflammation, have been significantly associated with coronary disease, myocardial ischemia and myocardial infarction, in association with IL-1, IL-1 receptor antagonist, IL-6, soluble IL-6 receptor, IL-18, TNF-α, serum amyloid A and soluble intercellular adhesion molecule 1 (ICAM-1) (Van Den Biggelaar et al., 2004).

Considering the critical role of oxidative stress in inflammation and consequently in the pathogenesis of different chronic diseases, numerous therapeutics have been developed, which incorporate antioxidants into the management of diseases (Valko et al., 2007). Many naturally occurring dietary supplements have been shown to mitigate low-grade inflammation by specific mechanisms.

Several studies reported that Vitamin C exhibited an important role in immune function and in various oxidative/inflammatory processes, such as scavenging ROS and RNS, preventing the initiation of chain reactions that lead to protein glycation and lipid peroxidation (Garcia-Bailo et al., 2011; Moore et al., 2010).

Table 6.1. Main agents involved in the inflammatory process, which are increased in inflammation

Agents involved in the inflammatory process
Inflammatory proteins
CRP
Pro-inflammatory mediators
Interleukin-1
Interleukin-4
Interleukin-6
Interleukin-12
Interleukin-15
Interleukin-18
Gamma-Interferon
Tumor Necrosis Factor, alfa, beta
Transforming Growth Factor
Chemokines
Interleukin-8
Monocyte chemoattractant protein-1 (MCP-1)
Anti-inflammatory mediators
Interleukin-1ra
Interleukin-10
Pro-inflammatory enzimes
Inducible nitric oxide synthase (iNOS)
Cyclooxygenase-2 (COX2)
Prostaglandin E2 (PGE2)
Adhesion molecules
Intracellular adhesion molecule-1 (ICAM-1)
Vascular cell adhesion molecule-1 (VCAM-1)
Hypoxic markers
Hypoxia inducible factor-1alpha (HIF-1 α)
Vascular endothelial growth factor A (VEGF-A)

Findings from epidemiologic studies show an inverse association between ascorbic acid and CRP, suggesting an anti-inflammatory effect of this micronutrient at the systemic level (Aggarwal et al., 2009). However, several intervention trials reported no association between vitamin C intake, circulating ascorbic acid and various inflammatory biomarkers (Ulrich et al., 2006; Casciari et al., 2005; Dworacki et al., 2007; Mikirova et al., 2012). In the following sections the effects of Vitamin C in different chronic diseases will be discussed.

3. VITAMIN C AND LOW GRADE SYSTEMIC INFLAMMATORY DISEASES

The necessity for looking for solutions to prevent diseases has become quite significant and the possibility of reducing the risk of diseases using vitamins has been instituted in literature (Keaney, 2000; Christen et al., 2000, Manson et al., 2012; Krishnan et al., 2012).

Vitamin C is very popular for its antioxidant properties and keeps having the "miracle-pill" denomination, being capable of acting as therapeutics or as a coadjuvant of the treatment in a variety of chronic inflammatory and non-transmissible diseases. However, many other important aspects of this multifaceted molecule are often underestimated or even ignored.

In the following sections the role of vitamin C in different low grade inflammatory diseases and conditons, such as atherosclerosis, diabetes, cancer and aging will be considered.

3.1. Atherosclerosis

Atherosclerosis is an inflammatory disease of the blood vessel wall, characterized in early stages by endothelial dysfunction, recruitment and activation of monocytes/macrophages, differentiation and migration of vascular smooth muscle cells (VSMCs) to later form the bulk of the atherosclerotic plaque (Hansson, 2005). Whereas inflammation may initiate the disease, it is likely that the resulting oxidative stress propagates it and worsens injury (Stocker and Keaney, 2004).

Considering the importance of oxidative stress and inflammation in the initiation and progression of atherosclerosis it is plausible that antioxidants such as ascorbate might mitigate the earliest stages of inflammatory atherosclerosis; nevertheless, vitamin C seems to have lesser effects on established lesions. In Table 6.2 some of the results obtained by administrating Vitamin C are summarized.

Table 6.2. Main effects of ascorbate on atherosclerosis

Different phases of the atherosclerotic process	Effects of vitamin C
Direct oxidation of LDL	↑
Endothelial cell dysfunction	
Nitric oxide generation	↑
Collagen synthesis	↑
Endothelial cell proliferation	↑
Endothelial cell death	↑
VSMC's	
Recruitment and proliferation	↓
Dedifferentiation	↓
Collagen synthesis	↑
Monocyte/macrophages	
Inflammatory markers	↓
Nitric oxide release	↓

↑ (prevents, enhances, stimulates); ↓ (inhibits).

Injury to the vascular endothelium represents a critical event for the initiation of atherosclerosis (Hansson, 2005), since endothelial denudation promotes VSMC activation, proliferation and migration to form the neointima (Seed et al., 2003). Reestablishing the endothelium prevents this response (Ulrich-Merzenich et al., 2004) and decreases neointimal mass (Stocker and Keaney, 2004).

Opposing the healing process of endothelial proliferation is the apoptosis of endothelial cells, which contributes to endothelial dysfunction (Rössig et al., 2001). Apoptosis in endothelial cells can be induced by a variety of factors, including hyperglycemia, oxidized low density lipoprotein (Ox-LDL), TNF-α and angiotensin II (Recchioni et al., 2002).

Vitamin C has long been known to protect the vascular endothelium. Ascorbate increases the synthesis and deposition of type IV collagen in the basement membrane, stimulates endothelial proliferation and inhibits apoptosis, scavenges radical species and spares endothelial cell-derived nitric oxide to modulate blood flow; it can also prevent the endothelial dysfunction that is the earliest sign of many vascular inflammatory diseases (Aguirre and May, 2008; May and Harrison, 2013). An important role for ascorbate in preventing vascular smooth muscle cells (VSMCs) proliferation/dedifferentiation is evidenced by the results obtained by Tomoda and co-workers (1996) in a clinical trial of restenosis after angioplasty, in which subjects receiving oral ascorbate supplements of 500 mg three times daily for 4 months had 25% larger luminal diameters compared to matched controls who did not receive ascorbate. Treated group also present a 50% decrease in the need for intervention compared to the control group (Tomoda et al., 1996). Resembling results were observed in studies of coronary restenosis in pigs using combinations of ascorbate and α-tocopherol (Orbe et al., 2003). Evidence also exists that ascorbate protects VSMCs from apoptosis/necrosis due to injury by oxidized LDL (Ulrich-Merzenich et al., 2002; Watanabe et al., 2001). In contrast to endothelial cells, where there is substantial support for a beneficial use of ascorbate, the results observed in macrophages are contradictory. More research should be done using better defined cellular models. Although there may be little benefit in increasing cellular ascorbate concentrations to near maximum values in normal people, many diseases and conditions have either systemic or localized cellular ascorbate deficiency as a cause for endothelial dysfunction, including early atherosclerosis, sepsis, smoking and diabetes (May and Harrison, 2013; Agarwal et al., 2012).

3.2. Type 2 Diabetes Mellitus

The incidence of type 2 diabetes mellitus (T2DM) is increasing worldwide and certain population subgroups are especially vulnerable to the disease, such as the Hispanics, Africans and Aboriginals, as well as children (Wild et al., 2004; Costan et al., 2010). T2DM is a multifactorial disease characterized by chronic hyperglycemia, altered insulin secretion and insulin resistance, a state of diminished responsiveness to normal concentrations of circulating insulin (Defronzo, 2009). T2DM is also defined by impaired glucose tolerance (IGT) that results from islet β-cell dysfunction, followed by insulin deficiency in skeletal muscle, liver and adipose tissues (Defronzo, 2009). In individuals with IGT, the development of T2DM is governed by genetic predisposition and environmental variables (a hypercaloric diet and the consequent visceral obesity or increased adiposity in liver and muscle tissues) and host-related factors (age, imbalances in oxidative stress and inflammatory responses) (AbdulGhani et al., 2009; Isharwal et al., 2009, Badawi et al., 2010).

A significant body of evidence highlights the key role of abnormal innate immune responses and chronic low-grade inflammation resulting from oxidative stress in obesity, metabolic syndrome and insulin resistance, which are critical stages in the development and progression of T2DM.

Therefore, inflammation may play a causal role in the pathogenesis of T2DM and reducing it via modulation of oxidative stress and the innate immune response could lead to a status of improved insulin sensitivity and delayed disease onset. Dietary supplementation with anti-inflammatory and antioxidant nutritional factors, such as micronutrients, might present a novel strategy toward the prevention and control of T2DM at the population level (Lamb and Goldstein, 2008).

As previously mentioned, vitamin C has an important role in immune function and various oxidative/inflammatory processes, such as scavenging ROS and RNS, preventing the initiation of chain reactions that lead to protein glycation (Calder et al., 2009). The oxidized products of vitamin C, ascorbyl radical and dehydroascorbic acid, are easily regenerated to ascorbic acid by glutathione, NADH or NADPH (Calder et al., 2009). In addition, ascorbate can recycle vitamin E and glutathione back from their oxidized forms (Bartlett et al., 2008). For this reason, determining if vitamin C can be used as a therapeutic agent against the oxidative stress and subsequent inflammation associated with T2DM has been an important area of interest. Several epidemiologic studies have assessed the effect of vitamin C on biomarkers of oxidation, inflammation and/or T2DM risk (Wannamethee et al., 2006; Hamer and Chida, 2007; Gao et al., 2004; García-Bailo, 2012).

The *European Prospective Investigation of Cancer - Norfolk Prospective Study* examined the association between fruit and vegetable intake and plasma levels of vitamin C and risk of T2DM. During a 12-year follow-up, 735 incident cases of diabetes were identified among nearly 21,000 participants. A significant inverse association was found between plasma levels of vitamin C and risk of diabetes. In the same study, a similar association was observed between fruit and vegetable intake and T2DM risk (Harding et al., 2008).

Although epidemiologic findings generally point towards an association between increased vitamin C and reduced oxidation and inflammation, intervention trials assessing the effect of vitamin C supplementation on various markers of T2DM have yielded inconsistent results. The trial conducted by Lu and colleagues (2005) reported no improvement in fasting plasma glucose and no significant differences in levels of CRP, IL-6, IL-1 receptor agonist or (Ox-LDL) after supplementation with 3000 mg/day of vitamin C for 2 weeks in a group of 20 T2DM patients, compared to baseline levels. Chen and colleagues (2006) performed a randomized, controlled, double-blind intervention on a group of 32 diabetic subjects with inadequate levels of vitamin C and found no significant changes in either fasting glucose or fasting insulin after intake of 800 mg/day of vitamin C for 4 weeks. Furthermore, Tousoulis et al (2007) reported that the treatment with 2000 mg/day for 4 weeks had no effect on levels of CRP, IL-6, TNF-α or soluble vascular cell adhesion molecule-1 in 13 T2DM patients.

On the other hand, the works of Wang et al. (1995) and Paolisso et al. (1995) showed an improvement on red blood cell sorbitol/plasma glucose ratio, in fasting plasma insulin, LDL and total cholesterol and free radicals. The results obtained by Wang et al. (1995) also suggest an inhibition of the polyol pathway by vitamin C.

The evaluation of the different results of intervention trials in T2DM using vitamin C whether as a supplement or as part of a diet rich in fruits and vegetables are conflicting. Small sample sizes, genetic variation, short intervention duration, insufficient dosage and disease status of the assessed cohorts may account for the lack of effect and the inconsistent outcomes observed in intervention studies. Therefore, further research and long-term prospective studies are needed to elucidate the role of vitamin C as a modulator of inflammation and T2DM risk and to evaluate its potential role as a preventive agent.

3.3. Cancer

Chronic inflammation has been linked to various steps involved in carcinogenesis. Inflammation plays a key role in tumor development, affecting tumor proliferation, angiogenesis, metastasis and resistance to therapy (Balkwill et al., 2005; Bartsch and Nair, 2006; Hussain and Harris, 2007). Key features of cancer-related inflammation (CRI) include leukocyte infiltration, cytokine build-up, tissue remodelling and angiogenesis. Infiltrating leukocytes such as tumor associated macrophages (TAMs), neutrophils, dendritic cells and lymphocytes establish an inflammatory microenvironment (Lu et al., 2006) and are key components in tumors of epithelial origin. These leukocytes secrete pro-inflammatory cytokines (IL-1, IL-6, TNF-α, TGF-β, fibroblast growth factor (FGF), epidermal growth factor (EGF) and hepatocyte growth factor (HGF21)), as well as chemokines (CCL2 and CXCL8) (Joyce and Pollard, 2009). While immune cells may suppress tumor growth in some cases, there is increasing concern that inflammatory microenvironments caused by infiltrating leukocytes can facilitate cancer development (Aggarwal et al., 2009; Zhang et al., 2004). In clinical studies, TAMs are associated with poor prognosis, while the use of anti-inflammatory agents is associated with reduced instances of certain cancers (Roxburgh and McMillan, 2010; Ulrich et al., 2006). Several studies indicate that inflammation is a marker of high cancer risk and poor treatment outcome (Moore et al., 2010).

Cancer is one of the diseases for which a beneficial role of vitamin C has been most frequently claimed. Dietary use of vitamin C has been proposed as part of cancer prevention for several years and is recently evidenced by Jansen and co-workers (2013). Apart from this nutritional side, an extensive and often confusing literature exists about the use of vitamin C in cancer that has considerably discredited its use. Emerging evidence indicates that ascorbate in cancer treatment deserves reexamination. Studies in healthy men and women show that ascorbate concentrations in plasma and tissue are tightly controlled as a function of oral dose. Pharmacokinetic facts suggest that this millimolar ascorbate concentrations obtained by oral administration are not usually considered 'physiological' and thus it does not have a therapeutic role in cancer. The effective concentrations only can be achieved if the vitamin is administered intravenously (i.v.) at high dose. Intravenous injection of ascorbate bypasses tight control and produces plasma concentrations as much as 70-fold greater than those produced by maximal oral dosing (Sebastian et al., 2004; Verrax and Calderon, 2008).

Intravenous vitamin C therapy has been used in the treatment of cancer (Riordan et al., 2005; Du et al., 2012; Chen et al., 2005). Rationales for intravenous vitamin C (IVC) therapy include preferential toxicity of ascorbate toward cancer cells (Casciari et al., 2001), potential benefits of ascorbate for immune cells (Riordan et al., 2005) and ascorbate inhibitory effect on angiogenesis (Mikirova et al., 2008; Mikirova et al., 2010). In a study with guinea pigs, tumor growth was significantly reduced in cases where intra-tumor ascorbate concentrations reached the millimolar level (Casciari et al., 2005). In addition, inflammation and oxidative stress can cause down-regulation of immune system associated with T cell dysfunction, which has been described in cancer, infectious and autoimmune diseases.

In addition, in cancer and other inflammatory conditions, the T-cell receptor (TCR) zeta chain is cleaved resulting in anergic T and Natural Killer (NK) cells (Dworacki et al., 2007).

As the *in vitro* tissue cultures have shown a reversal of TCR cleavage by antioxidants (Nambiar et al., 2002) the result of treatment by ascorbic acid may augment T-cell and NK cell immunity.

Vitamin C should be considered as a part of the treatment protocol for cancer therapy since it seems to improve quality of life and extend survival time (Vollbracht et al., 2011; Du et al., 2012). Nonetheless, further pharmacokinetic, pharmacodynamic and clinical studies are needed in order to understand the full potential of pharmacological vitamin C in cancer treatment.

3.4. Aging

Aging is a complex natural biological process characterized by a progressive declination of physiological functions that affects many tissues, with a more pronounced effect on brain functions; it is influenced by the individual's genetics, his lifestyle and environmental factors. Aging and especially human aging, can be explained by the emerging concept of para-inflammation-driven "inflammaging" a coinage of "inflammation" and "aging" (Franceschi et al., 2000; Franceschi, 2003). The characteristic consequence of aging in the immune system is the progressive filling of the immune system by activated lymphocytes, macrophages and dendritic cells in response to chronic/continuous subtle stress either due to pathological or physiological antigens/toxins. Therefore, the condition of inflammaging provides a continuous mild antigenic challenge leading to a pro-inflammatory condition associated with the progressive stimulation/depletion of the immune system and other systems of the organism (Franceschi and Bonafe, 2003; Franceschi et al., 2000; Giunta, 2006). This perspective fits with basic assumptions of the evolutionarily antagonistic pleiotropy theory regarding aging, which suggests that a trade-off between early beneficial effects and late negative outcomes can occur at the genetic and molecular level.

The aging process involves the deterioration of several organic systems and the appearance of different diseases that we may group as connective tissue disorders, endocrine metabolic disorders, immune disorders, neurodegenerative disorders, cancer, hypertension and atherosclerosis. All of these pathologies are associated with low chronic inflammation and thus vitamin C may act as previously mentioned.

Figure 6.2 summarizes both the major molecular pro-inflammatory pathways involved in chronic non-transmissible diseases associated with low grade systemic inflammation mentioned in this chapter and the possible sites where vitamin C can exert its effects.

4. PHARMACOLOGICAL APPROACH OF VITAMIN C

In order to address ascorbate therapeutic concentrations it is important to describe plasmatic and intracellular ascorbate availability, which will be focused in the present section.

For many years, the RDA for all vitamins was based on preventing deficiency, with a margin of safety. As previously mentioned there is great interest in the clinical roles of vitamin C because evidence suggests that inflammation and oxidative stress are a root cause of many non-transmissible diseases.

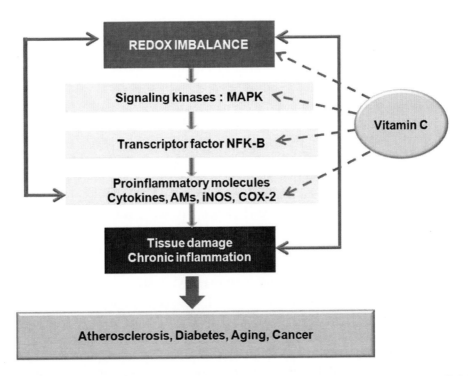

RS: reactive species; MAPK: mitogen-activated protein kinases, NIK, NFκ-B-induced kinase; IKK, IκB kinase; AMs, adhesion molecules; iNOS, inducible NO synthase; COX-2, cyclooxygenase.

Figure 6.2. Major molecular pro-inflammatory pathways involved in low chronic inflammatory diseases and the possible sites of action of vitamin C.

In fact, plasma ascorbic acid concentrations may be low in chronic or acute inflammatory states. The *Food and Nutrition Board (FNB) of the Institute of Medicine US National Academies* established in 2000 a system of dietary reference intake (DRI) values for the US population that, for the first time, provides advice on the safety of the nutrients. "Safety" is defined as presenting no "unreasonable risk of illness or injury" or "a reasonable certainty of no harm," under labeled or ordinary conditions of use, as set forth in US laws and regulations for dietary supplements and food additives.

The DRI system includes the estimated average requirement, the recommended dietary allowance (RDA) [or the acceptable intake for some nutrients] and the tolerable upper intake level (UL). In 2010 the FNB established a RDA for Vitamin C of: 90 mg/day for men; 75 mg/day for women; 85 mg/day during pregnancy and 120 mg/day for lactating women, with an upper limit (UL) of 2000 mg/day. In European countries, the average daily intakes reported in surveys are above the recommended daily intakes, with the 95th percentile intakes from food and supplements ranging up to about 1 g/day.

These dietary intakes do not represent a cause for concern. The *Expert Group on Vitamins and Minerals in the UK* (EGVM, 2003) has recommended an upper level of 2 g/day and a guidance level of 1 g/day, as a supplemental intake, respectively.

Despite the fact that vitamin C has a well known beneficial effect in preventing disease, the therapeutic effects of vitamin C are very hard to summarize mainly because:

i   ascorbate is added mostly in different combinations with other drugs, antioxidants, vitamins or other (natural) antioxidant diet constituents;
ii   several studies have an insufficient number of subjects, leading to equivocal results and consequently to conflicting conclusions;
iii the therapeutic use of ascorbate in everyday treatment by physicians is conflicting;
iv   there are major differences with respect to the oral and intravenous use of ascorbate. Ascorbate added intravenously is much more effective in elevating serum ascorbate levels, while several randomized clinical trials that have utilized oral administration of ascorbate have been unsuccessful (Padayatty and Levine, 2001)

In humans, the requirement for vitamin C is satisfied by natural sources and in some situations by supplements in the ordinary diet. Humans consume vitamin C orally with subsequent gastrointestinal absorption and distribution or they can receive it parenterally. The two major forms of vitamin C in the diet are L-ascorbic acid and L-dehydroascorbic acid (DHA). Both ascorbate and DHA are absorbed along the entire length of the human intestine, as shown by the measurement of transport activity in luminal (brush border) membrane vesicles (Wilson, 2005). Transporters for vitamin C and its oxidized form DHA are crucial to keep the optimal intracellular vitamin concentrations. In humans, cells may accumulate ascorbate by the Na^+-dependant vitamin C transporters SVCT1 (SLC23A1) and SVCT2 (SLC23A2) (Savini et al., 2008). SVCT1 is expressed in epithelial tissues such as the intestine, where it contributes to the maintenance of whole-body ascorbic acid levels, whereas the expression of SVCT2 is relatively widespread either to protect metabolically active cells and specialized tissues from oxidative stress or to deliver ascorbic acid to tissues that are in high demand of the vitamin for enzymatic reactions. DHA, the oxidized form of ascorbic acid, is taken up and distributed in the body by facilitated transport via members of the SLC2/GLUT family (GLUT1, GLUT3 and GLUT4). Absorption of vitamin C occurs in the small intestine via active transport through SVCT1. This receptor also exists in the renal proximal tubules, where it reabsorbs filtered ascorbate and is expressed throughout the body (Aguirre and May, 2008).

The characteristics of DHA uptake by luminal membranes of the human jejunum clearly differ from those of ascorbate uptake (Wilson, 2005). DHA is taken up by low-affinity (Km ~0.8 mM) sodium-independent facilitated diffusion. Glucose inhibits ascorbate uptake but not that of DHA. However, the transport inhibition profile ruled out the role of the sodium-dependent glucose co-transporter in ascorbate transport (Malo and Wilson, 2000). The transport protein responsible for the intestinal absorption of DHA has not yet been identified. Plasma concentrations of vitamin C are tightly controlled when the vitamin is taken orally. Peak plasma vitamin C concentration seemed to plateau with increasing oral doses (Padayatty et al., 2004). There are two simple reasons for this: on the one hand, as mentioned in the previous paragraph, the capacity of the transporters is limited; on the other hand, the two Na^+-dependent transporters can be subjected to fine tuned regulation by their own substrate. An elevated level of ascorbate in the intestinal lumen leads to down-regulation of SVCT1 mRNA in enterocytes (MacDonald et al., 2002). A similar self-regulatory role for ascorbate was demonstrated for SVCT2 in platelets (Savini et al., 2007).

Recently, it was shown that skeletal muscle cells modulated the expression of the SVCT2 carrier according to their redox balance. Both mRNA and protein levels of SVCT2 were up-regulated in hydrogen peroxide-treated myotubes, while antioxidant supplementation with LA lowered the expression of SVCT2 (Savini et al., 2007b). It seems likely that the redox state of the cell can influence the expression of SVCT2, thus regulating the transport and intracellular level of ascorbate. Plasma levels of vitamin C are not only limited by intestinal absorption, but also by reabsorption in the kidneys by SVCT1.

The works of Corpe and co-workers (2008) and those of Sotiriou and co-workers (2002) using knockout mice highlight the importance of the SVCT-type transporters to the maintenance of intracellular ascorbate concentrations in the low millimolar range. Knockout of the SVCT1 resulted in a normal appearing and fertile phenotype, but caused a 2 to 7-fold increase in the renal loss of ascorbate and a 50% decrease in plasma ascorbate (Corpe et al., 2008). This result clearly documents an important role for this transporter in ascorbate retention by the kidney. Knockout of the SVCT2 resulted in phenotypically normal and fertile heterozygotes with a 40-50% decrease in the ascorbate content of muscle and blood, despite the fact that these mice can still synthesize ascorbate (Sotiriou et al., 2002). Although there were no embryonic or fetal losses, homozygotes died at birth with cerebral hemorrhage and failure of the lungs to expand (Sotiriou et al., 2002). Ascorbate was very low in the brain, muscle tissue and liver (Sotiriou et al., 2002), indicating that SVCT2 is the only functional transporter in these tissues.

4.1. Vitamin C Concentration in Humans As a Function of Dose

Levine and co-workers (2001) clearly demonstrated that Vitamin C concentrations in plasma are tightly controlled as a function of dose. They observed healthy young women with a controlled intake of 30–2,500 mg of vitamin C from food and showed that in the women's plasma there was a steep sigmoidal relationship between vitamin C doses and resulting concentrations for doses of 30–100 mg daily, with an approximate 5-fold increase in plasma concentration over this dose range. At doses of 200 mg daily and higher, there was little change in plasma concentrations, with saturation between 200 and 400 mg daily. Circulating neutrophils, monocytes and lymphocytes contained 0.5–4.0 mM concentrations of vitamin C and also saturated between 200 and 400 mg daily. At doses of 400 mg daily and higher, vitamin C plasma concentrations did not increase, in part because of increasing vitamin C excretion in urine. At plasma concentrations less than 4 μM, symptoms of scurvy may occur. Doses of 30 mg daily yield steady-state plasma concentrations of approximately 7 μM for men and 12 μM for women. For both genders, there is a steep sigmoid relationship between dose and plasma concentrations at doses between 30 and 100 mg daily (Padayatty et al., 2003). At 100 mg daily steady-state plasma concentrations are slightly less than 60 μM for men and slightly greater than 60 μM for women. However, the dose-concentration curve between 30 and 100 mg daily is shifted to the left for women compared to men. At doses of 200 mg daily and higher, steady-state plasma values for both genders are similar. Plasma is completely saturated at doses of 400 mg daily and higher, producing a steady-state plasma concentration of approximately 80 μM (Calder et al., 2009). Accordingly, the maximum bioavailability of vitamin C is usually attained at lower doses and declines with the elevation of oral supplements (Levine et al., 1996).

Circulating concentrations of ascorbate in blood are considered adequate if they are at least 28 µM, but they are considerably higher in most cells due to active transport by SVCT2.

This observation was further confirmed by data from the three compartment pharmacokinetic model for vitamin C. According to this model, a single oral dose of 3 g – the maximum tolerated single dose – produces a peak plasma concentration of 206 mM, while the 1.25 g oral dose results in a slightly lower concentration of 187 mM (Padayatty et al., 2004). Hence, pharmacological plasma concentrations of vitamin C can only be reached through the intravenous administration of the vitamin (Padayatty et al., 2004). The only clinical benefit of ascorbate addition, with a proven mechanism of action, is the prevention of scurvy. However, intake of as little as 10 mg/day of vitamin C is appropriate for this purpose. This amount results in plasma vitamin C concentrations below 10 mM. When 'therapeutic' levels or even 'normal' levels of vitamin C are present in the diet, plasma ascorbate concentrations are at least one order of magnitude higher than that necessary to prevent scurvy (Padayatty et al., 2003).

The short half-life of vitamin C during the rapid excretion phase pointed out by Hickey and co-workers (Hickey et al., 2005) is sometimes ignored. Plasma levels above 70 µM have a half-life of approximately 30 minutes, so large doses taken several hours apart should be considered independent, as should their bioavailability. This cumulative pattern means that splitting a single large dose into several smaller ones, taken a few hours apart, increases the effective bioavailability of the large dose. This schedule-dependant phenomenon needs to be taken into consideration for any further interpretation of ascorbate pharmacokinetic and pharmacodynamic results.

The bioavailability of ascorbate is clearly different if administered i.v. or orally and this important point must be considered. Pharmacologic doses of ascorbate can produce plasma concentrations 70-fold higher than those possible with maximally tolerated oral doses (Chen et al., 2007). With infusion rates of 0.5–1 g/min plasma concentrations of 10 mmol/L (10,000 μmol/L) were predicted to be attainable for >3 h. For i.v. administration, plasma concentrations are expected to vary depending on the dose, rate and frequency of infusion. This was subsequently confirmed in animals and humans (Chen et al., 2008; Stephenson et al., 2013). In contrast to data from i.v. (parenteral) administration, maximal peak plasma concentrations from oral dosing were predicted and subsequently found by others to be <0.25 mmol/L (Park et al., 2009; Micallef et al., 2009). Although peak oral concentrations can possibly vary with the dose frequency, variations are minimal compared with concentrations attainable with i.v. administration.

Neutrophils, when exposed to bacteria, oxidize extracellular ascorbic acid to form dehydroascorbic acid, which is transported into the neutrophil and rapidly reduced to ascorbic acid by the protein glutaredoxin. As a result of this recycling of extracellular ascorbic acid, the neutrophil internal concentration of ascorbic acid increases 10-fold. Ascorbic acid may quench oxidants generated during phagocytosis and thus protect the neutrophil and surrounding tissues from oxidative damage (Padayatty and Levine, 2001).

Ascorbate appears in the urine at intakes of roughly 60 mg/day. However, in a depletion/repletion study in healthy young women, ascorbate plasma and white blood cell concentrations saturated at intakes of 200 mg/day or higher (Levine et al., 2001).

The plasma half-life of ascorbate is widely reported to be between 8-40 days (Kallner et al., 1979). However, this applies only to periods of deficient intake, when the renal transporters actively reabsorb the vitamin to prevent acute scurvy.

When intake levels are higher, more rapid excretion occurs. During this phase, ascorbate has a half-life of about 30 minutes (Kallner et al., 1979; Berger, 2009).

Tubular reabsorption is influenced by the concentration of ascorbic acid in the tubule. When the transport reabsorption mechanism approaches maximal velocity, additional vitamin C cannot be absorbed and is excreted in urine. The dose at which reabsorption saturates is the threshold dose for vitamin C excretion and occurs at an intake of 100 mg/day, corresponding to a plasma concentration of approximately 55 to 60 µmol/L. Maximal tubular reabsorption was shown to be 1.5 mg/ml of glomerular filtrate (Oreopoulos et al., 1993). Its reabsorption and excretion by the kidney play a key part in the tight control of vitamin C plasma and tissue concentrations in healthy humans. It is unclear, however, whether other mechanisms of regulation of ascorbic acid reabsorption exist and if there is a mechanism of an active secretion of ascorbic acid into the renal tubules.

4.2. Vitamin C: Use As a Pro-Drug and Safe Profile Evidences

The preponderance of scientific evidence, which has been thoroughly reviewed by several authors, consistently shows that vitamin C is safe at intakes of ≤2000 mg/d (*Jialal and Devaraj, 2003; Levine et al.,* 1999). Oral administration of vitamin C is limited by the saturation of osmotic intestinal absorption and diarrhea (Padayatty et al., 2004).

It is also known that high amounts of ascorbate can be harmful due to oxalate formation (*Levine et al., 1999). *Therefore, administration of high doses of vitamin C is contraindicative for patients with oxalate kidney stones or hyperoxaluria (Levine et al., 1999; *Schmidt et al.,* 1981, Siener and Hesse, 2002*). *In patients with renal failure, vitamin C is retained and converted to insoluble oxalate, which can accumulate in various organs. Subsequent to kidney transplantation, the administration of vitamin C (self-medication 2 g/day for 3 years while in dialysis) led to the development of renal failure due to the widespread deposition of calcium oxalate crystals (Nankivell and Murali, 2008). Therefore, high-dose vitamin C therapy should be avoided in patients with renal failure or renal insufficiency and in patients undergoing dialysis (Levine et al., 1999). Intravascular haemolysis occurred after high-dose vitamin C administration in patients with a deficiency in glucose-6-phosphate dehydrogenase (Levine et al., 1999). It is also contraindicated in patients with systemic iron overload (Rivers, 1987; Levine et al., 1999). Some studies have also observed increased uric acid concentrations (Stein et al., 1976), but others did not find increases of uric acid in either plasma or urine (Huang et al., 2005).

There are fears that vitamin C may have pro-oxidant (Podmore et al., 1998) or mutagenic (Lee et al., 2001*) *effects. In fact, the rationale for the use of vitamin C in cancer is based on its pro-oxidant effects (Hoffer et al., 2008; Vollbracht et al., 2011). In the biological milieu, pharmacologic ascorbate may set in motion a preponderance of reactions that favor formation of H_2O_2, the key cytotoxic effector species. Hydrogen peroxide was proposed to achieve effective steady-state concentrations of ≥25–50 μmol/L to elicit cell death (Chen et al., 2005 and 2008). However, the concentration of H_2O_2 induced by pharmacologic ascorbate is far higher, as much as 2 orders of magnitude, than those which regulate normal cellular processes (Stone and Yang, 2008).

It has been shown by Chen and co-authors (2005 and 2008) that extracellular ascorbate was able to selectively kill cancer cells by generating hydrogen peroxide. However, it is unknown why only cancer cells were affected.

There was no correlation with ascorbate-induced cell death and glutathione, catalase activity or glutathione peroxidase activity. The data presented by Chen and co-workers showed that ascorbate initiated H_2O_2 formation extracellularly, but H_2O_2 targets could be either intracellular or extracellular, because H_2O_2 is membrane permeant (Antunes and Cadenas, 2000; Chen et al., 2005). For example, extracellular H_2O_2 might target membrane lipids, forming hydroperoxides or reactive intermediates that are quenched or repaired in normal cells but not in sensitive cancer cells. In sensitive (but not resistant) cancer cells, intracellular H_2O_2 can target DNA, DNA repair proteins or mitochondria because of diminished superoxide dismutase activity (Oberley, 2001; Pani et al., 2004). New insights may follow from future studies of a very broad range of tumor cells or from microarray analysis of resistant and sensitive cells derived from the same genetic lineage.

If pharmacologic parenteral ascorbate is a pro-drug for selective H_2O_2 delivery to the extracellular space, then therapeutic use should consider a broader use of H_2O_2 in situations where it may have clinical benefit. In addition to cancer treatment, another potential therapeutic use is for treatment of infections. Pharmacological ascorbate administration was able to generate *in vivo* H_2O_2 concentrations of 25–50 µM that are bacteriostatic (Hyslop et al., 1995). Further research is needed to learn whether some bacteria are especially sensitive to clinically possible H_2O_2 concentrations, whether there is synergy with antibiotic therapy and whether such synergy can be used to treat problematic resistant species, such as *Acinetobacter* or methicillin-resistant *Staphylococcus aureus*. H_2O_2 concentrations only slightly higher than those presented in this paper are selectively toxic to hepatitis C virus replication in cell culture models (Choi et al., 2004). Other virally infected cells may also be candidates (Chen et al., 2005) and should be investigated, particularly those for which there are no current therapies.

Ascorbate administered intravenously has already been tested in a phase I clinical trial, is in wide use by complementary and alternative medicine (integrative medicine) practitioners and appears to have minimal side effects in patients who are properly screened. Nevertheless, more research should be done in order to enhance basic and clinical knowledge in these areas so that patients can benefit from it.

CONCLUSION

Given the diverse pathways it regulates and/or participates, as well as the beneficial effects presented throughout this chapter, ascorbic acid might be suitable for therapeutic use in various diseases as well as a preventive natural substance. Introducing novel and effective prevention strategies in a public health setting needs considering approaches with the least (if any) side effects and the maximal preventive efficacy and outcome.

In this context, applying nutritional intervention to attenuate inflammation and oxidative stress would be a feasible public health strategy for prevention of chronic low grade systemic inflammation, in various diseases and conditions, such as atherosclerosis, T2DM, cancer and aging.

There is evidence supporting the idea that vitamin supplementation can modify the innate immune response (i.e., the proinflammatory and inflammatory markers) and that it ameliorates oxidative stress and the subsequent proinflammatory signaling.

Taking this into account, the mechanism by which nutritional factors (such as vitamin C) prevent or delay disease development can be understood, allowing for its introduction and use in the general population, as well as in particularly susceptible subpopulations. However, new metabolic approaches may be useful and will help develop a more exhaustive portrait of the manifold roles of vitamin C in human nutrition in the next few years.

Future research focused on the potential of high-level therapy in particular cases, including treatment of cancer and in stem cell development, will yield a better understanding of potential vitamin C therapeutic benefit.

ACKNOWLEDGMENTS

The present chapter was reviewed by:

- Flávio Reis (PhD), Laboratory of Pharmacology and Experimental Therapeutics, Institute for Biomedical Imaging and Life Sciences (IBILI), Faculty of Medicine, University of Coimbra, Portugal
- João Páscoa Pinheiro (PhD), Rehabilitation Medicine and Sports Medicine, Faculty of Medicine, University of Coimbra, Portugal

REFERENCES

Abd, T. T.; Eapen, D. J.; Bajpai, A.; Goyal, A.; Dollar, A. and Sperling, L. (2011). The role of C-reactive protein as a risk predictor of coronary atherosclerosis: implications from the Jupiter trial. *Current Atherosclerosis,* 13(2), 154-61.

Abdul-Ghani, M. A.; Lyssenko, V.; Tuomi, T.; DeFronzo, R. A. and Groop, L. (2009). Fasting versus postload plasma glucose concentration and the risk for future type 2 diabetes: results from the Botnia Study. *Diabetes Care,* 32(2), 281-286.

Agarwal, M.; Mehta, P. K., Dwyer, J. H.; Dwyer, K. M.; Shircore, A. M.; Nordstrom, C. K.; Sun, P.; Paul-Labrador, M.; Yang, Y. and Merz, C. N. (2012). Differing Relations to Early Atherosclerosis between Vitamin C from Supplements vs. Food in the Los Angeles Atherosclerosis Study: A Prospective Cohort Study. *Open Cardiovasc. Med. J.,* 6, 113-21.

Aggarwal, B. B.; Vijayalekshmi, R. V. and Sung, B. (2009). Targeting inflammatory pathways for prevention and therapy of cancer: short-term friend, long-term foe. *Clin. Cancer Res.,* 15, 425-430.

Aguirre, R. and May, J. M. (2008). Lash Inflammation in the vascular bed: Importance of vitamin C. *Pharmacology and Therapeutics,* 119, 96–103.

Anderson, K. G.; Olson, J. E., Sinha, R. and Petersen, G. M. (2013). Nutrients from fruit and vegetable consumption reduce the risk of pancreatic cancer. *J. Gastrointest. Cancer,* 44 (2), 152-61.

Andrejus, K. and Burckhalter, J. H. (2008). *Química Farmacêutica.* Editora Guanabara Koogan, Rio de Janeiro.

Antunes, F. and Cadenas, E. (2000) Estimation of H_2O_2 gradients across biomembranes. *FEBS Lett.*, 475(2):121-6.

Badawi, A.; Klip, A. and Haddad, P. (2010). Type 2 diabetes mellitus and inflammation: prospects for biomarkers of risk and nutritional intervention. *Diabetes, Metabolic Syndrome and Obesity,* 3, 173–186.

Balkwill, F.; Charles, K. A. and Mantovani, A. (2005) Smoldering and polarized inflammation in the initiation and promotion of malignant disease. *Cancer Cell,* 7, 211-217.

Barabás J.; Nagy, E. and Degrell, I. (1995). Ascorbic acid in cerebrospinal fluid - a possible protection against free radicals in the brain. *Archives of Gerontology and Geriatrics Archives,* 21, 43-48.

Bartlett, H. E. and Eperjesi, F. (2008). Nutritional supplementation for type 2 diabetes: a systematic and protecting against lipid peroxidation. *Ophthalmic Physiology Optics,* 28(6), 503–523.

Bartsch, H. and Nair, J. (2006). Chronic inflammation and oxidative stress in the genesis and perpetuation of cancer: role of lipid peroxidation, DNA damage and repair. *Langenbecks Arch. Surg.*, 391, 499-510.

Berger, M. M. (2009). Vitamin C requirements in parenteral nutrition. *Gastroenterology,* 137, 70-78.

Block, G., Patterson, B. and Subar, A. (1992). Fruit, vegetables and cancer prevention: a review of the epidemiological evidence. *Nutrition and Cancer,* 18, 1–29.

Bürzle, M. and Hediger, M. A. (2012). Functional and physiological role of vitamin C transporters. *Curr. Top Membr.*, 70, 357-75.

Buyse, J.; Swennen, Q.; Niewold, T. A.; Klasing, K. C.; Janssens, G. P.; Baumgartner, M. and Goddeeris, B. M. (2007). Dietary L-carnitine supplementation enhances the lipopolysaccharide-induced acute phase protein response in broiler chickens. *Veterinary Immunol. Immunopathol.*, 118, 154-159.

Calder, P. C.; Albers, R.; Antoine, J. M.; Blum, S.; Bourdet-Sicard, R.; Ferns, G. A.; Folkerts, G.; Friedmann, P. S., Frost, G. S.; Guarner, F.; Løvik, M.; Macfarlane, S.; Meyer, P. D.; M'Rabet, L.; Serafini, M.; van Eden, W.; Van Loo, J.; Vaz Dias, W.; Vidry, S.; Winklhofer-Roob, B. M. and Zhao, J. (2009). Inflammatory disease processes and interactions with nutrition. *Br. J. Nutr.*, 101(Suppl. 1), 1–45.

Calder, P. C. and Kew, S. (2002). The immune system: a target for functional foods? *British Journal Nutrition,* 88, Suppl. 2, 165–177.

Calder, P. C., Albers, R. and Antoine, J. M. (2009). Inflammatory disease processes and interactions with nutrition. *British Journal Nutrition,* 101(Suppl. 1), 1–45.

Calder, P. C. and Jackson, A. A. (2000). Under-nutrition, infection and immune function. *Nutrition Research Reviews,* 13, 3–29.

Carr, A. C.; Bozonet, S. M; Pullar, J. M.; Simcock, J. W. and Vissers, M. C. (2013). Human skeletal muscle ascorbate is highly responsive to changes in vitamin C intake and plasma concentrations. *Am. J. Clin. Nutr.*, 97(4), 800-807.

Casciari, J. J.; Riordan, H. D.; Mirranda-Massara, J. R. and Gonzalez, M. J. (2005). Effects of high dose ascorbate administration on L-10 tumor growth in guinea pigs. *PR Health Sci. J.*, 145-150.

Casciari, J. J.; Riordan, N. H.; Schmidt, T. L.; Meng, X. L; Jackson, J. A. and Riordan, H. D. (2001). Cytotoxicity of ascorbate, lipoic acid and other antioxidants in hollow fiber in vitro tumors. *Br. J. Cancer*, 84,1544-1550.

Casciari, J. J.; Riordan, H. D.; Mirranda-Massara, J. R. and Gonzalez, M. J. (2005). Effects of high dose ascorbate administration on L-10 tumor growth in guinea pigs. *Puerto Rico Health Sciences Journal,* 24,145-150.

Cathcart, R. F. (1984). Vitamin C in the treatment of acquired immune deficiency syndrome (AIDS). *Med. Hypotheses.,* 14, 423-433.

Chen, Q.; Espey, M. G.; Krishna, M. C.; Mitchell, J. B.; Corpe, C. P.; Buettner, G. R.; Shacter, E. and Levine, M. (2005). Pharmacologic ascorbic acid concentrations selectively kill cancer cells: action as a pro-drug to deliver hydrogen peroxide to tissues. *Proc. Natl. Acad. Sci.* US;102, 13604–*13609*.

Chen, Q.; Espey, M. G.; Sun, A. Y.; Lee, J. H.; Krishna, M. C.; Shacter, E.; Choyke, P. L.; Pooput, C.; Kirk, K. L.; Buettner, G. R. and Levine, M. (2007). Ascorbate in pharmacologic concentrations selectively generates ascorbate radical and hydrogen peroxide in extracellular fluid in vivo. *Proc. Natl. Acad. Sci. US.,* 104, 8749–54.

Chen, Q.; Espey, M. G.; Sun, A. Y.; Pooput, C.; Kirk, K. L.; Kirshna, M. C.; Khosh, D. B.; Drisko, J. and Levine, M. (2008). Pharmacologic doses of ascorbate act as a prooxidant and decrease growth of aggressive tumor xenografts in mice. *Proc. Natl. Acad. Sci. US,* 105, 11105–11109.

Chen, H; Karne, R. J. and Hall, G. (2006). High-dose oral vitamin C partially replenishes vitamin C levels in patients with type 2 diabetes and low vitamin C levels but does not improve endothelial dysfunction or insulin resistance. *American Journal of Physiology - Heart and Circulatory Physiology;* 290(1), 137–145.

Choi, J.; Lee, K. J.; Zheng, Y.; Yamaga, A. K., Lai, M. M. and Ou, J. H. (2004). Reactive oxygen species suppress hepatitis C virus RNA replication in human hepatoma cells. *Hepatology*, 39(1), 81-9.

Christen, W. G.; Gaziano, J. M. and Hennekens, C. H. (2000). Design of Physicians' Health Study II—A Randomized Trial of Beta-Carotene, Vitamins E and C and Multivitamins, in Prevention of Cancer, Cardiovascular Disease and Eye Disease and Review of Results of Completed Trials. *Annals of Epidemiology*, 10, 125-134.

Coleman, J. W. (2001). Nitric oxide in immunity and inflammation. *International Immunopharmacology*, 1(8), 1397-1406.

Corpe, C.; Tu, H.; Wang, J.; Eck, P.; Wang, Y.; Schnermann, J.; Margolis, S.; Padayatty, S., Sun, H.; Wang, Y., Nussbaum, R. L.; Espey, M. G. and Levine, M. (2008). SVCT1 (Slc23a1) knockout mice: Slc23a1 as the vitamin C kidney reabsorptive transporter. *The FASEB Journal*, 21, LB111.

Da Costa, L. A.; Garcia-Bailo, B.; Badawi, A. and El-Sohemy, A. (2012). Genetic determinants of dietary antioxidant status. *Prog. Mol. Biol. Transl. Sci*, 108, 179-200.

Dagher, M. C. and Pick, E. (2007). Opening the black box: lessons from cell free systems on the phagocyte NADPH-oxidase. *Biochimie,* 89, 1123-1132.

Defronzo, R. A. and Banting, L. (2009). From the triumvirate to the ominous octet: a new paradigm for the treatment of type 2 diabetes mellitus. *Diabetes*, 58(4),773-795.

Dkhar, P. and Sharma, R. (2011). Amelioration of age-dependent increase in protein carbonyls of cerebral hemispheres of mice by melatonin and ascorbic acid. *Neurochemistry International,* 59(7), 996-1002.

Du, J.; Cullen, J. J. and Garry, R. B. (2012) Ascorbic acid: Chemistry, biology and the treatment of cancer. *Biochimica et Biophysica Acta,* 1826, 443–457.

Dworacki, G.; Meidenbauer, N.; Kuss, I.; Hoffmann, T. K.; Gooding, W.; Lotze, M. and Whiteside, T. L. (2007). Decreased zeta chain expression and apoptosis in CD3+ peripheral blood T lymphocytes of patients with melanoma. *Clinical Cancer Research,* 7, 947-957.

Expert Group on Vitamins and Minerals (convened and supported by the Food Standards Agency of the United Kingdom) (2003). Safe upper levels for vitamins and minerals. Accessed 2013 May 12. Available from http://www.foodstandards.gov.uk/multimedia/pdfs/vitmin2003.pdf

Famularo, G.; De Simone, C.; Trinchieri, V. and Mosca, L. (2004). Carnitines and its congeners: a metabolic pathway to the regulation of immune response and inflammation. *Annual N.Y. Academy Science,* 1033, 132- 138.

Fernandez-Real, J. M. and Pickup, J. C. (2007). Innate immunity, insulin resistance and type 2 diabetes. *Trend. Endocrin. Metabol.,* 19, 10-16.

Food and Nutrition Board, Institute of Medicine (2000). Dietary Reference Intakes for Vitamin C, Vitamin E, Selenium and Carotenoids. Washington, DC, US, National Academies Press.

Franceschi, C.; Bonafe, M.; Valensin, S.; Olivieri, F.; De Luca, M.; Ottaviani, E. and De Benedictis, G. (2000). Inflamm-aging: An evolutionary perspective on immunosenescence. *Ann. N Y Acad. Sci.* 2000, 908, 244-254.

Franceschi, C. and Bonafe, M. (2003) Centenarians as a model for healthy aging. *Biochemical Soc. Trans.,* 31, 457-461.

Franceschi, C. (2003). Continuous remodeling as a key to aging and survival. *Biogerontology,* 4, 329-334.

Gao, X.; Bermudez, O. I. and Tucker, K. L. (2004). Plasma C-reactive protein and homocysteine concentrations are related to frequent fruit and vegetable intake in Hispanic and non-Hispanic white elders. *Journal Nutrition,* 134(4), 913–918.

Garcia-Bailo, B.; El-Sohemy, A.; Haddad, P. S.; Arora, P.; BenZaied, F. and Karmali, M. (2011). Vitamins D, C and E in the prevention of type 2 diabetes mellitus: modulation of inflammation and oxidative stress. *Biologics,* 5, 7-19.

García-Bailo, B.; Roke, K.; Mutch, D. M.; El-Sohemy, A. and Badawi, A. (2012). Association between circulating ascorbic acid, α-tocopherol, 25-hydroxyvitamin D and plasma cytokine concentrations in young adults: a cross-sectional study. *Nutrition and Metabolism,* 9,(1),102-106.

Giunta, S. (2006). Is inflammaging an auto(innate)immunity subclinical syndrome? *Immunity Ageing,* 3, 2-3.

Gorren, A. C. and Mayer, B. (2002). Tetrahydrobiopterin in nitric oxide synthesis: a novel biological role for pteridines. *Current Drug Metabolism,* 3, 133-157.

Hallberg, L. and Hulthén, L. (2000). Prediction of dietary iron absorption: an algorithm for calculating absorption and bioavailability of dietary iron. *Am. J. Clin. Nutr.,* 71, 1147-1160.

Hamer, M. and Chida, Y. (2007). Intake of fruit, vegetables and antioxidants and risk of type 2 diabetes: systematic review and meta-analysis. *Journal of Hypertension,* 25(12), 2361–2369.

Hansson, G. K. (2005). Inflammation, atherosclerosis and coronary artery disease. *New England Journal of Medicine*, 352, 1685–1695.

Harakeh, S. and Jariwalla, R. J. (1995). Ascorbate effect on cytokine stimulation of HIV production. *Nutrition*, 11, 684-687.

Harding, A. H.; Wareham, N. J. and Bingham, S. A. (2008). Plasma vitamin C level, fruit and vegetable consumption and the risk of new-onset type 2 diabetes mellitus: the European prospective investigation of cancer–Norfolk prospective study. *Archives Internal Medicine,* 168(14), 1493–1499.

Harrison, F. E. and May, J. M. (2009). Vitamin C function in the brain: vital role of the ascorbate transporter SVCT2. *Free Radical Biology and Medicine*, 46, 719-730.

Hemilä, H. and Douglas, R. M. (1999). Vitamin C and acute respiratory infections. *Int. J. Tuberc. Lung Dis.*, 3(9), 756-61.

Hibbs, J. B. Jr. (2002). Infection and nitric oxide. *Journal Infectious Diseases*, 185, 9-17.

Hickey, D. S.; Roberts, H. J. and Cathcart, R. F. (2005). Dynamic Flow: A New Model for Ascorbate. *Journal of Orthomolecular Medicine*, 20(4), 237-244.

Hoffer, L. J.; Levine, M.; Assouline, S.; Melnychuk, D.; Padayatty, S. J.; Rosadiuk, K.; Rousseau, C.; Robitaille, L. and Miller, W. H. Jr (2008). Phase I clinical trial of i.v. ascorbic acid in advanced malignancy. *Ann. Oncol.,* 19, 1969–1974.

Hovi, T.; Hirvimies, A.; Stenvik, M.; Vuola, E. and Pippuri, R. (1995) Topical treatment of recurrent mucocutaneous herpes with ascorbic acidcontaining solution. *Antiviral Res.,* 27, 263-270.

Huang, H. Y.; Appel, L. J.; Choi, M. J.; Gelber, A. C.; Charleston, J. and Norkus, E. P. Miller (2005) The effects of vitamin C supplementation on serum concentrations of uric acid: results of a randomized controlled trial. *Arthritis Rheum.*, 52(6), 1843-7.

Huang, A.; Vita, J. A.; Venema, R. C. and Keaney, J. F. Jr. (2000). Ascorbic acid enhances endothelial nitric-oxide synthase activity by increasing intracellular tetrahydrobiopterin. *J. Biol. Chem.*, 275, 17399-17406.

Hurrell, R. and Egli, I. (2010). Bioavailability and dietary reference values. *Am. J. Clin. Nutr.,* 91(5), 1461-1467.

Hussain, S. P. and Harris, C. C. (2007). Inflammation and cancer: An ancient link with novel potentials. *Int. J. Cancer*, 121, 2373-2380.

Hyslop, P. A.; Hinshaw, D. B.; Scraufstatter, I. U.; Cochrane, C. G.; Kunz, S. and Vosbeck, K. (1995). Hydrogen peroxide as a potent bacteriostatic antibiotic: implications for host defense. *Free Radic. Biol. Med.*, 19(1), 31-37.

Isharwal, S.; Misra, A.; Wasir, J. S. and Nigam, P. (2009). Diet and insulin resistance: a review and Asian Indian perspective. *Indian Journal Medical Research*, 129(5), 485–499.

Izgüt-Uysal, V. N.; Agaç, A. and Derin, A. A. (2003). N. Effect of L-carnitine on carrageenan-induced inflammation in aged rats. *Gerontology*, 49, 287-292.

Izgüt-Uysal, V. N., Agaç, A., Karadogan, I. and Derin, N. (2003). Effects of Lcarnitine on neutrophil functions in aged rats. *Mechanisms of Ageing and Development,* 124, 341-347.

Izgüt-Uysal, V. N.; Agaç, A.; Karadogan, I. and Derin, N. (2004). Peritoneal macrophages function modulation by L-carnitine in aging rats. *Aging Clinical and Experimental Research*, 16, 337-341.

Jansen, R. J.; Robinson, D. P.; Stolzenberg-Solomon, R. Z.; Bamlet, W. R.; de Andrade, M.; Oberg, A. L.; Rabe, K. G.; Anderson, K. E.; Olson, J. E.; Sinha, R. and Petersen, G. M.

(2013). Nutrients from fruit and vegetable consumption reduce the risk of pancreatic cancer. *J. Gastrointest. Cancer,* 44(2), 152-61.

Kaelin, W. G. (2005). Proline hydroxylation and gene expression. *Annu. Rev. Biochem.,* 74, 115-128.

Kallner, A.; Hartmann, D. and Horning, D. (1979). Steady-state turnover and body pool of ascorbic acid in man. *Am. J. Clin. Nutr.,* 32, 530–539.

Keaney Jr, J. F. (2000). Atherosclerosis: from lesion formation to plaque activation and endothelial dysfunction. *Molecular Aspects of Medicine,* 21, 99–166.

Korhonen, R.; Lahti, A.; Kankaanranta, H. and Moilanen, E. (2005). Nitric oxide production and signaling in inflammation. *Current Drug Targets Inflamm. Allergy,* 4, 471-479.

Krishnan, A. V.; Swami, S. and Feldman, D. (2012). Equivalent anticancer activities of dietary vitamin D and calcitriol in an animal model of breast cancer: Importance of mammary CYP27B1 for treatment and prevention. *The Journal of Steroid Biochemistry and Molecular Biology. Epub ahead of print.*

Krone, C. A. and Ely, J. T. A. (2004). Ascorbic acid, glycation, glycohemoglobin and aging. *Medical Hypotheses,* 62, 275–279.

Lamb, R. E. and Goldstein, B. J. (2008). Modulating an oxidative-inflammatory cascade: potential new treatment strategy for improving glucose metabolism, insulin resistance and vascular function. *International Journal of Clinical Practice,* 62(7), 1087–1095.

Lee, S. H.; Oe, T. and Blair, I. A. (2001). Vitamin C-induced decomposition of lipid hydroperoxides to endogenous genotoxins. *Science,* 292, 2083– 2086.

Levine, M.; Conry-Cantilena, C.; Wang, Y.; Welch, R. W.; Washko, P. W.; Dhariwal, K. R.; Park, J. B.; Lazarev, A.; Graumlich, J. F.; King, J. and Cantilena, L. R. (1996). Vitamin C pharmacokinetics in healthy volunteers: evidence for a recommended dietary allowance. *Proc. Natl. Acad. Sci. US,* 93(8), 3704-3709.

Levine, M.; Rumsey, S. C.; Daruwala, R.; Park, J. B. and Wang, Y. (1999). Criteria and recommendations for vitamin C intake. *JAMA,* 281(15),1415-1423.

Levine, M.; Wang, Y.; Padayatty, S. J. and Morrow, J. (2001). A new recommended dietary allowance of vitamin C for healthy young women. *Proc. Natl. Acad. Sci. US,* 98, 9842-9846.

Loyd, D. O. and Lynch, S. M. (2011). Lipid-soluble vitamin C palmitate and protection of human high-density lipoprotein from hypochlorite-mediated oxidation. *Int. J. Cardiol.,* 152(2), 256-257.

Lu, H.; Ouyang, W. and Huang, C. (2006). Inflammation, a Key Event in Cancer Development. *Mol. Cancer Res.,* 4, 221-233

Lu, Q.; Bjorkhem, I.; Wretlind, B.; Diczfalusy, U.; Henriksson, P. and Freyschuss, A. (2005). Effect of ascorbic acid on microcirculation in patients with type II diabetes: a randomized placebo-controlled cross-over study. *Clinical Science,* 108(6), 507–513.

Macarthur, M.; Hold, G. L. and El-Omar, E. M. (2004). Inflammation and cancer. II. Role of chronic inflammation and cytokine polymorphisms in the pathogenesis of gastrointestinal malignancy. *Am. J. Physiol. Gastrointest. Liver Physiol.,* 286, 515-520.

Maggini, S.; Wintergerst, E. S.; Beveridge, S. and Hornig, D. H. (2007). Selected vitamins and trace elements support immune function by strengthening epithelial barriers and cellular and humoral immune responses. *British Journal Nutrition,* 98, Suppl. 1, 29-35.

Magnussen, C. G.; Koskinen, J.; Chen, W.; Thomson, R.; Schmidt, M. D.; Srinivasan, S. R.; Kivimäki, M.; Mattsson, N.; Kähönen, M.; Laitinen, T.; Taittonen, L.; Rönnemaa, T.;

Viikari, J. S.; Berenson, G. S.; Juonala, M. and Raitakari, O. T. (2010). Pediatric Metabolic Syndrome Predicts Adulthood Metabolic Syndrome, Subclinical Atherosclerosis and Type 2 Diabetes Mellitus – But Is No Better Than Body Mass Index Alone: The Bogalusa Heart Study and the Cardiovascular Risk in Young Finns Study. *Circulation,* 122(16), 1604-1611.

Mandl, J.; Szarka, A. and Bánhegyi, G. (2009). Vitamin C: update on physiology and pharmacology. *Br. J. Pharmacol.,* 157(7), 1097–1110.

Manson, J. E.; Bassuk, S. S.; Lee, I. M.; Cook, N. R.; Albert, M. A.; Gordon, D.; Zaharris, E.; Macfadyen, J. G.; Danielson, E.; Lin, J.; Zhang, S. M. and Buring, J. E. (2012). The Vitamin D and Omega-3 Trial: Rationale and design of a large randomized controlled trial of vitamin D and marine omega-3 fatty acid supplements for the primary prevention of cancer and cardiovascular disease. *Contemporary Clinical Trials*, 33, Issue 1, January 2012, 159-171.

Mast, J.; Buyse, J. and Goddeeris, B. M. (2000). Dietary L-carnitine supplementation increases antigen-specific immunoglobulin G production in broiler chickens. *British Journal Nutrition*, 83, 161-166.

May, J. M. and Harrison, F. E. (2013). Role of Vitamin C in the Function of the Vascular Endothelium. *Antioxidant Redox Signal.* (epub ahead of print)

McMillan, D. C. (2009). Systemic inflammation, nutritional status and survival in patients with cancer. *Curr. Opin. Clin. Nutr. Metab. Care*, 12, 223-226.

Merz, C. N. (2012). Differing Relations to Early Atherosclerosis between Vitamin C from Supplements vs. Food in the Los Angeles Atherosclerosis Study: A Prospective Cohort Study. *Open Cardiovasc. Med. J.*, 6, 113-21.

Micallef, J.; Attarian, S.; Dubourg, O.; Gonnaud, P. M.; Hogrel, J. Y.; Stojkovic, T.; Bernard, R.; Jouve, E.; Pitel, S.; Remec, J. F.; Jomir, L.; Azabou, E.; Al-Moussawi, M.; Lefebvre, M. N.; Attolini, L.; Yaici, S.; Tanesse, D.; Fontes, M.; Pouget, J. and Blin, O. (2009). Effect of ascorbic acid in patients with Charcot-Marie-Tooth disease type 1A: a multicentre, randomised, double-blind, placebo-controlled trial. *Lancet Neurol.*, 8(12), 1103–1110

Mikirova, N. A.; Casciari, J. J. and Riordan, N. H. (2010). Ascorbate inhibition of angiogenesis in aortic rings ex vivo and subcutaneous Matrigel plugs in vivo. *Journal of Angiogenesis Research*, 2, 2.

Mikirova, N. A.; Ichim, T. E. and Riordan, N. H. (2008). Anti-angiogenic effect of high doses of ascorbic acid. *J. Transl. Med.*, 6, 50.

Mikirova, N.; Casciari, J.; Rogers, A. and Taylor, P. (2012). Effect of high-dose intravenous vitamin C on inflammation in cancer patients. *Journal of Translational Medicine*, 10, 189.

Mizrahi, A.; Berdichevsky, Y.; Ugolev, Y.; Molshanski-Mor, S.; Nakash, Y.; Dahan, I.; Alloul, N.; Gorzalczany, Y.; Sarfstein, R.; Hirshberg, M. and Pick, E. (2006). Assembly of the phagocyte NADPH oxidase complex: chimeric constructs derived from the cytosolic components as tools for exploring structure-function relationships. *J. Leukoc. Biol.*, 79, 881-895.

Moore, M. M.; Chua, W.; Charles, K. A. and Clarke, S. J. (2010). Inflammation and cancer: causes and consequences. *Clinical Pharmacology and Therapeutics - Nature,* 87, 504-508.

Murphy, R. and De Coursey, T. E. (2006). Charge compensation during the phagocyte respiratory burst. *Biochim. Biophys. Acta.*, 1757, 996-1011.

Nagy, G.; Koncz, A.; Fernandez, D. and Perl, A. (2007). Nitric oxide, mitochondrial hyperpolarization and T cell activation. *Free Radical Biollogy Medicine,* 42(11), 1625-31.

Nagy, G.; Clark, J. M.; Buzás, E. I.; Gorman, C. L. and Cope, A. P. (2007). Nitric oxide, chronic inflammation and autoimmunity. *Immunology Letters,* 111(1), 1-5.

Nagy, G.; Clark, J. M.; Buzas, E.; Gorman, C.; Pasztoi, M.; Koncz, A.; Falus, A. and Cope, A. P. (2008). Nitric oxide production of T lymphocytes is increased in rheumatoid arthritis. *Immunology Letters,* 118(1), 55-58.

Nakai, K.; Urushihara, M.; Kubota, Y. and Kosaka, H. (2003). Ascorbate enhances iNOS activity by increasing tetrahydrobiopterin in RAW 264.7 cells. *Free Radic. Biol. Med.,* 35(8), 929-937.

Nambiar, M. P.; Fisher, C. U.; Enyedy, E. J.; Warke, V. G., Kumar, A. and Tsokos, G. C. (2002). Oxidative stress is involved in the heat stress-induced downregulation of TCR zeta chain expression and TCR/CD3-mediated [Ca(2+)](i) response in human T-lymphocytes. *Cell Immunol.,* 215, 151-161.

Nankivell, B. J. and Murali, K. M. (2008). Images in clinical medicine. Renal failure from vitamin C after transplantation. *N Engl. J. Med.,* 358(4), 4.

Oberley, L. W. (2001). Anticancer therapy by overexpression of superoxide dismutase. *Antioxid. Redox Signal.,* 3(3), 461-472.

Oeckinghaus, A.; Hayden, M. S. and Ghosh, S. (2011). Crosstalk in NF-κB signaling pathways. *Nat. Immunol.,* 12(8), 695-708.

Orbe, J.; Rodriguez, J. A.; Arias, R.; Belzunce, M.; Nespereira, B.; Perez-Ilzarbe, M.; Roncal, C. and Páramo, J. A. (2003). Antioxidant vitamins increase the collagen content and reduce MMP-1 in a porcine model of atherosclerosis: implications for plaque stabilization. *Atherosclerosis*, 167, 45–53.

Oreopoulos, D. G.; Lindeman, R. D.; Vanderlagt, D. J.; Tzamaloukas, A. H.; Bhagavan, H. N. and Garry, J. P. (1993). Renal excretion of ascorbic acid: Effect of age and sex. *J. Am. Coll. Nutr.,* 12, 537-542.

Padayatty, S. J. and Levine, M. (2001). New insights into the physiology and pharmacology of vitamin C. *CMAJ.,* 164(3), 353–355.

Padayatty, S. J.; Katz, A.; Wang, Y.; Eck, P.; Kwon, O.; Lee, J. H.; Chen, S.; Corpe, C.; Dutta, A.; Dutta, S. K. and Levine, M. (2003). Vitamin C as an antioxidant: evaluation of its role in disease prevention. *J. Am. Coll. Nutr.,* 22(1), 18-35.

Padayatty, S. J.; Sun, H.; Wang, Y.; Riordan, H. D.; Hewitt, S. M.; Katz, A.; Wesley, R. A. and Levine, M. (2004). Vitamin C Pharmacokinetics: Implications for Oral and Intravenous Use. *Annals of Internal Medicine*, 140, 533-537.

Paolisso, G.; Balbi, V.; Volpe, C.; Varricchio, G.; Gambardella, A.; Saccomanno, F.; Ammendola, S.; Varricchio, M. and D'Onofrio, F. (1995). Metabolic benefits deriving from chronic vitamin C supplementation in aged non-insulin dependent diabetics. *J. Am. Coll. Nutr.,* 14(4), 387–392.

Patel, K. B.; Stratford, M. R.; Wardman, P. and Everett, S. A. (2002). Oxidation of tetrahydrobiopterin by biological radicals and scavenging of the trihydrobiopterin radical by ascorbate. *Free Radicals Biology Medicine*, 32, 203-211.

Podmore, I. D.; Griffiths, H. R.; Herbert, K. E.; Mistry, N.; Mistry, P. and Lunec, J. (1998). Vitamin C exhibits prooxidant properties. *Nature*, 392(6676), 559.

Ramsay, R. R.; Gandour, R. D. and van der Leij, F. (2001). Molecular enzymology of carnitine transfer and transport. *Biochimica et Biophysica Acta,* 1546, 21-43.

Rebouche, C. J. (1991). Ascorbic acid and carnitine biosynthesis. *Am. J. Clin. Nutr.*, 54, 1147-1152.

Recchioni, R.; Marcheselli, F.; Moroni, F. and Pieri, C. (2002). Apoptosis in human aortic endothelial cells induced by hyperglycemic condition involves mitochondrial depolarization and is prevented by *N*-acetyl-L-cysteine. *Metabolism: Clinical and Experimental*, 51, 1384–1388.

Riordan, H. D.; Casciari, J. J.; González, M. J.; Riordan, N. H.; Miranda-Massari, J. R.; Taylor, P. and Jackson, J. A. (2005). A pilot clinical study of continuous intravenous ascorbate in terminal cancer patients. *P R Health Sci. J.*, 24(4), 269-276.

Rössig, L.; Hoffmann, J.; Hugel, B.; Mallat, Z.; Haase, A.; Freyssinet, J. M.; Tedgui, A.; Aicher, A.; Zeiher, A. M. and Dimmeler, S. (2001). Vitamin C inhibits endothelial cell apoptosis in congestive heart failure. *Circulation*, 104, 2182–2187.

Roxburgh, C. S. and McMillan, D. C. (2010). Role of systemic inflammatory response in predicting survival in patients with primary operable cancer. *Future Oncol.*, 6, 149-163.

Rumsey, S. C. and Levine, M. (1998). Absorption, transport and disposition of ascorbic acid in humans. *The Journal of Nutritional Biochemistry,* 9(3), 116-130.

Saeed, R. W.; Peng, T. and Metz, C. N. (2003). Ascorbic acid blocks the growth inhibitory effect of tumor necrosis factor-alpha on endothelial cells. *Exp. Biol. Med. (Maywood)*, 228, 855–865.

Savini, I.; Rossi, A.; Pierro, C.; Avigliano, L. and Catani, M. V. (2008). SVCT1 and SVCT2: key proteins for vitamin C uptake. *Amino Acids*, 34(3), 347-355.

Schmidt, T. S. and Alp, N. J. (2007). Mechanisms for the role of tetrahydrobiopterin in endothelial function and vascular disease. *Clinical Science,* 113, 47-63.

Scientific Panel on Dietetic Products, Nutrition and Allergies. (2004). Opinion of the Scientific Panel on Dietetic Products, Nutrition and Allergies related to the tolerable upper intake level of vitamin C (l-ascorbic acid, its calcium, potassium and sodium salts and l-ascorbyl-6-palmitate). *Eur. Food Safety Authority J.*, 59, 1–21.

Siddiq, A.; Aminova, L. R. and Ratan, R. R. (2008). Prolyl 4-hydroxylase activity-responsive transription factors: from hydroxylation to gene expression and neuroprotection. *Front. Biosci.*, 13, 2875- 2887.

Siener, R. and Hesse, A. (2002). The effect of different diets on urine composition and the risk of calcium oxalate crystallisation in healthy subjects. *Eur. Urol.*, 42(3), 289-96.

Sotiriou, S.; Gispert, S.; Cheng, J.; Wang, Y. H.; Chen, A.; Hoogstraten-Miller, S.; Miller, G. F.; Kwon, O.; Levine, M.; Guttentag, S. H. and Nussbaum, R. L. (2002). Ascorbic-acid transporter Slc23a1 is essential for vitamin C transport into the brain and for perinatal survival. *Nature Medicine*, 8, 514–517

Stein, H. B.; Hasan, A. and Fox, I. H. (1976). Ascorbic acid-induced uricosuria. *Ann. Intern. Med.,* 84, 385–8.

Stephenson, C. M.; Levin, R. D.; Spector, T. and Lis, C. G. (2013). Phase I clinical trial to evaluate the safety, tolerability and pharmacokinetics of high-dose intravenous ascorbic acid in patients with advanced cancer. *Cancer Chemother. Pharmacol.* Epub. ahead of print.

Stocker, R. and Keaney, J. F. Jr. (2004). Role of oxidative modifications in atherosclerosis. *Physiol. Rev.*, 84, 1381–1478

Stone, I. (1972). *The Healing Factor. Vitamin C Against Disease.* 1 ed. Putnam Publishing Group, New York, US.

Stone, J. R. and Yang, S. (2006). Hydrogen peroxide: a signaling messenger. *Antioxid. Redox. Signal*, 8, 243–70.

Sumimoto, H.; Miyano, K. and Takeya, R. (2005). Molecular composition and regulation of the Nox family NAD(P)H oxidases. *Biochem. Biophys. Res. Commun.*, 338, 677-686.

Tomoda, H.; Yoshitake, M.; Morimoto, K. and Aoki, N. (1996). Possible prevention of postangioplasty restenosis by ascorbic acid. *American Journal of Cardiology*, 78, 1284–1286.

Tousoulis, D.; Antoniades, C. and Vasiliadou, C. (2007). Effects of atorvastatin and vitamin C on forearm hyperaemic blood flow, asymmentrical dimethylarginine levels and the inflammatory process in patients with type 2 diabetes mellitus. *Heart,* 93(2), 244-246.

Ulrich, C. M.; Bigler, J. and Potter, J. D. (2006). Non-steroidal anti-inflammatory drugs for cancer prevention: promise, perils and pharmacogenetics. *Nat. Rev. Cancer*, 6, 130-140.

Ulrich-Merzenich, G.; Metzner, C.; Schiermeyer, B. and Vetter, H. (2004). Vitamin C and vitamin E antagonistically modulate human vascular endothelial and smooth muscle cell DNA synthesis and proliferation. *Eur. J. Nutr.*, 41, 27–34.

Valko, M.; Leibfritz, D.; Moncol, J.; Cronin, M. T.; Mazur, M. and Telser, J. (2007). Free radicals and antioxidants in normal physiological functions and human disease. *Int. J. Biochem. Cell Biol.,* 39(1), 44-84.

Van Den Biggelaar, A. H.; De Craen, A. J.; Gussekloo, J.; Huizinga, T. W.; Heijmans, B. T.; Frölich, M.; Kirkwood, T. B. and Westendorp, R. G. (2004). Inflammation underlying cardiovascular mortality is a late consequence of evolutionary programming. *FASEB J.,* 18, 1022-1024.

Verrax, J. and Calderon, P. B. (2008). The controversial place of vitamin C in cancer treatment. *Biochemical Pharmacology*, 76, 1644-1652.

Vissers, M. C. and Hampton, M. B. (2004). The role of oxidants and vitamin C on neutrophil apoptosis and clearance. *Biochem. Soc. Trans.,* 32, 499-501.

Vissers, M. C. and Wilkie, R. P. (2007). Ascorbate deficiency results in impaired neutrophil apoptosis and clearance and is associated with up-regulation of hypoxia-inducible factor 1alpha; *J. Leukoc. Biol.,* 81(5), 1236-1244.

Vollbracht, C.; Schneider, B.; Leendert, V.; Weiss, G.; Auerbach, L. and Beuth, J. (2011). Intravenous vitamin C administration improves quality of life in breast cancer patients during chemo-/radiotherapy and aftercare: results of a retrospective, multicentre, epidemiological cohort study in Germany. *In Vivo*, 25, 983-990.

Wan, F. and Lenardo, M. J. (2010). The nuclear signaling of NF-kappaB: current knowledge, new insights and future perspectives. *Cell Rearch,* 20(1), 24-33.

Wanden-Berghe, C. and Martín-Rodero, H. (2012). 25 Years in nutrition and food research in the Iberoamerican knowledge area. *Nutr. Hosp.*, 27 Suppl. 2, 26-33.

Wang, H.; Zhang, Z. B.; Wen, R. R. and Chen, J. W. (1995). Experimental and clinical studies on the reduction of erythrocyte sorbitol-glucose ratios by ascorbic acid in diabetes mellitus. *Diabetes Research Clinical Practice,* 28(1),1–8.

Wannamethee, S. G.; Lowe, G. D.; Rumley, A.; Bruckdorfer, K. R. and Whincup, P. H. (2006). Associations of vitamin C status, fruit and vegetable intakes and markers of inflammation and hemostasis. *American Journal Clinical Nutrition,* 83(3), 567–574.

Watanabe, T.; Pakala, R.; Katagiri, T. and Benedict, C. R. (2001). Lipid peroxidation product 4-hydroxy-2-nonenal acts synergistically with serotonin in inducing vascular smooth muscle cell proliferation. *Atherosclerosis*, 155, 37–44.

Webb, A. L. and Villamor, E. (2007). Update: effects of antioxidant and nonantioxidant vitamin supplementation on immune function. *Nutr. Rev.*, 65, 181-217.

White, L. A.; Freeman, C. Y.; Forrester, B. D. and Chappell, W. A. (1986). *In vitro* effect of ascorbic acid on infectivity of herpesviruses and paramyxoviruses. *J. Clin. Microbiol.*, 24, 527-531.

Wild, S.; Roglic, G.; Green, A.; Sicree, R. and King, H. (2004). Global prevalence of diabetes: estimates for the year 2000 and projection for 2030. *Diabetes Care,* 27(5), 1047–1053.

Wilson, J. X. (2005). Regulation of vitamin C transport. *Annu. Rev. Nutr.,* 25, 105-125.

Wintergerst, E. S.; Maggini, S. and Hornig, D. H. (2006). Immune-Enhancing Role of Vitamin C and Zinc and Effect on Clinical Conditions. *Ann. Nutr. Metab.,* 50, 85–94.

Wu, G. and Meininger, C. J. (2002). Regulation of nitric oxide synthesis by dietary factors. *Annual Review Nutrition,* 22, 61-86.

Young, I. S.; Tate, S.; Lightbody, J. H.; McMaster, D. and Trimble, E. R. (1995). The effects of desferrioxamine and ascorbate on oxidative stress in the streptozotocin diabetic rat. *Free Radical Biology Medicine,* 18(5), 833–840.

Zempleni, J.; Rucker, R. B.; McCormick, D. B. and Suttie, J. W. (2006). *Handbook of Vitamins.* 4th ed. CRC Press, Boca Raton, FL, US, 489–520.

Zhang, L.; Conejo-Garcia, J. R.; Katsaros, D.; Gimotty, P.A.; Massobrio, M.; Regnani, G.; Makrigiannakis, A.; Gray, H.; Schlienger, K.; Liebman, M. N.; Rubin, S. C. and Coukos, G. (2003). Intratumoral T cells, recurrence and survival in epithelial ovarian cancer. *N Engl. J. Med.*, 348(3), 203-13.

Zhou, Q., Mrowietz, U. and Rostami-Yazdi, M. (2009). Oxidative stress in the pathogenesis of psoriasis. *Free Radic. Biol. Med.,* 47(7), 891-905.

In: Vitamin C
Editor: Raquel Guiné

ISBN: 978-1-62948-154-8
© 2013 Nova Science Publishers, Inc.

Chapter 7

VITAMIN C DEFICIENCY ENHANCES DISRUPTION OF ADRENAL NON-ENZYMATIC ANTIOXIDANT DEFENSE SYSTEMS IN ODS RATS WITH WATER-IMMERSION RESTRAINT STRESS

Yoshiji Ohta[*] and Koji Yashiro[†]

Department of Chemistry, Fujita Health University
School of Medicine, Toyoake, Japan

ABSTRACT

In the present study, we examined whether and how vitamin C (VC) deficiency affects water-immersion restraint stress (WIRS)-induced disruption of adrenal non-enzymatic antioxidant defense systems in Osteogenic Disorder Shionogi (ODS) rats genetically unable to synthesize VC. Five-week-old male ODS rats received scorbutic diet with either distilled water containing VC (1 g/L) or distilled water not containing VC for 2 weeks, VC-deficient ODS rats (VC-D group) and VC-sufficient ODS rats (VC-S group) were exposed to WIRS for 1, 3 or 6 h. Before the onset of WIRS, serum VC concentration in the VC-D group was 31% of that concentration found in the VC-S group and serum lipid peroxide (LPO) concentration was higher in the VC-D group than in the VC-S group. The VC-D group had higher serum corticosterone (CORT), and glucose concentrations and higher adrenal CORT content than the VC-S group. The VC-D group had 21% of adrenal VC concentration in the VC-S group but there were no differences in adrenal LPO, vitamin E (VE), and reduced glutathione (GSH) concentrations between the two groups. When the VC-S group was exposed to WIRS, serum VC, CORT, and glucose concentrations increased in a stress time-dependent correlation, and serum LPO concentration started increasing after 3 h of WIRS and further increased thereafter. Regarding these serum concentrations in the VC-D group with WIRS, VC concentration further decreased at 6 h of the stress and decreases in increased CORT and glucose concentrations and further increase in increased LPO concentration occurred in a stress time-dependent manner.

[*] Yoshiji Ohta: E-mail: yohta@fujita-hu.ac.jp.
[†] Koji Yashiro: E-mail: yashiro@fujita-hu.ac.jp.

Moving forward to the variations in the adrenal gland in the VC-S group after being exposed to WIRS, it was observed that a decrease in VC concentration and an increase in CORT concentration occurred in a stress time-dependent manner, a decrease in GSH concentration and an increase in LPO concentration occurred after 6 h, and VE concentration increased after 1 h. The VC-D group with WIRS showed further reduction in adrenal VC concentration, decreases in adrenal CORT and GSH concentrations, and an increase in adrenal LPO concentration. These changes depended on stress time. The adrenal VE concentration increased at 1 h of WIRS but decreased stress time-dependently thereafter. After exposure to 6 h of WIRS, the VC-D group had higher serum and adrenal LPO concentrations and lower serum and adrenal VC and adrenal GSH concentrations than the VC-S group. These results indicate that VC deficiency enhances WIRS-induced disruption of adrenal non-enzymatic antioxidant defense systems in ODS rats.

1. INTRODUCTION

The adrenal gland is among the organs with higher concentration of vitamin C (VC) (or ascorbic acid) in the body. Both the adrenal cortex and the adrenal medulla accumulate such high levels of VC. VC present in the adrenal gland works as an important cofactor at its physiological functions (Patak et al., 2004). When compared with rat's main organs, including adrenal gland, brain, heart, kidney, liver, lung, skeletal muscle, spleen, and testis, the adrenal gland contains the highest concentrations of non-enzymatic antioxidants such as vitamin E (VE), reduced glutathione (GSH), and VC, which is the most abundant, non-enzymatic antioxidant present in rat's adrenal gland (Azhar et al., 1995). Comparatively, the content of lipid peroxide (LPO), which is generated via reactive oxygen species, in the adrenal gland of rats is the lowest among the main nine organs (Azhar et al., 1995).

VC is a water-soluble antioxidant and scavenges reactive oxygen species such as superoxide anion radical, hydroxyl radical, and peroxyl radical by itself (Rose and Bode, 1993). VC also supports the chain-breaking antioxidant action of VE by recycling VE radical to VE in the liquid/aqueous interface (Liebler, 1993). Oxidized VC (or dehydroascorbic acid) is returned to VC via reduced glutathione (GSH) itself in a non-enzymatic manner or via the enzymatic VC recycling system in which GSH participates as a cofactor (Winkler et al., 1994). Thus, VC exerts its antioxidant action by interacting with VE and GSH as well as by itself.

Water-immersion restraint stress (WIRS) is a test designed to induce emotional stress in the subject submitted to it, being considered a panoply of physical and psychological stressors. WIRS-induced gastric mucosal damage in experimental animals is widely used as a stress-induced gastric ulcer model (Jaggi et al., 2011). It has been shown in rats exposed to WIRS over a 6-h period that VC concentration decreases with a concomitant increase in LPO concentration and followed by a decrease in VE concentration in the gastric mucosa, although the concentration of non-protein sulfhydryl including GSH begins to decrease before the onset of decrease in VC concentration in the tissue (Ohta et al., 2005). It has also been shown that a decrease in VC concentration occurs with a concomitant decrease in GSH concentration and a concomitant increase in LPO concentration in rat's liver when exposed to WIRS over a 6-h period; however, VE concentration remains stable in the tissue (Ohta et al., 2007). It has also been reported that decreases in VC and GSH concentrations occur with a concomitant increase in LPO concentration followed by a decrease in VE concentration in the brain of rats exposed to WIRS over a 6-h period (Ohta et al., 2012). Furthermore, it has been reported that when rats with WIRS receive a single oral VC pre-administration, WIRS-induced disruption of non-enzymatic antioxidant defense systems in the gastric mucosa, liver, and brain is attenuated with the recovery of decreased VC content in those tissues (Kaida et al., 2010; Ohta et al., 2005, 2010, 2012). Thus, it has been suggested that VC plays an important role in WIRS-induced disruption of non-enzymatic antioxidant defense systems in the gastric mucosa, liver, and brain of rats.

In experimental animals with acute emotional stress, the stress response occurs mainly via the hypothalamic-pituitary-adrenal (HPA) axis and the sympathetic-adrenal system (Pignatelli et al., 1998). The HPA axis is a complex set of direct influences and feedback interactions among the hypothalamus, the pituitary gland, and the adrenal gland. Secretion of corticotropin-releasing hormone, adrenocorticotropic hormone (ACTH), and corticosteroids such as cortisol and corticsterone (CORT) via the HPA axis occurs in response to stress. The sympathetic-adrenal system is one of the major pathways mediating physiological responses and plays an important role in the regulation of blood pressure, glucose, sodium, and other key physiological and metabolic processes. Secretion of adrenaline and noradrenaline via the sympathetic-adrenal system occurs in response to stress. It has been reported that, in rats exposed to WIRS for a 6-h period, rapid increases in plasma adrenaline, noradrenaline, and glucose levels occur through activation of the sympathetic-adrenal system (Arakawa et al., 1997). It has also been reported that a single exposure of rats to WIRS for a 6-h period causes rapid increases in serum ACTH and CORT levels through activation of the HPA axis and serum glucose level through activation of the sympathetic-adrenal system (Ohta et al., 2012, 2013). It is known that a single treatment with ACTH causes a rapid reduction of VC level in the adrenal gland of rats (Lahiri and Lloyd, 1962; Overbeek, 1985). It is also known that ACTH inhibits the uptake of VC into isolated rat adrenal glands or isolated rat adrenocortical cells (Clayman et al., 1970; Leonard et al., 1983). In addition, it has been reported that human adrenal glands secrete VC in response to ACTH (Padayvatty et al., 2007). It has been shown that a single subcutaneous treatment of rats with sympathomimetic amines such as adrenaline and noradrenaline causes VC depletion in the adrenal gland (Nasmyth, 1949). Thus, it is implicated that VC depletion in the adrenal gland of stressed rats is closely associated with activation of the HPA system and the sympathetic-adrenal system. It has been reported that a single exposure of rats to immobilization (or restraint) stress over 4-h period causes a marked decrease in adrenal VC content with a concomitant increase in serum VC concentration (Nakano and Suzuki, 1984). Our recent report has shown that, in the adrenal gland of rats exposed to WIRS over a 6-h period, rapid VC depletion occurs at 0.5 h and further VC depletion continues followed by a decrease in GSH concentration and an increase in LPO concentration thereafter, although transient increases in GSH and VE concentrations occur at 1.5 h and that VC pre-administered to rats with 6 h of WIRS attenuates WIRS-induced disruption of adrenal non-enzymatic antioxidant defense systems with the recovery of decreased adrenal VC concentration (Ohta et al., 2013). Thus, it has been suggested that VC plays a critical role in WIRS-induced disruption of non-enzymatic antioxidant defense systems in the adrenal gland of rats.

The strain of Osteogenic Disorder Shionogi/Shi-od/od (ODS) rats is a colony of mutant Wistar rats defective in the ability to synthesize VC due to the loss of the gene that encodes for L-gulonolactone oxidase, an enzyme working at the final step of VC synthesis, in the liver tissue (Mizushima et al., 1984).

It is known that exposure of ODS rats to VC deficiency for more than 10 days causes a severe VC depletion in the plasma and tissues including adrenal gland and stomach (Tokumaru et al., 1998). Our previous study has shown that VC deficiency aggravates tissue damage by enhancing oxidative stress associated with disrupted non-enzymatic antioxidant defense systems in the gastric mucosa of ODS rats with WIRS (Ohta et al., 2006).

In the present study, therefore, we examined whether and how VC deficiency affects WIRS-induced disruption of non-enzymatic antioxidant defense systems in the adrenal gland of ODS rats unable to synthesize VC in order to further clarify the role of VC in WIRS-induced disruption of non-enzymatic antioxidant defense systems in the adrenal gland of rats.

2. MATERIALS AND METHODS

2.1. Materials

L-Ascorbic acid (VC), CORT, α,α'-dipyridyl, 5,5'-dithiobis(2-nitrobenzoic acid) (Ellman's reagent), ethylenediaminetetraacetic acid (EDTA), GSH, 2-thiobarbituric acid (TBA), tocopherol (Toc) standards (α-Toc and δ-Toc), and other chemicals were purchased from Wako Pure Chemical Ind., Ltd. (Osaka, Japan). All chemicals used were of reagent grade and were not further purified.

2.2. Animals

Male ODS rats aged five weeks were purchased from Nippon Clear Co. (Tokyo, Japan). The animals were housed in cages in a ventilated animal room with controlled temperature ($23 \pm 2°C$) and relative humidity ($55 \pm 5\%$) with 12 h of light (7:00 to 19:00). The animals were maintained with free access to rat chow, CL-1 (Nippon Clear Co., Tokyo, Japan) and distilled water with and without VC (1g/L) *ad libitum* for two weeks to make VC-sufficient and VC-deficient status, respectively, accordingly to the report of Tokumaru et al. (1996). VC-deficient ODS rats showed no clear signs of scurvy.

All animals received humane care in compliance with the Guidelines of the Management of Laboratory Animals in Fujita Health University. The animal experiment was approved by the Institutional Animal Care and Use Committee and its approved protocol number was M 14-02.

2.3. Induction of WIRS

It is known that WIRS causes a reliable severe stress in conscious rats under 24-h starvation, resulting in the reproducible occurrence of gastric mucosal damage (Landeria-Femandez, 2004). Therefore, all seven-week-old ODS rats used were starved for 24 h before the onset of WIRS but were allowed free access to water, The conscious starved ODS rats were restrained in wire cages and immersed up to the depth of the xiphoid process in a 23°C water bath to induce WIRS, as described in our previous reports (Kaida et al., 2010; Ohta et al., 2005, 2006, 2007, 2012, 2013). Exposure of VC-deficient and sufficient ODS rats to WIRS was started at 9:00 am and was lasted for 1, 3 or 6 h.

2.4. Assays of Adrenal and Serum Components

ODS rats were weighed and then sacrificed under ether anesthesia at 0, 1, 3 or 6 h after the onset of WIRS and blood samples were collected from the inferior vena cava. Immediately after sacrifice, adrenal glands were isolated, washed in ice-cold 0.9% NaCl, wiped on a filter paper, and then weighed. The collected blood was separated into serum by centrifugation. The collected adrenal glands and serum were stored at -80°C until use. Each adrenal gland was homogenized in 9 volumes of ice-cold 50 mM Tris-HCl buffer (pH 7.4) containing 1 mM EDTA to prepare 10% homogenate using a Physcotron handy microhomogenizer (Microtec Co., Funabashi, Japan). The adrenal homogenate was used for the assays of CORT VC, VE, GSH, and LPO. The serum was used for the assays of CORT, glucose, VC, VE, and LPO. CORT in the serum and adrenal homogenate was fluorometrically assayed by the method described by Guillemin et al. (1959) using authentic CORT as a standard. Serum glucose was assayed using a kit of Glucose CII-Test Wako (Wako Pure Chemical Ind., Ltd., Osaka, Japan). Serum LPO was assayed by the fluorometric TBA method of Yagi (1976) using tetramethoxypropane as a standard. The α,α'-dipyridyl method described by Zannoni et al. (1974) was used to determine serum and adrenal VC concentrations using authentic L-ascorbic acid as a standard. GSH in the adrenal homogenate was assayed by the method of Sedlak and Lindsay (1968) using Ellman's reagent and GSH as a standard. VE in the serum and adrenal homogenate was assayed by the method using high-performance liquid chromatography and electrochemical detection and δ-Toc was used as an internal standard as described in our previous report (Kamiya et al., 2005). The amount of VE in the serum and adrenal homogenate is expressed as that of α-Toc. LPO in the adrenal homogenate was assayed by the colorimetric TBA method of Ohkawa et al. (1979) using tetramethoxypropane as a standard except that 1 mM EDTA was added to the reaction mixture. The amount of LPO in the serum and adrenal homogenate is expressed as that of malondialdehyde (MDA) equivalents.

2.5. Statistical Analysis

All results obtained are expressed as means ± standard deviation (S.D.). The statistical analyses of the results were performed using a computerized statistical package (StatView). Each mean value was compared by one-way analysis of variance (ANOVA) and Bonferroni for multiple comparisons. The significance level was set at $p < 0.05$.

3. RESULTS

VC-deficient ODS rats (VC-D group) had significantly higher serum CORT and glucose concentrations than VC-sufficient ODS rats (VC-S group) before the onset of WIRS (Figure

7.1). When the VC-D group was exposed to WIRS for 1, 3 or 6 h, increased serum CORT concentrations in the VC-D group decreased stress time-dependently ((Figure 7.1A). In the VC-S group with the same period of WIRS, serum CORT and glucose concentrations increased stress time-dependently (Figure 7.1B). At 6 h of WIRS, there was no significant difference in serum CORT concentration between the VC-D and VC-S groups and the serum glucose concentration was 1.6-fold higher in the VC-S group than in the VC-D group (Figure 7.1A and B).

Before the onset of stress, body weight was significantly less in the VC-D group (121.3 ± 5.4 g, n = 32) than in VC-S group (154.1 ± 1.9 g, n = 20) ($p < 0.05$). Exposure to WIRS for 1, 3 or 6 h had no significant effect on the body weight in the VC-D and VC-S groups (data not shown).

There was no significant difference in adrenal weight between the VC-D and VC-S groups, while adrenal CORT concentration was significantly higher in the VC-D group than in the VC-S group (Figure 7.1C and D).

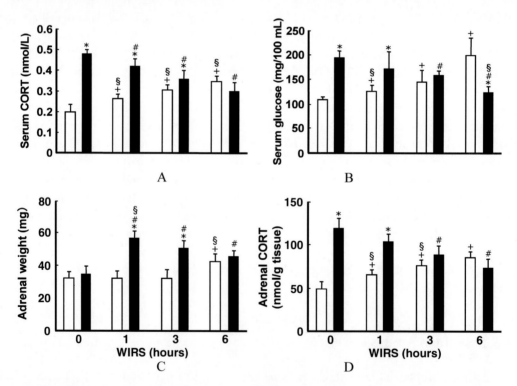

Figure 7.1. Stress time-related changes in serum CORT (A) and glucose (B) concentrations, adrenal weight (C) and adrenal CORT content (D) in VC-deficient and sufficient ODS rats with WIRS. Open bar, VC-sufficient ODS rats; closed bar, VC-deficient ODS rats. The weight of adrenal gland is expressed as the weight of the sum of both adrenal glands. Each value is a mean ± S.D. (n = 5 for each group at 0 h of WIRS; n = 7 for each group at 1, 3 or 6 h of WIRS). $^*p < 0.05$ (vs. the corresponding unstressed group); $^#p < 0.05$ (vs. the unstressed VC-deficient group) ; $^+p < 0.05$ (vs. the unstressed VC-sufficient group); $^§p < 0.05$ (vs. the value at the previous time point in the corresponding group).

The adrenal weight in the VC-D group exposed to 1 h of WIRS was significantly heavier than that found before the onset of stress and a reduction of the increased adrenal weight was observed until 6 h, while the adrenal weight in the VC-S group exposed to WIRS for 6 h of

WIRS was significantly heavier than that weight found before the onset of stress (Figure 7.1C). The increased adrenal CORT concentration in the VC-D group was significantly reduced by exposure to WIRS for 3 or 6 h and this reduction occurred in a stress time-dependent manner, while the adrenal CORT concentration in the VC-S group exposed to WIRS over a 6-h period increased significantly in a stress time-dependent manner (Figure 7.1D). After 6 h of WIRS, there were no significant differences in adrenal weight and adrenal CORT concentration between the two groups (Figure 7.1C and D).

Before the onset of stress, serum VC concentration in the VC-D group was 31% of that concentration in the VC-S group and serum VE concentration in the VC-D group was 78% of that concentration in the VC-S group (Figure 7.2). The decreased serum VC concentration in the VC-D group remained unchanged at 1 and 3 h of WIRS but further decreased significantly at 6 h, while the serum VC concentration in the VC-S group exposed to WIRS over a 6-h period increased in a stress time-dependent manner and this increase was statistically significant at 3 and 6 h (Figure 7.2A).

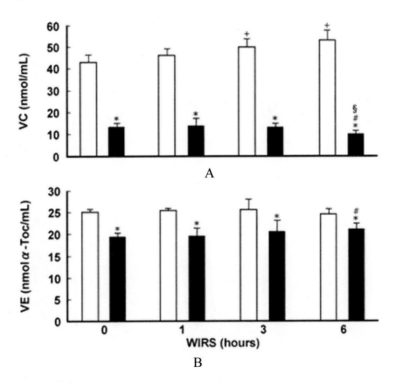

Figure 7.2. Stress time-related changes in serum VC (A) and VE (B) concentrations in VC-deficient and sufficient ODS rats with WIRS. Open bar, VC-sufficient ODS rats; closed bar, VC-deficient ODS rats with WIRS. Each value is a mean ± S.D. (n = 5 for each group at 0 h of WIRS; n = 7 for each group at 1, 3 or 6 h of WIRS). *p < 0.05 (vs. the corresponding unstressed group); #p < 0.05 (vs. the unstressed VC-deficient group) ; +p < 0.05 (vs. the unstressed VC-sufficient group); §p < 0.05 (vs. the value at the previous time point in the corresponding group).

When the VC-D group was exposed to WIRS, a gradual increase in the decreased serum VE concentration occurred in a stress time-dependent manner, being statistically significant after 6 h of WIRS, while exposure of the VC-S group to the same period of WIRS had no significant effect on the serum VE concentration (Figure 7.2B).

Before the onset of stress, serum LPO concentration was significantly higher in the VC-D group than in the VC-S group, while there was no significant difference in adrenal LPO content between the two groups (Figure 7.3). When the VC-D group was exposed to WIRS over a 6-h period, the increased serum LPO concentration further increased and the concentration found at 6 h of WIRS was 1.3-fold higher than that found before the onset of stress (Figure 7.3A). The serum LPO concentration in the VC-S group exposed to WIRS for the same period increased significantly at 6 h, although the serum LPO concentration in the VC-S group was significantly less than that in the VC-D group at 6 h of WIRS; the VC-S group had 87% of serum LPO concentration in the VC-D group at 6 h of WIRS (Figure 7.3A). The VC-D group exposed to WIRS over a 6-h period had a significant increase in adrenal LPO concentration in a stress time-dependent manner and the adrenal LPO concentration in the VC-D group with 6 h of WIRS was 3.2-fold higher than that concentration found before the onset of stress (Figure 7.3B).

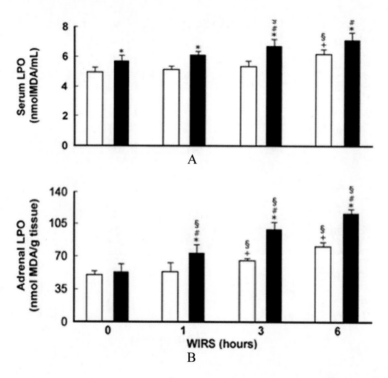

Figure 7.3. Stress time-related changes in LPO concentrations in the serum (A) and adrenal gland (B) of VC-deficient and sufficient ODS rats with WIRS. Open bar, VC-sufficient ODS rats; closed bar, VC-deficient ODS rats with WIRS. Each value is a mean ± S.D. (n = 5 for each group at 0 h of WIRS; n = 7 for each group at 1, 3 or 6 h of WIRS). *p < 0.05 (vs. the corresponding unstressed group); #p < 0.05 (vs. the unstressed VC-deficient group) ; +p < 0.05 (vs. the unstressed VC-sufficient group); §p < 0.05 (vs. the value at the previous time point in the corresponding group).

The VC-group exposed to WIRS for the same period had a gradual increase in adrenal LPO concentration in a stress time-dependent manner and a significant increase in adrenal LPO concentration was found at 3 or 6 h of WIRS, although adrenal LPO concentration in the VC-S group was 70% of that concentration in the VC-D group at 6 h of WIRS (Figure 7.3B)

Before the onset of stress, adrenal VC concentration was significantly less in the VC-D group than in the VC-S group; adrenal VC concentration in the VC-D group was 21% of that concentration in the VC-S group, while there were no differences in adrenal GSH and VE concentrations between the two groups (Figure 7.4).

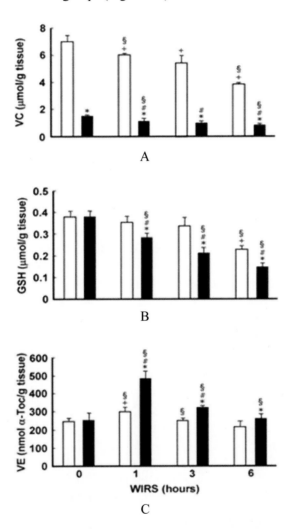

Figure 7.4. Stress time-related changes in adrenal VC (A), GSH (B), and VE (C) concentrations in VC-deficient and sufficient ODS rats with WIRS. Open bar, VC-sufficient ODS rats; closed bar, VC-deficient ODS rats with WIRS. Each value is a mean ± S.D. (n = 5 for each group at 0 h of WIRS; n = 7 for each group at 1, 3 or 6 h of WIRS). $^{*}p < 0.05$ (vs. the corresponding unstressed group); $^{#}p < 0.05$ (vs. the unstressed VC-deficient group) ; $^{+}p < 0.05$ (vs. the unstressed VC-sufficient group); $^{§}p < 0.05$ (vs. the value at the previous time point in the corresponding group).

Exposure of the VC-D group to WIRS over a 6-h period caused further reduction of the decreased adrenal VC concentration in a stress time-dependent manner and exposure of the VC-S group to the same period of WIRS caused a significant reduction of the adrenal VC concentration stress time-dependently (Figure 7.4A). The adrenal VC concentration in the VC-D group was 22% of that concentration in the VC-S group at 6 h of WIRS (Figure 7.4A). Adrenal GSH concentration in the VC-D group was significantly reduced by exposure to

WIRS over a 6-h period and this reduction occurred in a stress time-dependent manner, while a significant reduction of adrenal GSH concentration in the VC-S group exposed to WIRS for the same period occurred at 6 h, although the adrenal GSH concentration in the VC-S group was 1.6-fold higher than that concentration in the VC-D group at 6 h of WIRS (Figure 7.4B). The VC-D group exposed to WIRS over a 6-h period had a significant increase in adrenal VE concentration at 1, 3 or 6 h but the adrenal VE concentration found at 1 h of WIRS decreased stress time-dependently thereafter, while the VC-S group exposed to WIRS for the same period had a significant increase in adrenal VC concentration at 1 h, although the adrenal VE concentration in the VC-S group was significantly less than that concentration in the VC-D group at 1, 3 or 6 h of WIRS and the former group had 62% of adrenal VE concentration in the latter group at 1 h of WIRS (Figure 7.4C).

4. DISCUSSION

It has been shown that when Wistar rats which can synthesize VC in the liver are exposed to WIRS over a 6-h period, rapid increases in serum CORT, glucose, and ACTH concentrations occur and the increased levels are maintained thereafter (Ohta et al., 2012, 2013). Horio et al. (1985) have reported that when ODS rats unable to synthesize VC are fed a VC-deficient diet for 20 days, the serum and adrenal CORT levels are markedly higher than those in ODS rats fed a VC-sufficient diet for the same period. Ikeda et al. (1998) have reported that ODS rats given a VC-deficient diet over a 14-day period have a marked increase in serum CORT concentration and that serum CORT concentration in adrenalectomized ODS rats given a VC-deficient diet for 14 days does not differ from that concentration in adrenalectomized ODS rats and sham ODS rats without adrenalectomy which are given a VC-sufficient diet for the same period. Thus, continuous VC deficiency causes stress-like status in ODS rats. In the present study, serum CORT concentration in ODS rats with 14-day VC deficiency was significantly higher than that in ODS rats with the same period of VC sufficiency.

In addition, the VC-deficient ODS rats were found to have a higher serum glucose concentration than the VC-sufficient ODS rats. These findings suggest that VC deficiency should cause stress responses through activation of both the HPA axis and the sympathetic-adrenal system in ODS rats. When VC-deficient and sufficient ODS rats were exposed to WIRS over a 6-h period, the increased serum CORT and glucose concentrations in VC-deficient ODS rats decreased in a stress time-dependent manner, while those concentrations in VC-sufficient ODS rats increased in a stress time-dependent manner. The stress time-related changes in serum CORT and glucose concentrations in VC-sufficient ODS rats exposed to WIRS over a 6-h period were found to occur more slowly than those in Wistar rats exposed to WIRS for the same period (Ohta et al., 2012, 2013).

Thus, the increased serum CORT and glucose concentrations in VC-deficient ODS rats were found to be reduced by WIRS exposure unlike the case of VC-sufficient ODS rats, although there were no significant differences in serum CORT and glucose concentrations between VC-deficient and sufficient ODS rats after 6 h of WIRS. Hodges and Sadow (1967) have reported that when conscious rats are exposed to restraint stress just after subcutaneous injection of CORT (1 mg/100 g body weigh), the plasma CORT level is reduced with 1 h of lag time at which time the pituitary adrenocorticotropic activity is reduced. Similarly, Ginsberg et al. (2003) have reported that when conscious rats receive a single intraperitoneal (i.p.) administration of RU 28362, a selective glucocorticoid receptor agonist, (1 to 150 μg/kg body weight) at 1 h before the onset of 1-h immobilization stress, the increased plasma CORT level in stressed rats is reduced dose-dependently and corticotrophin-releasing hormone hnRNA expression in the paraventricular nucleus of stressed rats is reduced at a dose of 150 μg/kg body weight. The same authors have shown that pre-administered CORT (5 mg/kg body weight, i.p.) decreases the ACTH response to 1-h immobilization stress in conscious rats (Ginsberg et al., 2003). These findings may allow us to suggest that the reduction of increased serum CORT concentration found in VC-deficient ODS rats with WIRS is due to suppression of CORT secretion via the HPA axis. Kvetnanský et al. (1995) have shown that a single pre-administration of excessive cortisol (30 mg/kg body weight, i.p.) reduces increases in plasma adrenaline and noradrenaline levels in conscious rats with immobilization stress. It has been shown that the sympathetic-adrenal system is interacted with the HPA axis under stress conditions (Kvetnanský et al. 1995). These findings may allow us to assume that the reduction of increased serum glucose concentration in VC-deficient ODS rats with WIRS is due to suppression of adrenaline secretion via the sympathetic-adrenal system.

It is known that an increase in adrenal weight occurs in rats with repeated immobilization stress (Monteiro et al., 1989). Our recent report has shown that an increase in adrenal weight occurs in Wistar rats with 6 h of WIRS (Ohta et al., 2013). In the present study, VC-deficient ODS rats exposed to WIRS over a 6-h period showed an increase in adrenal weight at 1, 3 or 6 h, although it decreased stress time-dependently. In contrast, VC-sufficient ODS rats exposed to WIRS for the same period showed an increase in adrenal weight at 6 h as in the case of Wistar rats with WIRS (Ohta et al., 2013). However, there was no significant difference in the increased adrenal weight between VC-deficient and sufficient ODS rats with 6 h of WIRS. Akana et al. (1983) have reported that the adrenal weight of rats begins to increase when ACTH secretion reaches a certain level and is sustained. Therefore, it is suggested that the increase in adrenal weight in VC-deficient and sufficient ODS rats with WIRS could be due to long-lasting secretion of ACTH. In the present study, adrenal CORT concentration was much higher in VC-deficient ODS rats than in VC-sufficient ODS rats. The increased adrenal CORT concentration in VC-deficient ODS rats was reduced by exposure to WIRS over a 6-h period and this reduction occurred in a stress time-dependent manner. Therefore, it is suggested that the reduction of increased serum CORT concentration found in VC-deficient ODS rats with WIRS could be due to suppression of CORT synthesis and secretion in the adrenal gland by negative feedback via the HPA axis. In contrast, the adrenal CORT concentration in VC-sufficient ODS rats was increased by exposure to WIRS for the same period and this increase occurred in a stress time-dependent manner, although the stress time-dependent increase in adrenal CORT concentration in VC-sufficient ODS rats with WIRS proceeded more slowly than the case of Wistar rats with WIRS shown in our recent report (Ohta et al., 2013). However, there was no significant difference in adrenal CORT concentration between VC-deficient and sufficient ODS rats with 6 h of WIRS as in the case of the aforementioned serum CORT concentration. Taking into consideration the stress time-related changes in serum CORT and glucose concentrations in VC-deficient ODS rats with WIRS, it is suggested that ODS rats with VC deficiency have suppressive responses to WIRS which occur through the existence of increased serum CORT before the onset of stress.

In the present study, serum VC concentration was markedly lower in VC-deficient ODS rats than in VC-sufficient ODS rats, as reported previously (Tokumaru *et al.*, 1996). The serum VC concentration in VC-deficient ODS rats exposed to WIRS over a 6-h period remained unchanged until 3 h but was significantly, although slightly, reduced after 6 h. In contrast, serum VC concentration in VC-sufficient ODS rats exposed to WIRS over a 6-h period increased gradually in a stress time-dependent manner, although this increase was lower than in Wistar rats exposed to the same conditions (Ohta et al., 2013). In VC-deficient and sufficient ODS rats exposed to WIRS over a 6-h period, the stress time-related change in serum VC concentration was similar to those in serum CORT and glucose concentrations, although the stress time-related change in serum VC concentration was smaller than those in serum CORT and glucose concentrations.

These findings suggest that responses to WIRS via the HPA axis and the sympathetic-adrenal system affect serum VC concentration in VC-deficient and sufficient ODS rats in a different manner. Serum VE concentration in VC-deficient ODS rats was less than that in VC-sufficient ODS rats, as reported by Tanaka et al. (1997). VC-deficient ODS rats exposed to WIRS over a 6-h period maintained the serum VE concentration, although it increased significantly, but slightly, after 6 h of WIRS.

In contrast, there was no change in serum VE concentration in VC-sufficient ODS rats exposed to WIRS over a 6-h period as in the case of Wistar rats exposed to WIRS for the same period (Ohta et al., 2013).

Tanaka et al. (1997) have shown that ODS rats fed a VC-deficient diet for 21 days have higher plasma LPO level, an oxidative stress marker, than in ODS rats fed a VC-sufficient diet for the same period. In the present study, serum LPO concentration was significantly higher in ODS rats with 2-week VC deficiency than in ODS rats with the same period of VC sufficiency. However, there was no difference in adrenal LPO content between VC-deficient and sufficient ODS rats.

These results suggest that systemic oxidative stress occurring in VC-deficient ODS rats could not cause oxidative stress in the adrenal gland. When VC-deficient ODS rats were exposed to WIRS over a 6-h period, serum and adrenal LPO concentrations increased stress time-dependently.

Though VC-sufficient ODS rats exposed to WIRS for the same period showed increases in serum and adrenal LPO concentrations, the increases in serum and adrenal LPO concentrations occurred later than those in VC-deficient ODS rats with WIRS. In addition, the increased serum and adrenal LPO concentrations in VC-sufficient ODS rats with 6 h of WIRS were considerably less than those present in VC-deficient ODS rats submitted to the same conditions. The stress time-related changes in serum and adrenal LPO concentrations in VC-sufficient ODS rats with WIRS were similar to those in Wistar rats exposed to the same period of WIRS (Ohta et al., 2013). Accordingly, these findings indicate that VC deficiency enhances WIRS-induced oxidative stress associated with enhanced lipid peroxidation in the adrenal gland of ODS rats.

It is also suggested that systemic oxidative stress could contribute to the occurrence of oxidative stress in the adrenal gland of VC-deficient ODS rats with WIRS, because serum LPO concentration was higher in VC-deficient ODS rats than in VC-sufficient ODS rats at each period of WIRS, as described above.

In the present study, adrenal VC concentration was markedly less in VC-deficient ODS rats than in VC-sufficient ODS rats, as reported previously (Tokumaru et al., 1996).

Regarding adrenal GSH and VE concentrations, there were no differences between VC-deficient and sufficient ODS rats before the onset of stress. Thus, adrenal GSH and VE concentrations were found to be maintained in VC-deficient ODS rats. Such a maintenance of adrenal GSH and VE concentrations in VC-deficient ODS rats may contribute to the aforementioned no increase in adrenal LPO concentration. In VC-deficient ODS rats exposed to WIRS for a 6-h period, the decreased adrenal VC concentration was further reduced gradually in a stress time-dependent manner. The observed change in adrenal VC concentration in VC-deficient ODS rats with WIRS was similar to the above-described stress time-related change in serum VC concentration. VC-sufficient ODS rats exposed to WIRS for the same period also showed a stress time-dependent decrease in adrenal VC concentration, although the adrenal VC concentration in VC-sufficient ODS rats with 6 h of WIRS was much higher than that in VC-deficient ODS rats with the same stress exposure. This change in adrenal VC concentration in VC-sufficient ODS rats with WIRS was the reverse to the above-described stress time-related change in serum VC concentration. Such a reverse relationship between adrenal and serum VC concentrations has been shown in Wistar rats submitted to the same conditions (Ohta et al., 2013). These findings allow us to assume that VC in the adrenal gland of VC-sufficient ODS rats with WIRS not only is consumed in the tissue to protect against WIRS-induced oxidative stress but also is released from the tissue like the case of Wistar rats with WIRS. The decrease in adrenal VC concentration over time in VC-sufficient ODS rats exposed to WIRS over a 6-h period proceeded more slowly than the decrease found in Wistar rats with the same period of WIRS (Ohta et al., 2013). VC-deficient ODS rats exposed to WIRS over a 6-h period showed a stress time-dependent decrease in adrenal GSH concentration and a transient increase in adrenal VE concentration at 1 h of WIRS. The increased VE concentration was reduced to the initial level after 6 h of WIRS. Therefore, changes in adrenal GSH and VE concentrations in VC-deficient ODS rats submitted to WIRS seemed to occur in compensation for the induced disruption of non-enzymatic antioxidant status under continuous severe VC depletion in the tissue. VC-sufficient ODS rats exposed to WIRS over a 6-h period showed a decrease in adrenal GSH concentration at 6 h and a transient increase in adrenal VE concentration at 1 h, although the decrease in adrenal GSH concentration was much less than that in VC-deficient ODS rats with 6 h of WIRS and the transient increase in adrenal VE concentration was much lower than that in VC-deficient ODS rats with 1 h of WIRS. The transiently increased adrenal VE concentration in VC-sufficient ODS rats exposed to WIRS over a 6-h period was returned to the level found before the onset of stress at 3 h of WIRS, the returned adrenal VE conceentration being maintained until the 6th hour of WIRS. These changes were similar to those found in Wistar rats exposed to WIRS for the same period (Ohta et al., 2013), although a transient increase in adrenal GSH concentration was found in the stressed Wistar rats (Ohta et al., 2013) and was not observed in the stressed VC-sufficient ODS rats. Therefore, the stress time-related changes in GSH and VE concentrations in the adrenal gland of VC-sufficient ODS rats with WIRS seemed to occur in compensation for WIRS-induced disruption of non-enzymatic antioxidant status under continuous stress time-dependent VC reduction in the tissue as in the case of Wistar rats exposed to WIRS for the same period (Ohta et al., 2013). It is unclear how the transient increase in adrenal VE concentration occurs in VC-deficient and sufficient ODS rats with WIRS. Taking into consideration the above-described stress time-related changes in adrenal VC, VE, GSH, and LPO concentrations in VC-deficient ODS rats exposed to WIRS over a 6-

h period, it can be proposed that VC deficiency enhances WIRS-induced disruption of non-enzymatic antioxidant defense systems in the adrenal gland of ODS rats.

CONCLUSION

The results obtained from the present study indicate that VC deficiency enhances WIRS-induced disruption of non-enzymatic antioxidant defense systems in the adrenal gland of ODS rats unable to synthesize VC under suppressive stress responses possibly due to increased serum CORT existing before the onset of stress. In addition, the results allow us to confirm that VC plays a critical role in WIRS-induced disruption of non-enzymatic antioxidant defense systems in the adrenal gland of rats.

ACKNOWLEDGMENTS

The present chapter has been reviewed by:

- Herlander Daniel Silva (PharmD, MSc), CIandDETS, Centro de Investigação em Educação, Tecnologias e Saúde, Instituto Politécnico de Viseu, Portugal.
- Naheed Banu (PhD), Department of Biochemistry, Faculty of Life Sciences, A.M. University, Aligarh-202002, UP, India. Presently at- College of Medical rehabilitation, Qassim University, Buraydah, Kingdom of Saudi Arabia.

REFERENCES

Akana, S. F., Shinsako, J. and Dallman, M. F. (1993) Relationships among adrenal weight, corticosterone, and stimulated adrenocorticotropin levels in rats. *Endocrinology* 113, 2226-2231.

Arakawa, H., Kodama, H., matsuoka, N., and Yamaguchi, I. (1997) Stress increases plasma enzyme activity in rats: differential effects of adrenergic and cholinergic blockers. *Journal of Phamracology and Experimental Therapeutics* 280, 1296-303.

Azhar, S., Cao, L. and Reaven, E. (1995) Alteration of the adrenal antioxidant defense system during aging in rats. *Journal of Clinical Investigation* 96, 1414-1424.

Clayman, M., de Nicola, A. F. and Johnstone, R. M. (1970) Specificity of action of adrenocorticotrophin in vitro on ascorbate transport in rat adrenal glands. *Biochemical Journal* 118, 283-289.

Ginsberg, A. B., Campeau, S., Day, H. E., and Sprencer, R. L. (2003) Acute glucocorticoid pretreatment suppresses stress-induced hypothalamic-pituitary-adrenal axis hormone secretion and expression of corticotropin-releasing hormone hnRNA but does nor affect c-*fos* mRNA or Fos protein expression in the paraventricular nucleus of the hypothalamus. *Journal of Neuroendocrinology* 15, 1073-1083.

Guillemin, R., Clayton, G. W., Lipscomb, H. S., and Smith, J. G. (1959) Fluorometric measurement of rat plasma and adrenal corticosterone concentration. A note on technical details. *Journal of Laboratory and Clinical Medicine* 53, 830-832.

Hodges, J. R. and Sadow, J. (1967) Impairment of pituitary adrenocorticotrophic function by corticosterone in the blood. *British Journal of Pharmacology and Chemotherapy* 30, 385-391.

Horio, F., Ozaki, K., Yoshida, A., Makino, S., and Hayashi, Y. (1985) Requirement for ascorbic acid in a rat mutant unable to synthesize ascorbic acid. *Journal of Nutrition* 115, 1630-1640.

Ikeda, S., Horio, F. and Kakinuma, A. (1998) Ascorbic acid deficiency changes hepatic gene expression of acute phase proteins in scurvy-prone ODS rats. *Journal of Nutrition* 128, 832-838.

Jaggi, A. S., Bhaita, N., Kumar, N., Singh, N., Anand, P., and Dhawan, R. (2011) A review on animal models for screening potential anti-stress agents. *Neurological Sciences* 32, 993-1005.

Kaida, S., Ohta, Y., Imai, Y., and Kawanishi, M. (2010) Protective effect of L-ascorbic acid against oxidative damage in the liver of rats with water-immersion restraint stress. *Redox Report* 15, 11-19.

Kamiya, Y., Ohta, Y., Imai, Y., Arisawa, T., and Nakano, H. (2005) A critical role of gastric mucosal ascorbic acid in the progression of acute gastric mucosal lesions induced by compound 48/80 in rats. *World Journal of Gastroenterology* 11, 1324-1332.

Kvetnanský, R., Pacák, K., Furuhara, K., Viskupic, E., Hiremagalur, B., Nankova, B., Goldstein, D. S., Sabban, E. L., and Kopin, I. J. (1995) Sympathoadrenal system in stress. Interaction with the hypothalamic-pituitary-adrenocortical system. *Annals New York Academy of Sciences* 771, 131-158.

Lahiri, S. and Lloyd, B. B. (1962) The effect of stress and corticotrophin on the concentrations of vitamin C in blood and tissues of the rat. *Biochemical Journal* 84, 478-483.

Landeria-Fernandez, J. (2004) Analysis of the cold-water restraint procedure in gastric ulceration and body temperature. *Physiology and Behavior* 82, 827-833.

Leonard, R. K., Auersperg, N. and Parkes, C. O. (1983) Ascorbic acid accumulation by cultured rat adrenocortical cells. *In Vitro* 19, 46-52.

Liebler, D. C. (1993) The role of metabolism in the antioxidant function of vitamin E. *Critical Review of Toxicology* 23, 147-169.

Mizushima, Y., Harauchi, T., Yoshizaki, T., and Makino, S. (1984) A rat mutant unable to synthesize vitamin C. *Experientia* 40, 359-361.

Monteiro, F., Abraham, M. E., Sahakari, S. D., and Mascarenhas, J. F. (1989) Effect of immobilization stress on food intake, body weight and weights of various organs in rat. *Indian Journal of Physiology and Pharmacology* 33, 186-190.

Nakano, K. and Suzuki, S. (1984) Stress-induced change in tissue levels of ascorbic acid and histamine in rats. *Journal of Nutrition* 114, 1602-1608.

Nasmyth, P. A. (1949) The effect of some sympathomimeric amines on the ascorbic acid content of rats' adrenal glands. *Journal of Physiology* 110, 294-300.

Ohkawa, H., Ohishi, N. and Yagi, K. (1979) Assay for lipid peroxides in animal tissues with thiobarbituric acid reaction. *Analytical Biochemistry* 95, 351-358.

Ohta, Y., Chiba, S., Imai, Y., Kamiya, Y., Arisawa, T., and Kitagawa, A. (2006) Ascorbic acid deficiency aggravates stress-induced gastric mucosal lesions in genetically scorbutic ODS rats. *Inflammopharmacology* 14, 231-235.

Ohta, Y., Chiba, S., Tada, M., Imai, Y., and Kitagawa, A. (2007) Development of oxidative stress and cell damage in the liver of rats with water-immersion restraint stress. *Redox Report* 12, 139-147.

Ohta, Y., Imai, Y., Kaida, S., Kamiya, Y., Kawanishi, M., and Hirata, I. (2010) Vitamin E protects against stress-induced gastric mucosal lesions in rats more effectively than vitamin C. *Biofactors* 36, 60-69.

Ohta, Y., Kamiya, Y., Imai, Y., Arisawa, T., and Nakano, H. (2005) Role of gastric mucosal ascorbic acid in gastric mucosal lesion development in rats with water immersion restraint stress. *Inflammopharmacology* 13, 249-259.

Ohta, Y., Yashiro, K., Kaida, S., Imai, Y., Ohashi, K., and Kitagawa, A. (2013) Water-immersion restraint stress disrupts nonezymatic antioxidant defense systems through rapid and continuous ascorbic acid depletion in the adrenal gland of rats. *Cell Biochemistry and Function* 31, 254-262.

Overbeek, G. A. (1985) Hormonal regulation of ascorbic acid in the adrenal of the rat. *Acta Endocrinologica (Copenhagen)* 109, 393-402.

Padayvatty, S. J., Doppman, J. L., Chang, R., Wang, Y., Gill, J., and Papanicolatou, D. A., and Levine, M. (2007) Human adrenal glands secrete vitamin C in response to adrenocorticotrophic hormone. *American Journal of Clinical Nutrition* 86, 145-149.

Nasmyth, P. A. (1949) The effect of some sympathomimetic amines on the ascorbic acid content of rats' adrenal glands. *Journal of Physiology* 110, 294-300.

Patak, P., Willenberg, H. S. and Bornstein, S. R. (2004) Vitamin C is an important cofactor for both adrenal cortex and adrenal medulla. *Endocrine Research* 30, 871-875.

Pignatelli, D., Magalhães, M. and Mogalhães, M. C. (1998) Direct effects of stress on adrenocortical function. *Hormon and Metabolic Research* 30, 464-474.

Sedlak, J. and Lindsay, R. H. (1968) Estimation of total, protein-bound, and nonprotein sulfhydryl groups in tissues with Ellman's reagent. *Analytical Biochemistry* 25, 192-205.

Tanaka, K., Hashimoto, T., Tokumaru, S., Iguchi, H., and Kojo, S. (1997) Interactions between vitamin C and vitamin E are observed in tissues of inherently scorbutic rats. *Journal of Nutrition* 127, 2060-2064.

Tokumaru, S., Takeshita S., Nakata, R., Tsukamoto, I., and Kojo, S. (1996) Change in the level of vitamin C and lipid peroxidation in tissues of the inherently scorbutic rat during ascorbate deficiency. *Journal of Agricultural and Food Chemistry* 44, 2748-2753.

Winkler, B. S., Orselli, S. M. and Rex, T. S. (1994) The redox couple between glutathione and ascorbic acid: A chemical and physiological perspective. *Free Radical Biology and Medicine* 17, 333-349.

Yagi, K. (1976) A simple fluorometric assay for lipoperoxide in blood plasma. *Biochemia Medica* 15, 212-216.

Zannoni, V., Lynch, M., Goldstein, S., and Sato, P. (1974) A rapid micromethod for the determination of ascorbic acid in plasma and tissues. *Biochemia Medica* 11, 41-48.

In: Vitamin C
Editor: Raquel Guiné

ISBN: 978-1-62948-154-8
© 2013 Nova Science Publishers, Inc.

Chapter 8

VITAMIN C AND ERYTHROCYTES

Sambe Asha Devi[*] and
Challaghatta Seenappa Shiva Shankar Reddy[†]
Laboratory of Gerontology, Department of Zoology
Bangalore University, Bangalore, India

ABSTRACT

The myeloid produces about 2-3 million erythrocytes (red blood cells, RBCs) sec^{-1} amounting to 200 billion day^{-1} and replaces the ones that are lost. The main functions of RBCs are transportation of oxygen throughout the body, of carbon dioxide as carbamino–haemoglobin and maintenance of the acid-base status in the blood. The normal blood which is alkaline turns acidic under lowered pH. However, the functions of the erythrocytes may be disrupted prematurely under several environmental stressors including osmotic shock, oxidative stress (OS), ligation of cell membrane antigens and energy depletion, and may result in cell shrinkage, membrane blebbing, activation of proteases and phosphatidylserine (PS) exposure on the outer membrane leaflet. PS at the erythrocyte surface is recognised by macrophages which engulf and degrade the affected cells. Although eryptosis is envisaged as a mechanism of defective erythrocytes to escape, eryptosis in excess leads to altered physiological situations that reduce the normal life span of erythrocytes in circulation resulting in iron deficiency, sickle cell anemia, thalassemia, and glucose-6- phosphate dehydrogenase deficiency, malaria and infection with hemolysin-forming pathogens. However, antioxidants can regulate several cellular events by mechanisms related to their ability to clear free radicals and membrane stabilization. Vitamin C, also referred as L-ascorbic acid(ASC) is a well known water-soluble vitamin that is ingested through natural food or as dietary supplements. Further, deficiency of vitamin C is linked to premature eryptosis. This chapter presents a comprehensive report of *in vivo* and *in vitro* studies as well on how administration of vitamin C singly or co-administered with other antioxidants such as vitamin E (α-tocopherol) can impact erythrocyte function under OS, and surveys the advances in the field from a clinical perspective.

---

[*] E-mail: sambe.ashadevi@gmail.com.
[†] E-mail: ssreddy6@gmail.com.

1. INTRODUCTION

Erythrocytes (RBCs) are specialized cells for transporting oxygen, carbon dioxide and all essential nutrients due to their unique cellular and non-cellular components. They have an average life span of 120 days in humans and from 60 days to 90 days in mice and rats respectively following which they undergo apoptosis referred to as eryptosis and are subsequently cleared from the circulation by the macrophages. During their short stay in circulation, erythrocytes assist the vital functions of the body while simultaneously overcoming the various adverse conditions including oxidative stress (OS). However, erythrocytes have antioxidative mechanisms for defending not only themselves but also other tissues from the toxic effects of free radicals (FRs) in our body (Siem, 2000; Arbos et al., 2008). Being carriers of oxygen, erythrocytes are most susceptible to OS and are responsible for the progression of conditions such as diabetes, rheumatoid arthritis, dementia, Alzheimer's disease, Parkinson's disease, cataract and aging (Halliwell and Guterridge, 2007; Pandey et al., 2010, 2011).

It is widely known among health specialists and the general public that vitamin C is beneficial to health because of its protective effect against OS. Many cells have transporters for vitamin C unlike mature erythrocytes which cannot take up vitamin C from plasma (May, 1998). However, glucose transporter GLUT 1 permits efficient uptake of dehydroascorbic acid (DHA) (Montel-Hagen et al., 2008). In all the species examined DHA enters the erythrocyte considerably more rapidly than ascorbic acid (vitamin C). The uptake is pH-dependent and the rate of uptake of DHA is influenced by the activity of the erythrocyte DHA-reducing system. Dehydro-*iso* ascorbic acid (dehydro-d-araboascorbic acid) enters the erythrocyte considerably less rapidly than DHA. Ascorbic acid (ASC) is released from the erythrocyte at a slow rate (Hughes and Maton, 1968). Although human and animal studies are accumulating in support of vitamin C as an antioxidant, a number of scientists are apprehensive of its benefits due to the discrepant literature in the field because of the prooxidant and toxic effects of vitamin C in high doses. Therefore, our aim in this chapter is to present the current understanding of vitamin C as an antioxidant of erythrocytes from studies in our laboratory as well as of many scientists across the globe.

2. ERYTHROCYTES AND OXIDATIVE STRESS

Differentiation of erythrocytes starts from the hematopoietic stem cells in the bone marrow. As the erythrocytes are released from the bone marrow, they lose their nucleus, ribosomes and mitochondria. The mature erythrocyte is biconcave and of 5 to 8 microns and has a number of membrane proteins, most importantly the highly specialized spectrin network that renders high elasticity to overcome shear stress (An et al, 2002; Mozhanova et al., 2003; Dulinska et al., 2006), and a lipid bilayer (de Oliveira and Saldanha, 2010). Unlike the human and subhuman species, erythrocytes in the lower vertebrates, fishes, reptiles and aves are nucleated and have intracellular organelles such as mitochondria. The high arterial O_2 tension and heme Fe in the enucleated erythrocytes are responsible for the generation of reactive oxygen species (ROS) including the super oxide ($O_2 \cdot^-$), hydrogen peroxide (H_2O_2) and hydroxyl radical (OH^-)(Burak Çimen, 2008). Since erythrocytes lack mitochondria, glycolysis is the only source of ATP molecules and about 90% of influxed glucose is used by glycolysis while 10% is directed to the hexose monophosphate pathway, and the latter pathway is efficiently used for generating NADPH which are utilized by erythrocytes to reduce glutathione (GSH), an endogenous antioxidant (Sivilotti, 2004). Hemoglobin (Hb) is an abundant protein in erythrocytes that ferries high amounts of oxygen, its ferrous iron undergoing oxidation to methemoglobin (metHb) which is a non-carrier of oxygen. The human body contains an average of 750 g of Hb (Nagababu and Rifkind, 2004) most of which is contained in the erythrocytes. It is known that erythrocytes have about 270 million Hb molecules which comprise greater than 95% of the cytoplasmic proteins (Telen and Kaufen, 2004). Each Hb molecule can bind four oxygen molecules and hence enables each erythrocyte to carry about 1 billion oxygen molecules. It is therefore, not surprising that owing to their enormous capacity, erythrocytes are also subjected to Hb disorders. Oxidative injury to the erythrocytes affects the overall cellular structures of the erythrocyte and its Hb. The most striking aspect is that irrespective of the causes, all of these disorders are known to share the same characteristics of OS, lipid peroxidation (LPO) and protein oxidation of erythrocyte membrane, hemolysis and release of the denatured products into circulation (Stephen et al., 1985; Chaves et al., 2008). It is reported that under normal conditions, the concentration of metHb is about 1% and there is a several fold increase under OS (Arbos et al, 2008). Hemin, which is one of the denatured components of metHb, is demonstrated to intensify the inflammation reactions of endothelial cells and promote the progression of atherosclerosis by the oxidation of low density liporptoteins (Umbreit, 2007). Several *in vivo* and *in vitro* studies on OS have proven inactivation of membrane bound receptors and enzymes (Halliwell and Gutteridge, 2007), ionic balance (Maridonneau et al., 1983), intracellular pH (Asha Devi et al., 2009), increased oxidation of proteins and lipids (Pasini et al., 2006; Lykkesfeldt et al., 2007), and increased intracellular calcium and externalization of phosphatidyl serine (Figure 8.1) to signal irreversibly damaged cells to the reticulo-endothelial system for their removal (Kuypers, and de jong., 2004; Asha Devi et al., 2011). In diseases such as diabetes, uncontrolled hyperglycemia leads to increased binding of glucose to Hb and formation of glycated haemoglobin (HbA1C) which in Type-II diabetics is a reliable diagnostic marker of protein oxidation (Cakatay et al., 2004; Kostolanska et al., 2009). Hence, in diabetes, increased eryptosis is observed (Calderon-Salinas et al., 2011; Maellaro et al., 2011) due to increased stimulation of scrambling by glucose (Kucherenko et al., 2010). Excess eryptosis is also reported in hyperthermia resulting in fever (Foller et al., 2010) and in septic patients whose plasma has a factor that stimulates increased entry of calcium in their erythrocytes (Lang et al., 2010).

The effect of certain FRs such as peroxyl on erythrocytes is reported for varying atmospheric exposures of various organisms including humans. For instance, peroxyl-mediated increased hemolysis has been documented in studies on humans (Sandhu et al., 1992) and rat erythrocytes (Shiva Shankar Reddy et al., 2007). Figure 8.2 shows the irreversible membrane changes that occur in the presence of peroxyl radicals. ROS oxidized amino acid side chains form protein-protein cross-linkages, fragments and generate many products (Pandey et al, 2010). It is known that a step-wise oxidative attack on the peptide backbone is due to an .OH–dependent removal of α-hydrogen atom of an amino acid to form a carbon-centered radical. Alkoxyl radicals are responsible for the cleavage of peptide bond as a consequence of ROS interaction with glutamyl and aspartyl side chains. Few of the protein oxidation products include lipofuscin, advanced oxidation protein products and protein carbonyls and are recognized markers of OS due to their stability and early formation (Dalle-Donne et al, 2003).

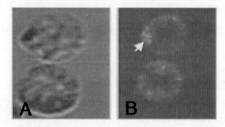

Figure 8.1. Externalization of phosphatidyl serine in rat erythrocytes as seen through annexin-V- Cy 3 binding. (A) Transmission (B) Fluorescence microscopy.

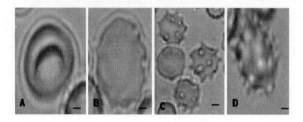

Figure 8.2. Morphological changes in rat erythrocytes exposed to peroxyl radicals induced by AAPH. A, normal erythrocyte; B, membrane invaginations; C, spheroechinocytes; D, membrane blebs over the cell surface, Scale = 2 μm.

Persisting with the idea of measuring OS in erythrocytes, our laboratory tested the impact of vitamin C in combination with vitamin E and carnitine in rats that were subjected to intermittent hypobaric hypoxia at 5,100 and 6,700 meters. The combined effects were more effective in terms of reduced LPO and protein oxidation in the erythrocytes (Vani et al., 2010) although single supplements of vitamin C and E were also effective (Asha Devi et al., 2007).

The life span of erythrocytes in different species are related to their antioxidant defense enzymes such as catalase (CAT), glutathione peroxidase (GSH-Px), superoxide disutase (SOD), glutathione S –transferase (GST), glutathione reductase (GR) and the ROS concentration (Kurata et al, 1993). A study conducted by Ozturk and Gumuslu (2004) on male *Wistar* rats of 1, 6 and 12 months of age reports age-related decreases in erythrocyte antioxidant, GSH, oxidized GSH (GSSG), total GSH and thiobarbituric acid reactive substance (TBARS) levels, GSH/GSSG ratio and the redox index.

It is well known that the FRs, moreso oxygen radicals, is related to the process of aging. Studies by Baur et al.(1982) on isolation of human erythrocytes as young, middle-age and senescent cells using continuous Percoll gradient have characterized highest activity of glucose-6-phosphate dehydrogenase, catalase (CAT), glutathione peroxidase (GSH-Px), glutathione reductase (GR) and GSH in the youngest cell compared to the senescent cells wherein, the enzymes decreased by about 20-30%. The malondialdehyde (MDA) content indicative of LPO increased by 35% in the eldest cell population. Erythrocytes from 10 anemic patients exhibited less GSH and also less MDA, while GSH-peroxidase and GSSG-reductase contents were higher proving that LPO is one of the causal events in erythrocytes aging.

Hence given that erythrocytes are associated with a plethora of OS-related pathological conditions, their morphology may serve as a useful indicator to detect inflammatory situations and atheroma progression in patients with coronary artery disease (Berliner et al., 2005). Figure 8.2 shows the normal discoid rat erythrocytes which when exposed to peroxyl radicals undergo irreversible membrane changes.

3. VITAMIN C AND ERYTHROCYTES: OBSERVATIONS IN ANIMALS AND HUMANS

Vitamin C is a vital antioxidant humans require and must be obtained from dietary sources unlike most vertebrates wherein vitamin C is synthesized de novo from glucose. It exists in two biological forms; the reduced form, ASC and oxidized form, DHA, and functions intracellularly through specific membrane transporters. Ascorbic acid is transported by the SVCT family of sodium-coupled transporters, with two isoforms molecularly cloned, the transporters SVCT1 and SVCT2, which exhibit differential tissue and cell expression. Recycling of ascorbic acid from its oxidized state assists in maintaining sufficient tissue levels of this vitamin in human erythrocytes. In order to determine the contribution of recycling from the ascorbate radical and dehydroascorbic acid May and his collaborators (2004) conducted a series of experiments using ferricyanide as an oxidant stress across the erythrocyte membrane. Ferricyanide was used to induce oxidant stress and quantify ascorbate recycling as well. Interestingly, their results showed that ferricyanide also generated DHA that accumulated in the cells. Further, ferricyanide-stimulated ascorbate recycling from DHA was dependent on intracellular GSH. However, in the absence of GSH, ferricyanide-stimulated ascorbate recycling from DHA was efficiently maintained at the expense of intracellular ascorbate reflecting on continued ascorbate radical reduction, independent of GSH. These studies suggested a two-tiered system wherein high affinity reduction of the ascorbate radical is itself sufficient to eliminate low levels of this radical that might be experienced by erythrocytes under non-oxidant conditions, with a supporting high capacity system for reducing DHA under severe oxidant stress. Further, in humans, the maintenance of a low daily requirement of vitamin C is reached through an efficient system for the recycling of the vitamin involving the two families of vitamin C transporters (Rivas et al., 2008). Similar concentrations of plasma and erythrocyte concentration are seen and the levels being lower than those of the nucleated cells (May et al., 2007). The low capacity of erythrocytes to concentrate ascorbate is related to low uptake rates of the molecule due to the absence of ascorbate transporter SVCT2 that is seen in the reticulocyte stage in the bone marrow. Johnston et al (1993) have shown that 500 mg/d of vitamin C supplementation increases plasma C level and also assists in the maintainence of reduced glutathione (GSH) levels in blood and thereby increase the plasma antioxidant capacity of the blood.

Erythrocytes undergo eryptosis when subjected to OS or when food in the form of glucose is depleted and vitamin C is known to protect the erythrocytes from premature cell death (Mahmud et al., 2010). Postaire and his co-workers (1995), while studying the effects of vitamins on human erythrocytes have demonstrated that vitamin E (15 mg/day) and vitamin C (30 mg/day) for 15 days can protect the erythrocytes from the singlet oxygen. Similarly, the oxidative process in human erythrocytes can be lowered by combined effects of vitamin C and E (Claro et al., 2006). A study by Garibella and his co-scientists (2013) on obese diabetic patients in the Arab populations, daily oral antioxidants supplementation comprising of 221 mg of α-tocopherol and 167 mg of vitamin C along with B-vitamins, 1.67 mg folic acid, 1.67 mg vitamin B-2, 20 mg vitamin B-6, 0.134 mg vitamin B-12 showed enhanced antioxidant capacity and anti-inflammatory effect. In vitro studies on rat (Figure 8.3) and duck (Figure 8.4) erythrocytes in our laboratory have shown 10 mM vitamin C treatment is effective in lowering oxidative injury induced by peroxyl radicals generated by 2,2'-azo-bis(2-amidinopropane) hydrochloride (AAPH).

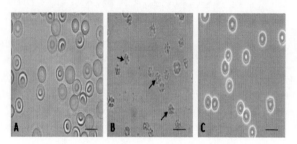

Figure 8.3. Normal rat erythrocytes (A), AAPH-exposed cells showing membrane vesciculations and shrinkage (B), cells treated with vitamin C+AAPH (C), Scale = 10 μm.

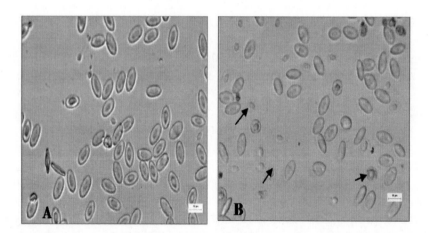

Figure 8.4. Bright field microphotographs of duck erythrocytes showing elliptical shape with distinct membrane and nucleus (A); cells treated with AAPH to induce oxidative stress(B). Arrow indicates membrane disruption under oxidative stress. Scale = 10 μm.

Although vitamin C is beneficial and non-toxic, it causes toxicity at high concentrations and is a pro-oxidant rather than an antioxidant (Duarte and Lunee, 2005; Markovic et al., 2010). *In vitro* studies on human erythrocytes have reported the oxidizing effect of vitamin C in high doses with high conductivity at increasing temperatures (Ibrahim et al., 2006).

Studies on erythrocytes in guinea pigs have shown that high levels of vitamin C, 30 mg/100 g body weight/day can increase the haemolytic and peroxidative effects of vitamin C and these effects could be overcome by vitamin E (Chen and Chang, 1979). Vitamin C exhibits a synergistic effect in inhibiting LPO when combined with phenolic compounds, catechin and epicatechin in human erythrocytes and liposomes as well (Liao and Yin, 2000).

Table 8.1. Few situations that generate oxidative stress in human and subhuman erythrocytes and the beneficial effects of vitamin C in alleviating the stress

Human/ Subhuman Erythrocyte	Oxidative stress Agents	Oxidative effects	Benefits of vitamin C	References
Human	Dimethoate(Dim) 0-20 mM Dim	Increased MDA levels	Significant protection against cytotoxic effects	Abdallah et al., 2011
Rats(*Wistar*)	Carbofuran Sub-acute dose	Increasesd membrane fragility, elevated SOD and CATactivities, diminished GST activity Increased LPO and reduced AOEs	Marked lowering of OS parameters	Rai et al., 2009
Rat (*Wistar*)	Chlorpyrifos-ethyl (CE) 41mg Kg^{-1} CE		Combined supplement of vitamin C and E at 200 and 150 mg kg^{-1} reduces lipoperoxidative effect	Gultekin et al., 2001
Human	Mercury as HgCl$_2$ 1.052 to 10.52M	Increased MDA levels, decreased SOD, CAT and GPx activities	Significant protection against LPO	Durak et al, 2010
Human	Chromate	Increased peroxidation	Vitamin C at 1 mM significantly increases chromate-induced Hb oxidation	Fernandes et al., 2000
Human	Acetaminophen 0.3-14.5 micromoles	Increased oxidation of metHb, increased SOD activity,lowered Na(+)-K(+) ATPase activity	Partial protection of Hb, SOD and ATPase by Vitamin C at 1mg/dl	Tükel, 1995
Domestic chick (*Nera black*)	Transportation	Increased osmotic resistance	650 mg Kg^{-1} diet. Antagonizing effect of vitamin C	Azeez et al., 2011
Rat (*Wistar*)	Intermittent hypobaric hypoxia(IHH) 5700 m and 6300 m	Increased MDA, lipofuscin-like substances	Alleviated LPO	Asha Devi et al., 2007
Guinea-pigs	Low vitamin E-fed 9-11 weeks	Low membrane fluidity Increased LPO	Supplements of 1, 10, and 100 mg/animal/ day. Dosage-dependent increase in fragility	Tatara and Ginter, 1994

AOEs, antioxidative enzymes; ATPase, adenosine triphosphatase; CAT, catalase ; GPx, glutathione peroxidase; GST, glutathione-S-transferase; Hb, hemoglobin; LPO, lipid peroxidation; MDA, malondialdehyde; metHb, methemoglobin; OS, oxidative stress; SOD, Superoxide dismutase.

3.1. Vitamin C and Storage of Human Erythrocytes

Few indexes such as ATP and SOD is higher than MDA and O_2^{-} levels in human RBCs stored in citrate-phosphate-dextrose (CPD) medium at 25^0 C in plastic bags containing vitamin C (Kanias and Acker., 2010; Zan et al., 2010). Long-term storage of erythrocytes for transfusion results in oxidative damage with changes to the structure of band 3 and LPO, apoptotic changes with racemisation of membrane phospholipids and loss of parts of the membrane through vesiculation (D'Allesandro et al., 2010). It is reported that glutathione-dependent enzymes such as GSH-Px, glutathione transferase (GSH-S-T) and glutathione are depleted in RBCs stored in citrate-phosphate-dextrose-adenine (CPDA) during long periods in plastic bags (Korgun et al., 2005). However, the blood undergoes peroxidative processes making it unsuitable for transfusion. Hence the length of storage is an important factor to be considered prior to transfusion since blood stored for 40 days in CPDA-1 with antioxidants have shown 25% increase in plasma MDA on day 15 and 27% decrease in plasma total antioxidant status (TAS). The same study showed decreases in SOD and CAT activities in the RBC depending on storage length. The study finally concluded that a 10 day period can be a safe limit for transfusion in relation to the oxidative stress the RBCs were subjected to in the storage medium (Ogunro et al., 2001). Despite recent advances in erythrocyte engineering from several stem cell sources, none of them have succeeded in the generation of functional erythrocytes in the absence of serum or plasma and feeder cells. It is well known that in the presence of serum and plasma, human erythrocyte engineering in a large scale is impossible, especially for the future bioreactor system. Kim and Baek (2012) have demonstrated through a combination of cost-effective and safe reagents, the terminal maturation of hematopoietic stem cells into enucleated RBCs, which are functional comparable to donated human erythrocytes. Interestingly, the viability of erythroid cells is higher in these serum- and feeder - free culture conditions than in the serum - containing condition and is made possible by supplementation with vitamin C in media and hypothermic conditions.

3.2. Vitamin C and Erythrocyte Diseases

Erythrocyte deformability resulting in negative variations under experimental osteoporosis resulting in reduced blood flow and hence lowered tissue perfusion affects bone metabolism. Interestingly, vitamin C supplementation has been shown to positively reverse the above variations in female *Wistar* rats (Arslan et al., 2011). In their studies on ischaemic rat model, Coban et al.(2005) have observed higher erythrocyte antioxidant capacity in vitamin C reperfusion after ischaemia. Similarly, dexmedetomidine, an anesthetic agent that is used in the intensive care units is known to cause disrupted erythrocyte deformability and experiments conducted on male rats have shown the reversibility of such changes by vitamin C (Kurtipek et al., 2012). However, these results need to be validated in clinical trials. Vitamin C is also shown to be effective in inhibiting metHb formation in human erythrocytes subjected to oxidative stress (Krukoski et al., 2009). One of the symptoms of the well known vitamin C deficiency disease, scurvy is reduced erythrocyte life span (Troadec and Kaplan, 2008). Combined supplements of vitamin C and E with beta-carotene in 300 elderly subjects ranging between 60 and 75 years of age are reported to result in a regain of membrane fluidity lost from H_2O_2-induced oxidative stress (Li et al., 2008). Similarly, combined vitamin C and vitamin E are effective in decreasing OS effects in human erythrocytes resulting from the oxidative action of phenylhydrazine hydrochloride (Claro et al., 2006). Organophosphate and carbamate pesticides that are extensively used are known to cause OS resulting in increased osmotic fragility of the erythrocytes (Table 8.1). Heme (irom protoporphyrin IX) is a functional group in many proteins, including hemoglobin and myoglobin. Under pathological conditions, such as thalassemia, sickle cell anemia, glucose 6-phosphate dehydrogenase deficiency which are among the more frequent genetic anomalies accompanied by OS, and hemorrhage and muscle injury, hemin is released and an excess of hemin can interact with erythrocyte cell membranes resulting in the generation of ROS and cellular injury (Wagener et al., 2001). The toxic effects of hemin on erythrocytes are manifested in the form of enzyme inhibitions, and dissociation of erythrocyte skeletal structures. Further hemin is known to cause hemolysis by a colloid-osmotic mechanism that is charactertized by loss of potassium from erythrocytes followed by hemolysis. However, ASC can inhibit hemin-induced hemolysis only if glutathione is present (LI et al., 2006). Vitamin C inhibits PS externalization at the erythrocyte surface in clinical conditions such as immunosuppressive drug treatments causing anemia in patients wherein the clearance of erythrocytes is greater than its turnover. In sickle ghosts exposed to H_2O_2, ascorbate at low concentrations, 20 μM, can inhibit LPO, whereas it increases LPO at high concentrations, >50 μM (Repka et al., 1991). OS contributes to the sickle process of the erythrocytes and one of the factors that predispose them to the hemolytic process is the oxidative degradation of the hemoglobin S and deoxygenation leading to hemichrome formation and precipitation as Heinz bodies (Chaves et al., 2008). Vitamin C also protects membrane α-tocopherol in *Plasmodium vinckei*-infected erythrocytes (Stocker et al., 1986).

CONCLUSION

Currently, vitamin C is an indisputable essential vitamin for erythrocytes. Although erythrocyte hypothermic storage is successful, it is still not devoid of oxidative injury since *ex vivo* storage has compromised antioxidant enzymes, high glucose levels in the storage media and high concentrations of molecular oxygen. Further, for an effective treatment of patients, it is necessary to use the right dose of vitamin C. The ongoing trends in the field are applications of the antioxidant functions of vitamin C in erythrocyte storage with an ultimate aim of quality erythrocyte transfusions.

ACKNOWLEDGMENTS/REVISION

One of the authors (S.Asha Devi) acknowledges LSRB (LSRB-32/2002/EPB) and DST (SR/SO/AS-58/2004), Govt.of India, New Delhi for providing financial assistance during which period the present review article was conceived.
The present chapter has been reviewed by:

- Sumathi Swaminathan (PhD), St.John's National Academy of Health Sciences, Sarjapur Road, Bangalore 560 034, Karnataka, India
- M.V.V. Subramanyam (PhD), Laboratory of Physiology, Department of Life Sciences, Bangalore University, Bangalore 560 056, Karnataka, India

REFERENCES

Abdallah, F.B.; Gargourim, B.; Bejaoui, H.; Lassoued, S. & Ammar-Keskes, I. Dimethoate-induced oxidative stress in human erythrocytes and the protective effect of vitamin C and E in vitro. *Environ Toxicol.*, 23, 287-281.

An, X.; Lecombte, M.C.; Chasis, J.A.; Mohandad, N. & Grutzer, W.(2002). Shear stress response of the spectrin dimer-tetramer equilibrium in the red blood cell membarne. *J.Biol Chem.*, 277, 31796-317800.

Arbos, K.A.; Claro, L.M.; Borges, L.; Santos, C.A. & Weffort-Santos, A.M.(2008). Human erythrocytes as a system for evaluating the antioxidant capacity of vegetable extracts. *Nutr Res.*, 28, 457-463.

Arslan, A.; Aydin, G.; Keles, I.; FM, C. & Arslan, M. (2011). Evaluation of erythrocyte deformability in experimentally induced osteoporosis in female rats and the effects of vitamin C supplementation on erythrocyte deformability. *Bratisl Lek Listy*, 112, 605-609.

Asha Devi, S.; Shiva Shankar Reddy, C.S. & Subramanyam, M.V.V.(2009). Oxidative stress and intracellular pH in the young and old erythrocytes of rat. *Biogeron.*, 10, 659-669.

Asha Devi, S.; Shiva Shankar Reddy, C.S. & Subramanyam, M.V.V. (2011). Peroxyl-induced oxidative stress in aging erythrocytes of rat. *Biogeron.*, 12, 283-292.

Asha Devi, S.; Vani, R. & Subramanyam, M.V.V.; Reddy, S.S. & Jeevaratnam, K.(2007). Intermittent hypobaric hypoxia-induced oxidative stress in rat erythrocytes: protective effects of vitamin E, vitamin C and carnitine. *Cell Biochem Funct.*, 25, 221-231.

Azeez, O.I.; Oyagbemi, A.A. & Oyewale, J.O. (2011). Erythrocyte membrane stability after transportation stress in the domestic chicken as modulated by pretreatment with vitamins C and E. *J Animal Vet Adv.*, 10, 1273-1277.

Baur, G.; Jung, A. & Wendel, A. (1982). Activity of the glutathione redox system in human erythrocytes at various ages. *Klin Wochenschr.*, 60, 867-869.

Berliner, S; Rogowski, O.; Aharonov, S; Mardi, T.; Tolshinsky, T.; Rozenblat, M.; Justo, D.; Deutsch, V.; Serov, J.; Shapira, I. & Zeltzer, D. (2005). Erythrocyte adhesiveness/aggregation: a novel biomarker for the detection of low-grade internal inflammation in individuals with atherothrombotic risk fcators and proven vascular disease. *Am Heart J*, 149, 260-267.

Burak Çimen, M.Y. (2008). Free radical metabolism in human erythrocytes. *Clinica Chim.Acta*, 390, 1-11.

Cakatay, U. (2005). Protein oxidation parameters in type 2 diabetic patients with good and poor glycaemic control. *Diabetes Metab.*, 31, 551–557.

Calderon-Salinas, T.V.; Munas-Reiyes, E.H.; Guerrero-Romero, J.F.; Rodriguez-Moran, M.; Bracho-Riqulam, R.I.; Carrera-Gracia, M.A. & Quintanar-escorza, M.A. (2011). Eryptosis and oxidatiev damage in type 2 diabetic mellitus patient with chronic kidney disease. *Mol Cell Biochem.*, 357, 3171-3179.

Chaves, M.A.F.; Leonart, M.S.S. & Nascimento, A.J. (2008). Oxidative process in erythrocytes of individuals with with hemoglobin S. *Hematology*, 13, 187-192.

Chen, L.H. & Chang, H.M. (1979). Effects of high level of vitamin C on tissue antioxidant status of guinea pigs. *Int J Vitam Nutr Res.*, 49, 87-91.

Coban, Y.K.; Bulbuloglu, E.; Polat, A. & Inanc, F. (2005). Improved preservation of erythrocyte antioxidant capacity with ascorbic acid reperfusion after ischemia: A comparative study in a rat hindlimb model. *The Internet J Alternative Med.,* 2(1). DOI: 10.5580/c56.

Claro, LM; Leobart, MSS; Comar, SR; do Nascimento, AJ. (2006). Effcet of vitamins C and E on oxidative processes in human erythrocytes. *Cell Biochem Funct.,* 24, 531-535.

Dalle-Donne, I.; Rossi, R.; Giustarini, D.; Milzani, A. & Colombo, R. (2003). Protein carbonyls as markers of oxidative stress. *Clinica Chimica Acta* 329, 23– 8

de Oliveira, S. & Saldanha, C. (2010). An overview about erythrocyte membrane. *Clin Hemorheol Microcirc*, 44, 63-74.

D'Allesandro, A.; Liumbruno, G.; Grazzini, G. & Zolla, L. (2010). Red blood storage: the story so far. *Blood Transfus.* 8, 82–88.

Duarte, T.L. & Lunec, J. (2005). When is an antioxidant not an antioxidant? A review of novel actions an dreactions of vitamin C. *Free Rad Res.,* 39, 671-686.

Dulinska, I.; Targosz, M.; Strojny, W.; Lekka, M.; Czuba, P.; Balwierz, W. & Szymonski, M. (2006). Stiffness of normal and pathological erythrocytes studied by means of atomic force microscopy. *J Biochem Biophys Meth.* 66, 1–11.

Durak, D.; Kalender, S.; Uzun, F.G.; Demýr, F. & Kalender, Y. (2010). Mercury chloride-induced oxidative stress in human erythrocytes and the effects of vitamins C and E in vitro. *African J Biotech.,* 9, 488-495.

Fernandes, M.A.; Geraldes, C.F.; Oliveira, C.R. & Alpoim, M.C. (2000). Chromate-induced human erythrocyte haemoglobin oxidation and peroxidation: influence of vitamin E, vitamin C, salicylate, deferoxamine, and N-ethylmaleimide. *Toxicol Letts.,* 114, 237-243.

Foller, M., Braun, M., Qadri , S.M., Lang, E., Mahmud, H & lang, F. (2010). Temperature sensitivity of suicidal erythrocyte death. *Eur J Clin Invest.,* 40, 534-540.

Garibella, S.; Afandi, B.; AbuHalten, MN.; Yassin, J.; Habib, H. & Ibrahim, W. (2013).. Oxidative damage and inflammation in obese diabetic Emirati subjects supplemented with antioxdiants and B-vitamins: a randomized placebo-controlled train*. Nutr. Metabolism.* 10, 21.

Gultekin, F.; Delibas, N.; Yasar, S. & Kilinic, A. (2001). In vivo changes in antioxdiant systems and protective role of melatonin and a combination of vitamin C and vitamin E on oxidative damage in erythrocytes induced by chlorpyrifos-ethyl in rats. *Arch.Toxicol.*75, 88-96.

Halliwell, B. & Gutteridge, J.M.C. (2007). Cellular responses to oxidative stress: adaptation, damage, repair, senescence and death. In: *Free Radicals in Biology and Medicine.* 4th ed. New York: Oxford University Press, 187-267.

Hughes, R.E. & Maton, S.C. (1968). The passage of vitamin C across the erythrocyte membrane. *Brit J Haematology,* 14, 247–253.

Ibrahim, I.H.; Sallam, S.M.; Omar, H. & Rizk, M. (2006). Oxidative hemolysis of erythrocytes onduced by various vitamins. *Int J Biomed Sci.,* 2, 295-298.

Johnston, C.S.; Meyer, C.G. & Srilakshmi, J.C. (1993). Vitamin C elevates red blood cell glutathione in healthy adults. *Amer J Clin Nutr*, 58, 103-05.

Johnston CS, Meyer CG, Srilakshmi JC. (2005). Vitamin C elevates red blood cell glutathione in healthy adults. *J.Exp. Haematology*, 13, 1106-1108.

Kanias, T. & Acker, J.P. (2010). Biopreservation of red blood cells – the struggle with hemoglobin oxidation. *FEBS J.,* 277, 343-356.

Kim, H.O.& Baek, E.J. (2012). Red blood cell engineering in stroma and serum/plasma-free conditions and long term storage. *Tissue Engineering* Part A, 18, 117-126

Korgun, DK; Bilmen, S; Yesilkaya, A. (2005). Alterations in the erythrocyte antioxidant system of blood stored in blood bags. *Clin.Biochem.,* 38, 1009-1014.

Kostolanska, J.; Jakus, V. & Barak, L. (2009). HbA1c and serum levels of advanced glycation and oxidation protein products in poorly and well controlled children and adolescents with type 1 diabetes mellitus. *J Pediatr Endocrinol Metab.,* 5, 433–442

Krukoski, D.W.; Comar., S.R.; Claro, L.M.; Leonart., M.S. & do Nascimento, A.J. (2009). Effect of vitamin C, deferoxamine, quercetin and rutin against tert-butyl hydroperoxide oxidative damage in human erythrocytes. *Hematology.* 14, 168–172.

Kucherenko, Y.U.; Bhauser, S.F.; Grischenko, V.I.; Fischer, U.R.; Huber, S.H.& Lang, F.(2010). Increased cation conductance in human erythrocytes artificially aged by glycation. *J Membr Biol.,* 235, 177-189.

Kurata, M,, Suzuki, M. & Agar, N.S. (1993). Antioxidant systems and erythrcoyte life-span in mammals. *Comp Biochem Physiol B.,* 106, 477-87.

Kurtipek, O.; Comu, F.N.; Ozturk, L.; Alkan, M.; Pampal, K. & Arslan, M. Does vitamin C prevent the effects of high dose dexmedetomidine on rat erythrcpyte deformability? *Bratislavské lekárske listy* PMID 22428760.

Kuypers, F.A. & de Jong, H. (2004). The role of phosphatidylserine in recognition and removal of erythrocytes. *Cell Mol Biol.,* 50, 147-158.

Lang, F.; Gulbins, E.; Lang, P.A.; Zappulla, S.& Foller, M. (2010). Ceramide in suicidal death of erythrocytes. *Cell Physiol Biochem.,* 26, 21-28.

Li, Y; Ma, A; Shao, X. & Du, Z. (2008). Study the effect of antioxidant vitamin E, vitamin C and beta-carotene supplement on erythrocyte functions in elderly persons. *Wei sheng Yan Jiu,* 37, 305-308.

LI, S; Su, Y; LO, M. & Zou, C. (2006). Hemin-mediated hemolysis in erythrocytes: effects of ascorbic acid and glutathione. *Acta Biochimica et Biophysica Sinica,* 38, 63-69.

Liao, K. & Yin, M. (2000). Individual and combined antioxidant effects of seven phenolic agents in human erythrocyte membrane ghosts and phosphatidylcholine liposome systems: importance of the partition coefficient. *J Agric Food Chem.,* 48, 2266-2270.

Lykkesfeldt, J. (2007). Malondialdehyde as biomarker of oxidative damage to lipids caused by smoking. *Clin Chim Acta,* 380, 50-58.

Mahmud, H.; Qadri, S.M.; Foller, M.& Lang, F. (2010). Inhibition of suicidal erythrocyte death by vitamin C. *Nutrition,* 26, 671-676.

Maellaro, E.; Leoncini, S.; Boretti, D., Del Bello, B.; Tanganelli, I.; De Felica, C. & Cilcdi, L. (2011). Erythrocyte caspase-3 activation and oxidative imbalance in erythrocytes and in plasma of type 2 diabetic patient. *Acta Diabetol.* DOI 10.1007/s00592-011-0274-0.

Markovic; S.D.; Dacic; D.D.; Cvetkovic., D.M.; Obradovic., A.D.; Zizic., J.B.; Ognjanovic., B.I.; Stajn, A.S.; Saicic., Z.S. & Spasic, M.B. (2010). Effects of acute treatment of vitamin C on redox and antioxidative metabolism in plasma and red blood cells of rats. *Kragujevac J. Sci.,* 32, 109-116.

Maridonneau, I.; Barquet, P. & Garay, R.P. (1983). Na+ K+ transport damage induced by oxygen free radicals in human red cell membranes. *J Biol Chem.,* 258, 3107-3117.

May, J.M. (1998). Ascorbate function and metabolism in human erythrocyte. *Front Biosci.,* 3, 1-10.

May, J.M..; Qu, Z. & Cobb, C.E. (2004). Human erythrocyte recycling of ascorbic acid. *J Biol Chem.,* 279, 14975-14982.

May, J.M.; Qu, H. & Koury, M.J. (2007). Maturational loss of the vitamin C transporter in erythrocytes. *Biochem Biophys Res Commun.*, 360, 295-298.

Montel-Hagen, A.; Kinet, S.; Manel, N.; Mongellaz, C.; Prohaska, R.; Battini, J.L.; Delaunay, J.; Sitbon, M. & Taylor, N. (2008). Erythrocyte GLUT 1 triggers dehydroascorbic acid uptake in mammals unable to synthesize vitamin C. *Cell*, 132, 1039-1048.

Mozhanova, A.A.; Nurgazizov, N.I. & Bukharaev, A.A. (2003). Local elastic properties of biological materials studied by SFM. SPM-2003. In: *Proceedings Nizhni Novgorod*, March 2–5, 266–267.

Nagababu, E. & Rifkind J.M. (2004). Heme degradation by reactive oxygen species. *Antioxid Redox Signal*, 6, 967-978.

Ogunuro, P.S.; Ogungbamigbe, T.O. & Muhibi, M.A. (2001). The influence of storage period on the antioxidants level of red blood cells and the plasma before transfusion. *Res Commun Mol Pathol Pharmacol.*, 109, 357-363.

Oztürk, O. & Gümüşlü, S. (2004). Changes in g;ucose-6-phosphate dehydrogenase, copper, zinc-superoxide dismutase and catalase activities, glutathione and its metabolizing enzymes, and lipid peroxidation in rat erythrocytes with age. *Exp Gerontol.*, 39, 211-216.

Pandey, K.B. & Rizvi, S.I. (2011). Biomarkers of oxidative stress in red blood cells. *Biomed Pap Med Fac Univ Palacky Olomouc Czech Repub.*, 155, DOI 10.5507/bp.2011.027

Pandey, K.B. & Rizvi, S.I. (2010). Markers of oxidative stress in erythrocytes and plasma during aging in humans. *Oxid Med Cell Longev.*, 3, 2-12.

Pasini, E.M.; Kirkegaard, M.; Mortensen, P.; Lutz, H.U.; Thomas, A.W. & Mann, M. (2006). In-depth analysis of the membrane and cytosolic proteome of red blood cells. *Blood*, 108, 791-801.

Postaire, E.; Regnault, C.; Simone, L.; Rousset, G. & Bejot, M. (1995). Increase of singlet oxygen protection of erythrocytes by vitamin E, vitamin C, and beta carotene intakes. *Biochem Mol Biol Int.*, 35, 371-374.

Rai, D.K.; Rai, P.K.; Rizvi, S.I.; Watal, G. & Sharma, B.(2009). Carbofuran-induced toxicity in rats: protective role of vitamin C. *Exp Toxicol Pathol.*, 61, 531-535.

Repka, T & Hebbel, R.P., (1991). Hydroxyl radical formation by sickle erythrocyte membranes: Role of pathological iron deposits ad cytoplasmic reduicng agents. *Blood*, 87, 2753-2758.

Rivas, C.I.; Zuniga, F.A.; Salas-Burgos, A.; Mardones, L.; Ormazabal, V. & Vera, J.C.(2008). Vitamin C transporters. *J Physiol Biochem.*, 64, 357-375.

Sandhu, I.S.; Yadav, R.; Trivedi. & Bhatnagar, D.J. (1992). Peroxyl radical–mediated hemolysis : role of lipid, protein and sulfhydryl oxidation. *Free Radic.Res.*. 16, 111-122.

Shiva Shankar Reddy, C.S.; Subramanyam, M.V.V.; Vani, R. & Asha Devi, S. (2007). In vitro models of oxidative stress in rat erythrocytes. Effect of antioxdiant supplements. *Toxicol. In Vitro.* 21, 1355-1364.

Siems, W.G.; Sommerburg, O. & Grune, T.(2000). Erythrocyte free radical and energy metabolism. *Clin Nephrol*, 53, S9-S17.

Sivilotti, M.L (2004). Oxidant stress and haemolysis of the human erythrocyte. *Toxicol Rev.* 23, 169–188

Stephen, M.W. & Philips, L.(1985). Hemicrome binding to band 3: Nucleation of Heinz bodies on the erythrocyte membrane. *Biochem.*, 24, 34-39.

Stocker, R.; Hunt, N.H; Weidemann, M.J & Clark, I.A. (1986). Protection of vitamin E from oxidation by incrased ascorbic acid ciontent within *Plasmodium vinckei*-infected erythrocytes. *Biochimica et Biophysica Acta*. 876, 294-299.

Tatara, M. & Ginter, E. (1994). Erythrocyte membrane fluidity and tissue lipid peroxides in female guinea-pigs on graded vitamin C intake. *Physiol.Res.*, 43, 101-105.

Telen, M.J. & Kaufman, R.E (2004). Part II: Normal hematologic system, the mature erythrocyte. In *Wintrobes Clinical Hematology* (Greer JP, Foerster J, Lukens JN, Rodgers GM, Paraskevas F, Glader B eds), pp.217-248. Lippincott Williams & Wilkins, Philadelphia.

Tükel, S.S. (1995). Effects of acetaminophen on methemoglobin, superoxide dismutase and Na(+)-K(+) ATPase activities of human erythrocytes. *Exp.Toxicol Pathol.*, 61, 531-535

Umbreit, J. (2007). Methemoglobin – it's not just blue: a concise review. *Am J Hematol.*, 82, 134-144.

Vani, R.; Shiva Shankar Reddy, C.S. & Asha Devi, S. (2010). Oxidative stress: a study on the effect of antioxidant mixtures during intermittent exposures to high altitude. *Int J Biometeorol,* 54, 553-562.

Wagener, F.; Eggert, A.; Boerman, O.C.; Oyen, W.J.G.; Verhofstad, A.; Abraham, N.G. & Aedema, G. Heme is a potent inducer of inflammation in mice and is counteracted by hemeoxygenase. *Blood*, 98, 1802-1811.

Zan, T.; Tao, J.; Tang, R.C.; Liu, Y.C.; Liu, Y.; Huang, B.; Zhou, J.Y.; Wu, M.H. & Liu, H.L.(2010). Effect of vitamin C antioxidative protection in human red blood cells. *J.Exp.Haematology,* 39, 99-104.

In: Vitamin C   ISBN: 978-1-62948-154-8
Editor: Raquel Guiné   © 2013 Nova Science Publishers, Inc.

Chapter 9

VITAMIN C: LOSS THROUGH COOKING AND CONSERVATION METHODS AND SYMPTOMS OF DEFICIENCY

Marcela A. Leal[*] and Ivana Lavanda[†]
School of Nutrition Director, Faculty of Health Sciences,
Maimonides University, Buenos Aires City, Argentina

ABSTRACT

Humans are unable to synthesise L-ascorbic acid (L-AA, ascorbate, vitamin C), and are thus entirely dependent upon dietary sources to meet needs. Vitamin C (ascorbic acid) is a water-soluble vitamin, necessary for the formation of collagen in bones, cartilage, muscle, and blood vessels; it is also required for the conversion of ferric iron to ferrous iron, which enables the organism to better absorb this mineral. In addition, this vitamin plays an important antioxidant role, contributing to the prevention of degenerative diseases. Human organisms cannot synthesize ascorbic acid; this is why its incorporation through food is essential. Vitamin C requirements vary throughout different stages of life. As years pass by, the recommendations for this vitamin increase and men usually require higher intakes than women. An adult man needs a 90mg daily intake of vitamin C while an adult woman needs a 75mg intake per day.

Vitamin C is mostly found in fresh fruits and vegetables: rosehip, green peppers, citric fruits, strawberries, cabbage, spinach, broccoli, Brussels sprouts, potatoes, amongst other food products. In case of deficient vitamin C consumption, the following symptoms might appear: overall weakness, irritability, pain in muscles and joints, weight loss, weariness, gum bleeding, hemorrhages apparition under the skin, difficulty for wound healing, anaemia.

Vitamin C is easily destroyed by the following factors: heat, contact with oxygen, alkali presence, and dissolution in water. In order to prevent vitamin C loss, foods containing this nutrient must be prepared and served as soon as possible.

---

[*] Marcela A. Leal: School of Nutrition Director, Faculty of Health Sciences, Maimonides University, Buenos Aires, Argentina. E-mail: leal.marcela@maimonides.edu.
[†] Ivana Lavanda: E-mail: nutricion@maimonides.edu.

1. Introduction

The content of vitamin C in fruits and vegetables can be influenced by various factors such as genotypic differences, preharvest climatic conditions and cultural practices, maturity and harvesting methods, and postharvest handling procedures (Seung KL, Kader AA, 2000).

It is important to note that fresh produce, like manufactured foods also undergoes post-harvest change during distribution, marketing and in-home storage, as well as during end-cooking. These changes are such that the nutritional value of the fresh produce as eaten is often quite different to that of the fresh product.

Vitamin C is an important nutrient that carries out several key functions in the organism. Deficiency is not commonly manifested through clinical signs or symptoms or biochemical analysis of nutritional status. The most frequently observed signs of impairment are manifested in dentistry. This chapter explains functions of this nutrient as well as sources of increased consumption.

Finally, it collects information about the most frequent signs of its deficiency as well as usual sources of supplementation and food fortification.

2. Vitamin C: Loss through Cooking and Conservation Methods and Symptoms of Deficiency

2.1. Sources of Vitamin C

Ascorbate is found in many fruits and vegetables. Citrus fruits and juices are particularly rich sources of vitamin C but other fruits including cantaloupe and honeydew melons, cherries, kiwi fruits, mangoes, papaya, strawberries, tangelo, tomatoes, and water melon also contain variable amounts of vitamin C. Vegetables such as cabbage, broccoli, Brussels sprouts, bean sprouts, cauliflower, kale, mustard greens, red and green peppers, peas, and potatoes may be more important sources of vitamin C than fruits, given that the vegetable supply often extends for longer periods during the year than does the fruit supply. The vitamin C content of food is thus strongly influenced by season, transport to market, length of time on the shelf and in storage, cooking practices, and the chlorination of the water used in cooking (WHO -FAO, 2004).

Fruits and vegetables provide different amounts of vitamin C, considering that fruits containing a greater proportion can be consumed raw, which maintains the initial content of vitamin C. Tables 9.1 and 9.2 show several fruits and vegetables that are richest in vitamin C; the values are expressed for each 100 g of food product.

2.2. Function

The biological functions of ascorbic acid are based on its ability to provide reducing equivalents for a variety of biochemical reactions. Because of its reducing power, the vitamin can reduce most physiologically relevant reactive oxygen species.

Table 9.1. L-Ascorbic acid content of selected fruits and vegetables

Source in fruit	mg/100gr
Acerola (west Indian cherry)	1300
Avocado	15-20
Banana	10-30
Blackcurrant	200-210
Redcurrant	40
Passion fruit	25
Grapefruit	40
Guava	230-300
Kiwi	60
Lemon	50
Lychee	45
Melon	10-35
Orange/Organe juice	50
Tangerine	30
Peach	7-31
Pineapple	12-25
Raspberry	25
Rosehip	1000
Strawberry	59-60
Tomato/Tomate juice	25/16

Adapted of: Davey et al., 2000.

Table 9.2. L-Ascorbic acid content of selected vegetables

Source in vegetable	mg/100gr
Brocoli/ Brocoli cooked	113/ 90
Brussels sprouts	87-109
Cabbage (raw)	46-47
Cauliflower / Cauliflower cooked	72/ 55
Horseradish	120
Kale/ Kale cooked	186/ 62
Potato (new)	30
Potato (oct, Nov)	20
Potato (Dec)	15
Potato (Jan, Feb)	10
Potato (Mar, May)	5
Potato (boiled)	16
Spinach/ Spinach cooked	51/28
Waltercress	68-79

Adapted of: Davey et al., 2000.

As such, the vitamin functions primarily as a cofactor for reactions requiring a reduced iron or copper metalloenzyme and as a protective antioxidant that operates in the aqueous phase both intra- and extracellularly. Both the one- and the two-electron oxidation products of the vitamin are readily regenerated in vivo—chemically and enzymatically—by glutathione, nicotinamide adenine dinucleotide (NADH), and nicotinamide adenine dinucleotide phosphate (NAD-PH) dependent reductases.

Vitamin C is known to be an electron donor for eight human enzymes. Three participate in collagen hydroxylation; two in carnitine biosynthesis; and three in hormone and amino acid biosynthesis. The three enzymes that participate in hormone and amino acid biosynthesis are dopamine-β-hydroxylase, necessary for the biosynthesis of the catecholamines norepinephrine and epinephrine; peptidyl-glycine monooxygenase, necessary for amidation of peptide hormones; and 4-hydroxyphenylpyruvatedioxygenase, involved in tyrosine metabolism. Ascorbate's action with these enzymes involves either monooxygenase or dioxygenase activities.

As a cofactor for hydroxylase and oxygenase metalloenzymes, ascorbic acid is believed to work by reducing the active metal site, resulting in reactivation of the metal-enzyme complex, or by acting as a co-substrate involved in the reduction of molecular oxygen. The best known of these reactions is the posttranslational hydroxylation of peptide-bound proline and lysine residues during formation of mature collagen.

In these reactions, ascorbate is believed to reactivate the enzymes by reducing the metal sites of prolyl (iron) and lysyl (copper) hydroxylases Evidence also suggests that ascorbate plays a role in or influences collagen gene expression, cellular procollagen secretion, and the biosynthesis of other connective tissue components besides collagen, including elastin, fibronectin, proteoglycans, bone matrix, and elastin-associated fibrillin). The primary physical symptoms of ascorbic acid's clinical deficiency disease, scurvy, which involves deterioration of elastic tissue, illustrate the important role of ascorbate in connective tissue synthesis.

Ascorbic acid is involved in the synthesis and modulation of some hormonal components of the nervous system. The vitamin is a co-factor for dopamine-β-hydroxylase, which catalyzes hydroxylation of the side chain of dopamine to form norepinephrine, and α-amidating monooxygenase enzymes, involved in the biosynthesis of neuropeptides. Other nervous system components modulated by ascorbate concentrations include neurotransmitter receptors, the function of glutamatergic and dopaminergic neurons, and synthesis of glial cells and myelin.

Because of its ability to donate electrons, ascorbic acid is an effective antioxidant. The vitamin readily scavenges reactive oxygen species (ROS) and reactive nitrogen species (RNS) (e.g., hydroxyl, peroxyl, superoxide, peroxynitrite, and nitroxide radicals) as well as singlet oxygen and hypochlorite. The one- and two-electron oxidation products of ascorbate are relatively nontoxic and easily regenerated by the ubiquitous reductants glutathione and NADH or NAD-PH.

The relatively high tissue levels of ascorbate provide substantial antioxidant protection: in the eye, against photolytically generated free-radical damage; in neutrophils, against ROS produced during phagocytosis; and in semen, against oxidative damage to sperm deoxyribonucleic acid (DNA). Ascorbic acid protects against plasma and low-density lipoprotein (LDL) oxidation by scavenging ROS in the aqueous phase before they initiate lipid peroxidation and possibly by sparing or regenerating vitamin E.

Evidence suggests that ascorbate also provides antioxidant protection indirectly by regenerating other biological antioxidants such as glutathione and α-tocopherol back to their active state (FNB, 2000).

Table 9.3 shows the daily recommended intakes of Vitamin C, according to biological group and age group. As shown in the table, the values slightly vary according to each submitting entity. However, after analysis, the main result shows a very high upper limit intake; making it impossible to reach these higher values through food fortification.

2.3.1. Potential for Maintaining Levels Found in the Fresh Produce

All foods are complex mixtures of components that have the potential to react and interact with each other. In broad terms the milder the treatment and the lower the temperature the better the retention of the vitamin, but there are a host of interacting factors which affect ascorbic acid retention. Firstly, the rates of loss from raw (unprocessed) fruits and vegetables differ widely (Shewfelt RL et al., 1990), and are affected by such factors as surface area (spinach more vulnerable than sprouts), pH (stability in citrus fruits), exposure (peas in pod), protection by other oxygen scavengers (broccoli), and also enzyme (AO, ascorbic acid oxidase) activity.

Table 9.3. Recommended intakes of Vitamin C (mg/day)

	Life stage –Group	EAR (IOM)	RDA (IOM)	UL (IOM)	RNI[a] (FAO)
Infants	0 to 6 mo		40	ND	25
	6 to 12 mo		50	ND	30[b]
Children	1-3y	13	15	400	30[b]
	4-8y	22	25	650	30[b]/35[b]
Males	9-13 y	39	45	1200	40[b]
	14-18 y	63	75	1800	40[b]
	19-30 y	75	90	2000	45
	31-50 y	75	90	2000	45
	51-70 y	75	90	2000	45
	>70 y	75	90	2000	45
Females	9-13 y	39	45	1200	40[b]
	14-18 y	56	65	1800	40[b]
	19-30 y	60	75	2000	45
	31-50 y	60	75	2000	45
	51-70 y	60	75	2000	45
	>70 y	60	75	2000	45
Pregnancy	14-18 y	66	80	1800	55
	19-30 y	70	85	2000	55
	31-50 y	70	85	2000	55
Lactation	14-18 y	95	115	1800	70
	19-30 y	100	120	2000	70
	31-50 y	100	120	2000	70

aAmount required to half saturade body tissues with vitamin C in 97.5% of the population. Larger amount may often be required to ensure an adequate absorption of non-haem iron.
bArbitrary values.

The mechanisms of such losses have not been established for specific fruit and vegetables, and are likely to involve some or all of these processes to varying extents. Storage temperature however is a factor common to all the above mechanisms. Thus, storage at ambient temperatura (20°C) results in greater losses than at chilling temperatures (4°C), which in turn has higher losses than deep frozen (-20°C) produce. Cut spinach deteriorates very rapidly at ambient temperature, with most of ascorbic acid lost in two days, whilst broccoli and podded peas retain their quality for a week at ambient temperature and for several weeks at chill temperature. Not all fruit and vegetable produce is acceptable after freezing but for those that can tolerate it, both ascorbic acid and overall quality can be maintained for a few months. However, losses cannot be eliminated, and for long-term storage, some form of processing is necessary.

Processing, such as blanching and canning, involves heat and water, and with ascorbic acid being heat-sensitive and water-soluble, losses are inevitable. The crucial factor is the time/temperature integral needed to inactivate the key enzymes. Thus, ideally, the fruit or vegetable produce should attain the inactivation temperature rapidly, in the minimum of water, and be held at this temperature for the minimum amount of time possible. It should then be rapidly cooled with the minimum of contact with water. Inevitably compromises have to be made and it is virtually impossible to avoid some loss. The trade-off is that there is minimal further loss from the processed product during long-term storage.

2.3.2. Effects of Processing

The different conservation methods and the following cooking methods applied to different foods determine, in great measure, the specific nutrient content at the moment of food consumption. This particularly happens in vegetables and its relation with certain vitamins' stability. The processing techniques most relevant to fruits and vegetables are canning, freezing and dehydration.

These techniques have been important during the past 50 to 100 years, and will continue to be important in helping to provide all-year-round availability of these foods. All fruits and vegetables are `seasonal', and all, with the exception of certain root crops (eg potatoes), undergo progressive and in some cases quite rapid changes if stored untreated at ambient temperature. These changes are brought about by the various enzymes in the fruit/vegetable in the presence of air, and can affect colour, taste and hence overall palatability, in addition to having profound effects on nutritive values. Vitamin C is used as a marker of deterioration, but as one of the most susceptible nutrients during processing of food. Therefore, eliminate enzyme activity, is essential to to ensure the long-term storage stability (months rather than days) of fruits and vegetables (Breene 1994, Clydesdale 1991, Favel 1998)

The food conservation conventional methods through heat, lead to physicochemical reactions that deteriorate their nutritional value.

In order to guarantee the microbiological security and stability in food, currently there are combined conservation methods that are employed through a sum of obstacles that reduce the intensity of the thermic treatment and maintain the sensory and nutritional characteristics of food products (Fernandez de Rank et al., 2005, Sluka, E. et al., 2004).

In fact, the combined methods application makes it possible to preserve elaborated products, in a secure way at room temperature. In case of vegetables, the microbiological stability is affected by the pH parameter. In this case, the addition of acidifiers is used, amongst which we can find citric, ascorbic and lactic acids.

This addition as an objective to take the pH to values under 4,6 in vegetables that will be heat processed, considering clostridium botulinum as the indicator for microbiological security. This microorganism grows in pH higher than 4,6.

During the canning process, this involves high-temperature treatment (sterilisation) and sealing to exclude air; the freezing process involves a blanching stage, prior to freezing to below -20°C; and dehydration involves hot air treatment to drive off the water. In all cases the temperature and time of treatment reduce unwanted enzyme activity to an acceptable minimal level. Unsurprisingly, this heat treatment also has consequences or labile nutrients and in particular for ascorbic acid (Breene 1994, Clydesdale 1991, Favel 1998).

2.3.3. Industrial Processing

The care to be taken during harvesting of food, as the time it takes place, will have a direct impact on the nutritional quality of the food, like during processing.

Green leafy vegetables, peas (ex-pods), and green beans are particularly vulnerable in the immediate post-harvest period and losses of over 20% of ascorbic acid can occur The thermal treatments (sterilisation in the canning process, blanching in the freezing process, fuidised-bed hot air treatment for the dehydration process, result in further losses which can be particularly significant during canning and dehydration. However, the extent of these losses is highly variable, and during canning is reported to be dependent on such factors as container construction (glass, metal etc.), pH of the food, type of steriliser (batch, continuous, ultra-high temperature) and conduction versus convection heating (Ang CYW and Livingstone GE, 1974). Losses of well over 50% are typical for vegetables, but are much less for most fruits and in particular acid fruits because of the stabilising effects of low pHs.

The dehydration process, which is generally more widely applied to potatoes than to fruit and vegetables, can be very destructive to ascorbic with losses of 75% being reported (Mishkin M, Saguy I and Karel M,, 1984).

The losses that occur during the freezing process occur mainly at the blanching stage, again due to thermal degradation, but also through leaching of nutrients into the blanching medium. In a detailed laboratory study (Klein BP, 1997), ascorbic acid losses during blanching were found to be 10% for sweetcorn, 20% for Green beans and 30% for broccoli. In other work by the same autor (Wu Y, 1992) blanching losses of 20% and 40% were found for green beans and broccoli, respectively. In a more recent study on commercially frozen produce (Favell DJ, 1998) average of ascorbic acid losses during the freezing process were reported to be 30% for peas, 10% for green beans, and 20% for broccoli and in three individual studies on peas, blanching losses were between 26% and 37%, illustrating the extent of variation in a well-controlled commercial system. Such losses will additionally depend on such factors as harvest damage, cutting/slicing, particle size, and type of blancher (steam/water, rotary/cabin). Thus for vegetables, losses through the freezing process are typically in the range of 10 to 40%.

In a study that was focused on capsicum, green beans, and eggplant; applied combined techniques: conservation, based on heat and acid application through scalding with subsequent packing in acid solution, without use of preservatives or sterilization during the elaboration. The conservation process for these vegetables consisted in washing, cutting and scalding at 82°C, during two minutes in citric, lactic and acetic acids solution. The following step consisted in placing them in glass jars with filling solution until they are covered.

This solution has the acids that were mentioned before; ascorbic acid was added at the end of the scalding to avoid losses by heat (Fernandez de Rank et al., 2005).

Through analysis in fresh vegetables and conserved vegetables at 48hs, 3 months and 6 months after elaboration, vitamin C was assessed with the iodine solution qualification method. The analysis showed that the pH values in fresh vegetables are higher than the conserved products values. The reason is the addition of acids in the scalding and filling solution. There are no significant differences for this variable at 48hs, 3 or 6 months of elaboration. Regarding vitamin C, the values in vegetables are higher in conserved products, due to the filling solution composition, which contributes positively to their nutritional value. However, there are significant differences in the storage time, presenting a vitamin C decrease at 3 and 6 months. It is important to point out that even though the decrease in the vitamin C content occurs during storage, the final product is enriched with this vitamin, in relation to the fresh vegetable (Table 9.4) (Fernandez de Rank et al., 2005).

As a conclusion of this study, it needs to be pointed out that the use of combined conservation methods, as the ones previously presented allows the preservation of food products at room temperature and maintains the microbiological safety. Regarding the vegetables that were previously mentioned, fresh green beans and eggplant do not have vitamin C, which means that the use of the filling solution incorporates this nutrient, improving their nutritional quality. Even though the pepper already contains vitamin C, the content of this nutrient was increased through the presented method (Fernandez de Rank et al., 2005).

The low temperature conservation methods (refrigeration and freezing) promote a better vegetable conservation, because they slow down and inhibit enzymatic, respiration and bacterial multiplication activity.

It is important to point out that previousto freezing, vegetables require blanching. This procedure is responsible for the enzymatic inactivation, microorganism elimination and color fixation.

Table 9.4. Vitamin C content in fresh vegetables and conserved vegetables by combined methods (CCM) in capsicum, green beans and eggplant

VEGETABLE	VITAMIN C mg/100gr
Fresh Capsicum	$160 \pm 0,75$
Capsicum 48hs CCM	$290 \pm 0,82^a$
Capsicum 3 months CCM	$250 \pm 0,92^b$
Capsicum 6 months CCM	$234 \pm 0,49^c$
Fresh Green Beans	$19 \pm 0,75$
Green Beans 48hs CCM	$348 \pm 0,85^a$
Green Beans 3 months CCM	$255 \pm 0,90^b$
Green Beans 6 months CCM	$220 \pm 0,75^c$
Fresh Eggplant	$6,0 \pm 0,75$
Eggplant 48 hs CCM	$295 \pm 0,82^a$
Eggplant 3 months CCM	$188 \pm 1,43^c$
Eggplant 6 months CCM	$158 \pm 1,00^b$

*abc Different literals in the same column for the same vegetable differ, P < 0,05.
Adapted of: Fernández de Rank, E. et al., 2005.

One freezing technique is super-freezing, a method that is usually employed in the processed foods elaboration, which combines short time factors and very low temperatures. Food is submitted to a -40°C temperature, and then conserved at -18°C, which allows the conservation of the nutritional and sensory characteristics, and consequently, its quality.

Nevertheless, there is an existent consumer tendency to consider that food products that were submitted to these techniques are of a lower quality, prioritizing the consumption of fresh foods.

Studies that analyze the ascorbic acid content in fresh and ultra-frozen broccoli and cauliflower, and then are submitted to different standardized cooking methods in time, show nutritional quality differences in relation to the techniques that were employed.

Studies that were made in the cruciferous vegetable family or *Brassica oleracea*, and their ascorbic acid content, in relation to the used conservation and post-cooking methods. Through particularly analyzing broccoli and cauliflower, it is observed that they present high respiration rates and sensitivity to heat, highly impacting in considerable loss of nutritional characteristics. In a research carried out in Sao Paulo City, the ascorbic acid in fresh and ultra-frozen broccoli and cauliflower was determined, before and after each cooking method, through spectrophotometers, detecting differences in the content of this vitamin (Borges, R.M. et al., 2004).

In both fresh broccoli and two brands of ultrafrozen broccoli, the major loss is due to boiling, obtaining relevant differences only in ultrafrozen broccoli (in comparisson to the fresh broccoli), and the minor loss is obtained through microwave use. Regarding the cauliflower, in an ultrafrozen brand of this vegetable, the major loss happens during boiling and in the other brand through steam. It can be observed that the ascorbic acid content in fresh broccoli and cauliflower was higher than in the respective samples that were put down through ultra-freezing. Broccoli presents significant differences ($p \leq 0.05$), whereas fresh cauliflower is not significantly different from one of the analyzed ultra-frozen brands. This vitamin instability, followed by the processing of vegetables, such as blanching, freezing and type of cooking, has a repercussion in the difference regarding the vitamin C content. Considering the cooking methods of ultra-frozen broccoli, we can observe significant differences between them ($p \leq 0.05$), in which cooking through boiling lead to a higher loss of vitamin C. In the other cooking methods for broccoli and cauliflower no significant differences were observed. Regarding the methods that best preserve the content of vitamin C in raw vegetables compared to their final content after each cooking method, it can be observed that the steam and microwave methods are the ones that mostly preserve the ascorbic acid. This higher retention of the vitamin is because vegetables are not in contact with water during cooking, avoiding solubility losses. When buying fresh and ultra-frozen vegetables, it is observed that after cooking the first ones present a higher ascorbic acid retention that the second ones (Figure 9.1) (Borges, R.M. et al., 2004).

This difference between fresh and ultra-frozen vegetables can also be attributed to the juice loss, due to cell precipitation, as a consequence of processing, with the following loss of nutrients.

In this way, it can be observed that the fresh vegetables' nutritional quality is higher than in the ultra-frozen, taking the ascorbic acid as an indicator. Nevertheless, this quality can be lower if vegetables are not consumed right after their purchase. Considering this last characteristic and the fact that fresh vegetables are stored before their consumption, the ultra-frozen vegetables' nutritional quality does not compromise the diet's nutritional value.

On the other hand, the time/temperature relation, and the water volume that is employed in vegetables' cooking will determine, more or less, the losses of vitamins, and consequently these food product's nutritional quality. The consumer's capacity to control the parameters that were previously mentioned will determine their election between fresh or processed vegetables (Borges RM et al., 2004 ; Leja M et al. 2001; Barret, D.M. et al., 2000; Marrizal, M.A. et al., 1997).

The *Eugenia stipitata* or araza, known as guava, is a bush that belongs to the Myrtaceae family, which is continuously cultivated, with great adaptation capacities. Nevertheless, because of its short life, when the fresh fruit is stored, it shows antioxidant substances losses, like the ascorbic acid.

Several food products, such as nectar, juices, marmalades and yoghurt, are elaborated from the azara fruit. Considering its application and the fact that this is a very perishable fruit, there is a need to look for alternatives for the conservation of its pulp. One of these alternatives is the pulp freezing to increase its shelf life.

This method, along with scalding, and the control of the freezing and defrosting speed, can contribute to longer product duration. The scalding function is to inactivate enzymes such as catalase, lipase, lipoxygenase, among others, contributing to the decrease of ascorbic acid loss. Nevertheless, this technique, being a thermic treatment, must be properly controlled to avoid a cooked flavor, texture damages and ascorbic acid degradation (Millán, E. et al., 2007).

Studies show that the slow freezing at -20°C maintains the sensory features during the first month of storage. The nutritional quality half-life (time required for the degradation of 50% of the ascorbic acid content) is 80 days.

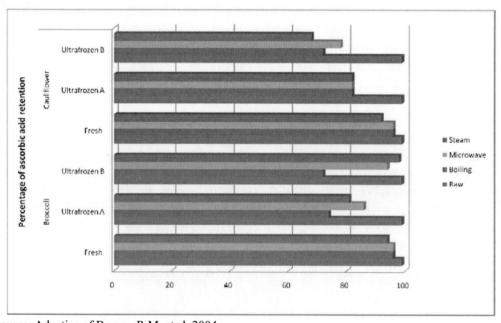

Source: Adaption of Borges, R.M. et al. 2004.

Figure 9.1. Percentage of ascorbic acid retention in fresh and ultrafrozen broccoli and cauliflower submitted to several cooking methods.

The difference between slow freezing and fast freezing is in the size, shape and position of ice crystals. The first ones give the formation of big, extracellular crystals, which cause membrane breaking, deteriorating the plant tissue. On the other hand, the fast freezing leads to the intracellular microcrystal formation that cause less damage to membranes, increasing the food product's shelf life. Regarding the defrosting speed, in fruits and vegetables, its cooking is recommended without previous defrosting.

A study carried out in Bogotá evaluated the effect of scalding, freezing speed and defrosting speed over the nutritional quality of the araza frozen pulp, taking the ascorbic acid as a quality indicator. The scalding was evaluated; two types of defrosting were tested: slow and fast, and short 15 day storage at -20°C. This research shows that de freezing speed and the type of defrosting used do not have an influence on the ascorbic acid stability. However, this stability is decreased, by comparing the ascorbic acid levels in the non-frozen pulp in comparison to the frozen stored pulp after 15 days.

In relation to scalding, it is observed that when the pulp wasn't scalded, the degradation due to the frozen storage effect was increased. At the same time, the degradation during freezing is lower as the scalding time is higher. As a result of what was observed in this study, the araza pulp scalding at times equal or over 7 minutes is a good alternative as a pre-freezing treatment, because as it destroys part of vitamin C, by the effect of heat, it avoids its future degradation during the freezing storage. This is due to the inactivation of enzymes that participate in the degradation of ascorbic acid (ascorbate peroxidase and ascorbate reductase). Less time of scalding will not inactivate these enzymes, with which, during frozen storage, the ascorbic acid degradation would be continuous and higher each time (Millán, E. et al., 2007).

In conclusion, implementing the scalding technique for at least 7 minutes (Temperature in the center equal to 72°C), followed by a fast freezing and slow defrosting is the best combination to control de ascorbic acid degradation, while it alleviates the deterioration of other parameters such as fluid retention, firmness, viscosity index, cohesivity and consistence (Mejía HLJ, 2006, Vargas AM et al. 2005, Zhang M et al. 2004).

In potato strips was evaluated the effect of cutting and storage in air (AIR), modified atmosphere packaging (MAP) and deep-freezing (DF) on the vitamin C content. The L-ascorbic acid content of potato strips derived from five potato cultivars ('Agria', 'Cara', 'Liseta', 'Monalisa' and 'Spunta') previously held in long-term storage was determined. In a second experiment, new-season potato tubers of 'Agria' and 'Spunta' cvs were used. Fresh-cut potato strips were stored for 6 days at 4°C while DF strips were evaluated up to 5 weeks upon storage at −22°C.

All fresh-cut samples stored in AIR showed an increase in ascorbic acid content (16–108%) after 2–4 days at 4°C. At the end of storage, all fresh-cut potatoes stored in AIR had ascorbic acid contents at or above initial concentrations, except new-season 'Spunta' tubers which experienced a 26% decrease. Moreover, potato strips from new-season 'Agria' tubers increased in vitamin C content after 6 days by 12%. Steady state MAP conditions were reached after 2 days with concentrations of 8.2–9.8 kPa CO_2 and 3.1–3.8 kPa O_2 within the packages. Potato strips stored in MAP decreased in ascorbic acid content by 14–34% compared to samples held in AIR.

Frozen storage resulted in a reduced vitamin C content (23%) of 'Spunta' potato strips after 5 weeks while 'Agria' tubers did not show any change. A general increase over time in the respiration rate of potato strips was observed during storage at 4°C.

As a conclusion, vitamin C content of fresh-cut potatoes was retained in AIR storage after 6 days at 4°C while it was reduced in MAP storage and frozen storage at −22°C (Tudela et al., 2002). In general, losses of ascorbic acid are greatest during dehydration, are substantial but slightly less during canning, and are lowest during freezing. These conclusions need however to be viewed in the context of subsequent storage and end-cooking (Davey MW et al., 2000).

2.3.4. Losses during Storage

All raw fruits and vegetables undergo a series of postharvest changes, and the key to the stability of ascorbic acid is the enzyme-catalysed oxidation reactions. As such the composition of the fruit or vegetable, its pH, as well as its integrity (eg whole or chopped, the extent of damage etc) all have a bearing on ascorbic acid retention. As might be expected, the vulnerability of different vegetables and fruits to oxidative loss of ascorbic acid varies greatly, as indeed do general quality changes (ie spoilage). Low pH fruits (citrus fruits) are relatively stable, whereas soft fruits (strawberry, raspberry) undergo more rapid changes. Leafy vegetables (eg spinach) are very vulnerable to spoilage and ascorbic acid loss, whereas root vegetables (eg potatoes) retain quality (and ascorbic acid) for many months. However, with all these products, there is a progressive loss of ascorbic acid with time and the extent of loss is profoundly affected by temperature. Reducing the temperature from ambient (20°C) to chill (4°C) significantly reduces losses in peas, broccoli and spinach, and further temperature reduction to freezer temperatures (ie -18°C) will additionally reduce the rate of loss. Even at these temperatures however, losses of ascorbic acid and overall quality continue to occur. The enzyme catalysed oxidation reactions responsible for this spoilage can be eliminated by thermal treatment and as a result of processing, frozen and canned vegetables and fruits do survive subsequent long-term storage with little or no further loss of ascorbic acid (Favell DJ 1998).

2.3.5. Conservation and Domestic Cooking

In-home freezing of vegetables and fruit is often used to extend the storage life of seasonally available fruit and vegetable produce. There is little reported literature on the nutritional value of such products, but where the methods employed mimic the corresponding commercial processes, then losses during processing can be expected to be much the same. Differences arise when the vegetable produce is not blanched, and in this case, while losses during the freezing process would be expected to be small, the storage capabilities of the product will be much reduced and the rate of loss of ascorbic acid much higher. In-home cooking can have quite a significant effect on the ultimate nutrient delivery to the consumer, particularly that of the labile, water-soluble ascorbic acid. The losses of ascorbic acid that occur during the cooking of fresh fruits and vegetables are as high, if not higher, than those that occur during the cooking of processed produce (Davey MW et al., 2000).

In a study on fresh vegetable produce average losses from spinach were reported to be 60% through boiling, 46% through steaming, and 58% through pressure cooking (Rumm-Kreuter D and Demmel I, 1990). The same authors conformed that in the cooking of broccoli and green beans, the largest losses occurred during boiling and the smallest during steaming. Surprisingly the paper also reported that large losses occur during microwave cooking, but the inference from the paper was that the microwave cooking was done in the same ratio of wáter to vegetable as boiling.

This contrasts markedly with a cooking study on six different frozen vegetables (Gould M and Golledge D 1989) which reported that significantly higher levels of ascorbic acid were retained in microwave cooking versus conventional boiling; in this case minimal water was added to vegetables during the microwave cooking.

In a study (Novello B, 1999) the retention of ascorbic acid in cooked frozen spinach and the losses of the nutrients in the cooking water were examined. The study showed the importance of the ratio of water to vegetable employed, with most of the cooking loss from the vegetable being due to leaching into the water rather than thermal degradation. Again the losses were lowest with microwave cooking in minimal water.

In other study, fresh spinach was assayed for total reduced ascorbic acid content, before and after cooking by a microwave and conventional method. Mean ascorbic acid content of raw, microwave cooked and conventionally cooked spinach was 26.5 mg/lOOg, 13.5 mg/100g, and 17.0 mg/lOOg, respectively. Ascorbic acid content was decreased significantly by both cooking methods; retention was 47% in microwave and 51% in conventionally cooked spinach (Klein BP et al., 1981).

In a study on the nutrient quality of vegetables prepared by conventional and cook-freeze methods, four selected vegetables prepared by boiling were frozen and stored for six months at -18°C. Ascorbic acid was determined on the raw vegetables, again immediately after cooking (boiling), and then after microwave heating of the stored produce. The greatest loss of ascorbic acid occurred during boiling, with only small further losses during storage and microwave re-heating.

Losses during re-heating of canned produce are generally small, as are the losses during the reconstitution of dehydrated vegetables. However, as with all vegetables ascorbic acid contents will decrease if the produce is maintained at an elevated temperature, for instance if food is placed in a `bain-marie' for a long time prior to serving and ascorbic acid losses of 40% have been reported for cooked mashed potatoes held on a "steam table" for a period of 1h (Augustin J et al. 1977).

2.4. Symptoms of Deficiency of Vitamin C

2.4.1. Evidence on Dental Health and Vitamin C

Vitamin C can intervene in the periodontal disease through one or more mechanisms (Castro Porras I, 2009):

1   Vitamin C low levels affect the collagen metabolism of periodontum, which affects the tissue capacity for its regeneration and repair. At the cellular level, the deficiency is shown as the lack of collagen formation that affects the proline hydroxylation.
2   Vitamin C deficiency intervenes with bone formation and leads to alveolar bone loss (Klokkevold et al., 2004; Staudte et al., 2005).
3   Vitamin C deficiency increases the permeability oral mucous and the gum line epithelium for endotoxins (Klokkevold et al., 2004). Some studies show that it can increase significantly the non-keratinized oral mucous epithelium for bacterial endotoxins; this is why vitamin C might play an important role in the gum epithelium decreased permeability and in preventing the penetration of these toxic substances towards the periodontal tissues (Nishida et al., 2000).

4   Low vitamin C levels decrease the neutrophil chemotaxis, which affects the microorganisms' oxidative destruction. In addition, the neutrophil and the host's tissue integrity preservation is altered to neutralize the neutrophil oxidation products during the respiration metabolic process (Nishida et al., 2000).

5   If vitamin C does not achieve its optimum values, the periodontal microvessels' integrity is altered as well as the vascular response towards the bacterial irritation and the wound healing process (Klokkevold et al., 2004).

6   The vitamin C depletion may interfere with the ecological balance of dental plaque and increase its pathogenicity (Klokkevold et al., 2004). As it is a physiological antioxidant, it may generate an unfavorable environment for the presence and optimum P. gingivalis growth. It is possible that its extreme deficiency increases the P. gingivalis colonization, which can also affect the periodontal tissue's healing.

In senior citizens (ages 50 years old and over) that participated in the third National Health and Nutrition Examination Survey (NHANES III) survey (5,958 participants), the associations between the number of posterior occlusal pairs of teeth and the nutritional status was examined. Impaired dentition was assessed by number of posterior occluding pairs of teeth (grinding teeth, n_8 pairs), and complete denture status. Nutritional status was measured by nutrient intake, Healthy Eating Index (HEI) score, serum values, and body mass index (BMI). The results indicated that the subjects that had more dental occlusions presented lower HEI scores: lower consumption of servings of fruits, lower serum values of beta carotene and ascorbic acid.

At the same time, participants in one or more groups with impaired dentition had lower dietary intake levels of vitamin A, carotene, folic acid, and vitamin C, and presented a lower score in diet variety, cholesterol, and sodium components of the HEI. Among dentate individuals over age 65, more than 50% had at least one missing premolar or molar tooth. Replacement of missing posterior teeth is not a universally accepted practice. The cost of prosthetics may be an important issue for elderly people, many of whom do not have dental insurance or do not make regular visits to the dentist. This suggests that tooth loss prevention is important. It also indicates that dental health should be obtained as an integral component of nutrition assessment and be acknowledged as part of nutrition counseling (Sahyoun et al., 2003).

In Brazil, the relationship between inadequate nutrient intake and oral health was evaluated in a sample of 887 non-institutionalized elderly people. Oral examination was performed by trained and calibrated examiners and three measurements were considered: number of posterior occluding pairs of natural teeth (POP), number of teeth and overall dental status. Nutrient intake was assessed by a 24-hour diet recall interview. People with no POP were more likely to have inadequate intake of vitamin C (OR = 2.79; 95% CI: 1.16-6.71) than those with 5 or more POP. In conclusion, this study showed that oral health was related to inadequate intake of important nutrients among non-institutionalized elderly people (Andrade et al., 2011).

In an elderly Japanese population, the relation between dental and nutritional status was assessed. The subjects were 182 individuals, aged 65-85 years, who voluntarily participated in a health seminar at Kyoto Prefectural University of Medicine. These subjects were divided into two groups according to the occlusion.

The subjects in the retained contact group were those who had retained molar occlusion with natural teeth. The lost contact group were those who retained molar occlusion with removable partial dentures. The lost contact group reported significantly lower consumption of vegetables and higher consumption of confectionaries (foods rich in sugar) than the retained contact group (P < 0.05); and therefore had significantly lower intake of vitamin C and dietary fibre (P < 0.05). It can be concluded that natural tooth contact loss in the posterior region affects the intake of vitamins and dietary fibre (Yoshida et al., 2011).

The relationship between vitamin C and the severity of periodontitis was studied in the Java project on periodontal diseases. The assessed population consisted on subjects from the Malabar/Purbasari tea estate on West Java, Indonesia. Clinical measurements were performed in 123 subjects, including evaluation of plaque, bleeding on probing, pocket depth and attachment loss. Plasma levels of vitamin C were between 0.02 to 34.45 mg/l with a mean of 7.90 mg/l (±5.35). The coefficient correlation between plasma vitamin C level and periodontal attachment loss was −0.199 (p<0.05); stepwise linear regression revealed that vitamin C levels explained 3.9% of the variance in periodontal attachment loss. Subjects with vitamin C deficiency (14.7% of the study population) had more attachment loss compared with those with depletion or normal plasma vitamin C values. Therefore, the negative association between plasma vitamin C levels and periodontal attachment loss suggests that vitamin C deficiency may contribute to the severity of periodontal breakdown (Amaliya et al., 2007).

The relation between vitamin C and periodontitis has been shown with higher evidence in a random sample that included 431 men, 194 from Finland and 237 from Russia. The plasma vitamin C concentration was determined by o-phtaldialdehyde–fluorometry, and serum immunoglobulin G antibodies to Actinobacillus actinomycetemcomitans and Porphyromonas gingivalis were determined by a multiserotype enzymelinked immunosorbent assay (ELISA). In the combined Finnish and Russian population, the antibody levels to P. gingivalis were negatively correlated with vitamin C concentrations (r = -0.22; P < 0.001); this association remained statistically significant (P = 0.010) in a linear regression model after adjustment for confounding factors. The proportion of P. gingivalis-seropositive subjects decreased while increasing vitamin C concentrations (P for trend, <0.01), but no trend was seen among A. actinomycetemcomitans-seropositive subjects. In this way, authors conclude that P. gingivalis infection is associated with low concentrations of vitamin C in plasma, which may increase colonization of P.gingivalis or disturb the healing of the infected periodontium (Pussinen et al., 2003). A research evaluated the vitamin C plasma levels and inflammatory measures in periodontitis patients before and after the consumption of grapefruit. Fifty-eight patients with chronic periodontitis were assigned to the test group (non-smokers n=21, smokers n=17) and a diseased control group (non-smokers n=11, smokers n=9). Furthermore, 22 healthy subjects were recruited to compare vitamin C plasma levels between periodontally diseased and healthy subjects. Clinical evaluations, including plaque index (PI), sulcus bleeding index (SBI), probing pocket depths (PPD) and plasma vitamin C levels, were performed at baseline, and after two weeks of grapefruit consumption. Significantly reduced plasma vitamin C levels in the test group and diseased controls were observed in comparison to the healthy controls. Firstly, smokers showed lower levels of vitamin C (mean 0.39±0.17 mg dl-1) than non-smokers (mean 0.56±0.29 mg dl-1). After grapefruit consumption, the mean plasma vitamin C levels rose significantly in the test group compared to the diseased controlled group (non-smokers: 0.87±0.39 mg dl-1, smokers: 0.74±0.30 mg dl-1).

Furthermore the SBI was reduced in the test group (non-smokers: from 1.68±0.6 to 1.05±0.6, p<0.001), whereas PI and PPD were unaffected. The present results show that periodontitis patients are characterised by plasma vitamin C levels below the normal range, especially in smokers. The intake of grapefruit leads to an increase in plasma vitamin C levels and improves sulcus bleeding scores. Longer term studies are necessary to determine whether other periodontal outcomes improve with such supplementation, particularly in smokers. It is possible that the recommendation of vitamin C rich foods could support the management of periodontal disease (Staudte et al., 2005).

2.4.2. Vitamins and the Treatment of Oral and Dental Diseases

While vitamin therapies are important in the treatment of vitamin deficiencies, current literature reveals only limited success of vitamin therapies in the treatment of oral and dental diseases. Furthermore, vitamin therapy has potential toxicity issues. A review evaluated the relevance of vitamin therapy regarding oral and dental conditions. There are a number of nutritional deficiencies that are manifested within the oral cavity. Therefore, the inference of nutritional deficiencies may be first discovered upon an oral examination and often by dentists. Any utilization of pharmacotherapy must begin with a risk-benefit analysis. If the risk/benefit appraisal is within a grey area, it is then necessary for the clinician to educate the patient and allow the patient to be part of the discussion and decision.

It is established that several water soluble vitamins have relatively low toxicity levels and at least a premise for successful therapy (Brown et al., 2010).

A new therapy that has been tested was the vitamin C incorporation in chewing gum. To indicate the effectiveness of its use and as a prophylaxis for the plaque formation prevention, a study took place to assess the release of vitamin C from chewing gum and its effects on supragingival calculus formation. It was evaluated whether vitamin C in chewing gum, alone or in combination with carbamide, (i) influences calculus formation, and (ii) whether carbamide affects the release, stability and uptake of vitamin C in chewing gum. A significant reduction in the total calculus score was observed after the use of vitamin C (33%) and vitamin C + carbamide (12%) gums compared with no gum use; this reduction was mostly pronounced in the heavy calculus formers. A reduced amount of visible plaque was also observed after use of vitamin C and non-vitamin C gum, but only the vitamin C gum reduced the number of bleeding sites (37%). In a separate study, the release, stability and uptake of vitamin C were evaluated using the iodine titration method in both saliva and urine after exposure to the following gums: vitamin C + carbamide (30 mg + 30 mg) and vitamin C (30 mg). There was no indication that carbamide affected the release, stability or uptake of vitamin C when used in a chewing gum (Lingström et al., 2005).

CONCLUSION

Fruits and vegetables are the major food source of vitamin C, but it is necessary to consider a number of factors that modify its contents from the moment of harvest and since ascorbic acid is one of the more reactive compounds it is particularly vulnerable to treatment and storage conditions.

In broad terms the milder the treatment and the lower the temperature the better the retention of the vitamin, but there are a host of interacting factors which affect ascorbic acid retention. In general, losses of ascorbic acid are greatest during dehydration, are substantial but slightly less during canning, and are lowest during freezing.

Previous studies demonstrate a relationship between the lack of vitamin C and an increased risk of periodontal disease. Vitamin C is involved in immunological functions, for eg. Phagocytosis, wound healing and it also presents antioxidant properties. These functions make periodontal therapy and prevention relevant.

ACKNOWLEDGMENTS

The present chapter has been reviewed by:

- María Elisa Zapata (MSc), School of Nutrition, Faculty of Chemistry, Latin-American Educational Centre University (UCEL), Rosario, Santa Fe, Argentina.
- Liliana B. Ascaino, School of Nutrition, Faculty of Health Sciences, Adventista Del Plata University (UAP), Entre Rios, Argentina.

REFERENCES

Amaliya, M. F., Timmerman, F., Abbas, B. G., Loos, G. A., Van der Weijden, A. J., Van Winkelhoff, E. G., Winkel, U., Van der Velden. (2007) Java project on periodontal diseases: the relationship between vitamin C and the severity of periodontitis. *Journal of Clinical Periodontology,* Volume 34, Issue 4, pages 299–304

Andrade, Fabiola Bof; de França Caldas Junior, Arnaldo; Kitoko, Pedro Makumbundu; Zandonade, Eliana. (2011) The relationship between nutrient intake, dental status and family cohesion among older Brazilians. *Cad. Saúde Pública, Rio de Janeiro,* 27(1):113-122.

Ang, C. Y. W. and Livingstone, G. E. (1974). *Nutritive losses in the home storage and preparation of raw fruits and vegetables, in Nutritional Qualities of Fresh Fruits and Vegetables*, Ed. by White, P. L. and Selvey, N., Futura Publishing Co, Mount Kisco, pp. 121-132

Arroqui, C., et al. (2001) Effect of different soluble solids in the water on the ascorbic acid losses during water blanching of potato tissue. *Journal of Food Engineering* Vol. 47, pp. 123-126.

Augustin, J., Toma, R. B., True, R. H., Shaw, R. L., Teitzel, C., Johnson, R. S., and Orr, P. (1977). Composition of raw and cooked potato peel and Fresh: Proximate and vitamin composition. *J. Food Sci.* 44:805-806

Baduí, S. (2006) Química de los alimentos. *Pearson Educación.* México, pp. 25, 387- 395.

Barret, D. M., et al. (2000) Blanch time and cultivar effects on quality of frozen and stored corn and broccoli. *Journal of Food Science* Vol. 65 (3), pp. 534-539,

Borges, R. M., et al. (2004) Análisis sensorial y ácido ascórbico de hortalizas en fresco y ultracongeladas. *Cienc. Tecnol. Aliment.* Vol. 4, N°4 pp. 240-245.

Borutta, A. (2005) Vitamin C intake and periodontal disease. Director of the WHO Collaboration Centre, Prevention of oral diseases. doi: 10.1038/sj.bdj.4812616. *Br. Dent. J.* 199: 210

Breene, W. M. (1994). Healthfulness and nutritional quality of fresh versus processed fruit and vegetables: A review. *J. Foodservice Systems* 8:1-45

Brown, R. S., Glascoe, A., Feimster, T., Lawrence, L. M., Marshall, K., Harland, B. (2010) Vitamins and the Treatment of Oral and Dental Diseases. *Dent. Today.* Dec.;29(12):51-2, 54, 56; quiz 57, 50.

Castro Porras, I. (2009) Vitamina C y enfermedad periodontal. *Publicación Científica Facultad de Odontología • UCR • N°11*

Clydesdale, F. M., Ho, C. T., Lee, C. Y., Mondy, N. I., and Shewfelt, R. L. (1991). The effects of post-harvest treatment and chemical interactions on the bio-availability of ascorbic acid, thiamin, vitamin A, carotenoids, and minerals. *CRC Crit. Rev. Food Sci. Nutr.* 30:599-638

Davey, M. W., Van Montagu, M., Inze, D., Sanmartin, M., Kanellis, A., Smirnoff, N., Benzie, I. J. J., Strain, J. J., Favell, D., Fletcher, J. (2000) Plant L-ascorbic acid: chemistry, function, metabolism, bioavailability and effects of processing. *J. Sci. Food Agric.* 80:825-860

Favell, D. J. (1998). A comparison of the vitamin C content of fresh and frozen vegetables. *Food Chem.* 62:59-64

Fernández de Rank, E., et al. (2005) Tecnologías de conservación por métodos combinados en pimiento, chaucha y berenjena. *Rev. FCA* UNCuyo. *Tomo XXXVII. N°2*, pp. 73-81.

Food an Nutrition Board (2000). Institute of Medicine. Doetary Reference Intakes for Vitamin C, Selenium and Carotenoids.

Gould, M. and Golledge, D. (1989) Ascorbic acid levels in conventionally cooked versus microwave oven cooked frozen vegetables. *J. Food Sci. Nutr.* 42:145-152

Klein, B. P., Kuo, C. H. Y., Boyd, G. 1981. Folacin and Ascorbic Acid Retention in Fresh Raw, Microwave, and Conventionally Cooked Spinach. *Journal of Food Science*, 46(2): 640–64.

Klein, B. P. (1997). Stability of nutrients in fresh and processed vegetables. *Pillsbury Product Communication*

Klokkevold, P. R., Mealey, B. L. y Carranza, F. A. (2004). *Influencia de enfermedades y trastornos sistémicos sobre el periodoncio. En S. K. Haake (Ed.), Periodontología Clínica* (pp. 218-220). México: Mc. Graw Hill Interamericana.Staudte y col., 2005

Lee, C. Y., Massey, L. M. and Van Buren, J. P., (1983).Effects of post-harvest handling and processing on the vitamin contents of peas. *J. Food Sci.* 47:961-964

Leja, M., et al. (2001) Antioxidant ability of broccoli flower buds during short-term storage. *Food Chemistry.* Vol. 72, pp. 219-222.

Davey, M. W., Van Montagu, M., Inze, D., Sanmartin, M., Kanellis, A., Smirnoff, N., Benzie, I. J. J., Strain, J. J., Favell, D., and Fletcher, J. (2000) Plant L-ascorbic acid: chemistry, function, metabolism, bioavailability and effects of processing. *J. Sci. Food Agric.* 80:825±860.

Marrizal, M. A., et al. (1997) Retention of vitamin C, iron and beta-carotene in vegetables prepared using different cooking methods. *Journal of Food Quality.* Vol. 20(5), pp. 403-418.

Mejía, H. L. J., et al. (2006) Cambios físicos, químicos y sensoriales durante el almacenamiento congelado de pulpa de arazá (Eugenia stipitata Mc Vaught). *Agronomía Colombiana* 24, pp. 87-95.

Millán, E., et al. (2007) Efecto del escaldado, de la velocidad de congelación y de descongelación sobre la calidad de la pulpa congelada de azará (Eugenia stipitata Mc Vaught). *Agronomía Colombiana* 25 (2), pp. 333-338.

Mishkin, M., Saguy, I. and Karel, M. (1984). A dynamic test for kinetic models of chemical changes during processing: Ascorbic acid degradation in dehydrated potatoes. *J. Food Science* 49:1276-1274

Monserrat, S., et al. (2001). Mango: conservación por métodos combinados. *Rev. de la Asoc. Argentina de Horticultura.* Vol. 20 (48), pp. 79, 2001.

Nishida, M., Grossi, S. G., Dunford, R., Ho, A. W., Trevisan, M., Genco, R. (2000) Dietary Vitamin C and the Risk for Periodontal Disease. *J. Periodontology Aug.;* 71 (8): 1215-1223.

Novello, B. 1999 Ascorbic acid and folate retention in cooked spinach.:(unpublished).

Parrott, D. L. (1992) Use of ohmic heating for aseptic processing of food particulates. *Food Technol.* 46:68-72.

Pussinen, Pirkko J.; Laatikainen, Tiina; Alfthan, Georg; Asikainen, Sirkka and Jousilahti, Pekka (2003). Periodontitis Is Associated with a Low Concentration of Vitamin C in Plasma. *Clinical And Diagnostic Laboratory Immunology, Sept.* Vol. 10, No. 5 ,p. 897–902

Rees, J. and Bettison, J. (1994) *Procesado térmico y envasado de los alimentos.* Zaragosa. Acribia, pp. 288.

Rumm-KreuterDand Demmel, I. (1990) Comparison of vitamin losses in vegetables due to various cooking methods. *J. Nutr. Sci. Vitaminol.* 36:S7-S15.

Sahyoun, Nadine R.; Lin, Chien-Lung; Krall, Elizabeth (2003) Nutritional status of the older adult is associated with dentition status. *J. Am. Diet Assoc.;*103:61-66

Sauer, F. (1971). Vitamin fortification of dehydrated potato products. *Proc. 20th Ann. National Potato Utilisation Conf., ARS,*

Seung, K. L., Kader, A. A. 2000 Preharvest and postharvest factors influencing vitamin C content of horticultural crops. *Postharvest Biology and Technology.,* 20(3):207-220.

Shewfelt, R. L. (1990). Sources of variation in the nutrient content of agricultural commodities from the farm to the consumer. *J. Food Qual.* 13:34-54.

Sluka, E., et al. (2004) Incidencia de factores combinados en la conservación de pulpa de ají. *La Alimentación Latinoamericana.* Vol. 249, pp. 62-65.

Staudte, B. W. Sigusch and Glockmann E. Grapefruit consumption improves vitamin C status in periodontitis patients (2005). *Br. Dent. J.* 199: 213–217

Tudela, J. A., Espin, J. C., Gil, M. I. 2002 Vitamin C retention in fresh-cut potatoes. *Postharvest Biology and Technology.,* 26(1): 75-84.

Vargas, A. M., et al. (2005) Capacidad antioxidante durante la maduración del azará (Eugenia stipitata Mc Vaught). *Rev. Col. Quím.* 34, pp. 7-65.

World Health Organization and Food and Agriculture Organization of the United Nations. (2004) Vitamin and mineral requirements in human nutrition.

Wu, Y., Perry, A. K. and Klein, B. P. (1992). Vitamin C and b-carotene in fresh and frozen green beans and broccoli in a simulated system. *J. Food Qual.* 15:87-96

Zhang, M., et al. (2004) Effects off freezing conditions on quality of areca fruits. *J. Food eng.* 61, pp. 393-397.

In: Vitamin C
Editor: Raquel Guiné

ISBN: 978-1-62948-154-8
© 2013 Nova Science Publishers, Inc.

Chapter 10

PHARMACOLOGICAL EFFECTS OF ASCORBIC ACID

Muhammad Ali Sheraz,[*] Marium Fatima Khan,[†]
Sofia Ahmed[‡] and Iqbal Ahmad[§]

Departments of Pharmaceutics and Pharmaceutical Chemistry, Institute of
Pharmaceutical Sciences, Baqai Medical University, Karachi, Pakistan

ABSTRACT

Ascorbic acid (also known as vitamin C) is one of the most widely used vitamin both
medically and pharmaceutically. Since its discovery, ascorbic acid (AA) has been found
to be of great importance due to its effectiveness and antioxidant properties in various
clinical applications. Scurvy was the first disease condition that was effectively cured by
using AA. However, since then a number of investigations have been made to further
evaluate the effectiveness of this vitamin in different clinical symptoms. Based on the
recent literature findings, the pharmacological applications of AA in various conditions
such as osteoarthritis, common cold, heart diseases, hypertension, cancer, diabetes
mellitus, asthma, pregnancy, wound healing, gout, cataract and glaucoma, depression,
Parkinsonism, schizophrenia, Alzheimer disease, and urinary tract infections have been
reviewed along with the adverse effects and some contraindications associated with the
vitamin.

1. INTRODUCTION

L-ascorbic acid (or simply ascorbic acid) is also known as Vitamin C, antiascorbutic
vitamin, cevitamic acid, L-xyloascorbic acid, Acidum ascorbicum, 3-oxo-L-gulofurano-
lactone, L-threo-hex-2-enonic acid γ-lactone, etc. (O'Neil, 2013; Sweetman, 2009; Moffat et

---

[*] Muhammad Ali Sheraz: Department of Pharmaceutics, Institute of Pharmaceutical Sciences, Baqai Medical
University, Toll Plaza, Super Highway, Gadap Road, Karachi-74600, Pakistan. E-mail: ali_sheraz80@hotmail.
com.
[†] Marium Fatima Khan: E-mail: marium87@gmail.com.
[‡] Sofia Ahmed: E-mail: sofia.ahmed@baqai.edu.pk.
[§] Iqbal Ahmad: E-mail: iqbal.ahmed@baqai.edu.pk.

al., 2004; Rowe et al., 2009). It is a well-known vitamin, with people claiming it as a cure for almost many diseases and problems such as from cancer to the common cold. Ascorbic acid (AA) is water soluble and is easily destroyed by oxidation (Rowe et al., 2009; Ahmad et al., 2010, 2011, 2012a,b; Sheraz et al., 2011).

Plants and most animals synthesize their own AA but humans are unable to synthesize it. They lack this ability due to the deficiency of an enzyme, L-gulono-gamma-lactone oxidase, which catalyzes the terminal step in AA biosynthesis (Nishikimi et al., 1994). AA is extensively used in its native or in the form of a derivative such as sodium ascorbate and ascorbyl palmitate as an ingredient in variety of pharmaceutical and anti-aging cosmetic products (Rowe et al., 2009; Ahmad et al., 2011, 2012a,b; Sheraz et al., 2011).

2. PHARMACOLOGICAL UTILIZATION OF AA

A number of pharmacological effects in addition to the treatment of scurvy have been identified for AA since its discovery. Majority of these findings are still under investigation and needs further evaluation before being recommended clinically. The well-recognized biological activities of AA are as follows:

2.1. Scurvy

The most common disease resulting with the deficiency of AA is scurvy. Early symptoms associated with scurvy may be non-specific such as weakness and muscular pain. Other clinical indications may include keratosis of hair follicles with 'corkscrew' hair, spontaneous and / or perifollicular hemorrhages, swollen and spongy gums with bleeding and infection, loosening of teeth, bruising, anemia, delayed wound healing, etc. (Kumar and Clark, 2009).

The treatment includes administration of AA in a divided dose of 250 mg per day for few days. Daily intake of fresh fruits and vegetables is also recommended (British National Formulary, 2011; Porter, 2011; Kumar and Clark, 2009).

2.2. Osteoarthritis

AA is involved in the synthesis of collagen, which helps in the formation of cartilage. Osteoarthritis is a disease condition which affects cartilages and exerts pressure on bones and joints. Similarly, formation of free radicals in the body is also considered to be involved in the destruction of cartilage along with the damage to the cells and DNA. The use of AA in the treatment of osteoarthritis is not fully understood and clinically supported.

However, few studies have reported the beneficial role of AA in the treatment, whereas some other studies have shown no significance of the use of this vitamin in the treatment of osteo- or any other type of arthritis (Frech and Clegg, 2007; Peregoy and Wilder, 2011; Canter et al., 2007; Rosenbaum et al., 2010).

2.3. Common Cold

AA in the treatment of common cold has been recommended and used for almost six decades. However, some controversy has so far been accumulated regarding its clinical effectiveness in the treatment of common cold. Various workers have reported it to be of significance but similarly many studies have rejected it to be of any value in common cold (Nahas and Balla, 2011; Uchide and Toyoda, 2011; Audera et al., 2001; Douglas et al., 2004, 2007; Maggini et al., 2012). Recently, Hemila and Chalker (2013) have extensively reviewed the use of AA in common cold. After reviewing a number of studies, they concluded that AA supplementation had failed to reduce the incidence of common cold in general population but it still might be useful for people exposed to brief periods of severe physical exercise. However, few studies have shown the effectiveness of this vitamin but others failed to reproduce those clinical findings. Therefore, more trials are needed to be carried out to further understand the importance of AA in the treatment of common cold (Hemila and Chalker, 2013).

2.4. Heart Diseases

Consumption of fruits and vegetables has been associated with reduced risk of cardiovascular diseases but there is no consistent data available regarding the therapeutic use of various vitamins in heart diseases (Block et al., 2001; Michels et al., 2005; Pfister et al., 2011; Riccioni et al., 2012). The plasma concentration of AA is considered as a biomarker which reflects fruits and vegetables consumption (Michels et al., 2005; Harding et al., 2008; Pfister et al., 2011).

In the study performed on healthy men and women an inverse relationship was observed between the plasma AA concentration and risk of heart failure (Pfister et al., 2011). Oral intake of AA has been found to improve sympathetic functioning of patients with myocardial infarction that resulted in better exercise capacity (Kato et al., 2006). Its higher intake is also associated with a decreased risk of angina in drinkers due to a biological interaction between AA and alcohol (Simon and Hudes, 1999). In contrast, some workers have reported no beneficial effect of AA in heart diseases (Gomes et al., 2011; Bjordahl et al., 2012; Riccioni et al., 2012).

2.5. Hypertension

Like heart diseases, various studies have also shown an inverse relationship between plasma AA concentrations and hypertension. A reduction of both systolic and diastolic blood pressure has been reported by the intake of AA (Lee et al., 2010; Mohammad et al., 2010; Donpunha et al., 2011; Fernandes et al., 2011; Myint et al., 2011; Juraschek et al., 2012).

In addition, restoration of the peripheral vasodilation response in mentally stressed obese children was also noted (Fernandes et al., 2011). Majority of these findings are based on several short term trials, therefore, it has been recommended to carry out trials on large population groups before recommending this vitamin in the prevention of hypertension (Juraschek et al., 2012).

2.6. Cancer

AA is known to have potent antioxidant and pro-oxidant properties that reduces or neutralizes the oxidative stress by scavenging reactive oxygen species (ROS). The formation of ROS is associated with the nucleic acid damage and carcinogenesis (Crott and Fenech, 1999; Mamede et al., 2011; Du et al., 2012; Kim et al., 2012; Ullah et al., 2012; Putchala et al., 2013).

A number of *in vitro* and *in vivo* studies involving both animals and humans have shown the potential of this vitamin in the treatment of melanoma, lung cancer, thyroid cancer, breast cancer, oesophageal and colorectal adenocarcinoma, gastric cancer, pancreatic cancer, prostate cancer, bladder cancer, B-cell lymphoma, etc. (Lukic et al., 2012; Mamede et al., 2012; Mikirova et al., 2012; Nagappan et al., 2012; Cha et al., 2013; Putchala et al., 2013). In some cancer patients, intravenous use of high dose of AA is associated with the reduction in the tumor size.

Its intravenous administration is generally considered safe if the patient does not have any history of stone formation in the kidney (Riordan et al., 2005). Oral intake of AA is generally not preferred in cancer patients as it fails to yield high plasma concentration (Cullen, 2010), whereas same intravenous dose was reported to give 25-folds higher blood plasma concentrations of the vitamin (Padayatty et al., 2006).

Intravenous administration of high dose of AA is also known to reduce inflammation in cancer patients by affecting C-reactive protein level and pro-inflammation cytokines (Mikirova et al., 2012). In spite of these outcomes, the use of AA in the treatment of cancers requires further trials and reassessment (Grober, 2009; Padayatty et al., 2006; Hoffer et al., 2008; Ohno et al., 2009).

2.7. Diabetes Mellitus

Some studies have reported a correlation between fruits and vegetables consumption and the incidence of diabetes mellitus. However, like heart diseases, no conclusive evidence has been provided (Ford and Mokdad, 2001; Liu et al., 2004; Harding et al., 2008; Kurotani et al., 2013). In some studies, a lower level of AA has been observed in diabetic patients (Harding et al., 2008; Shim et al., 2010; Dakhale et al., 2011) whereas some others have reported beneficial effect of AA supplementation in type 2 diabetes (Mazloom et al., 2011; Odum et al., 2012; Franke et al., 2013). Extensive study performed on US oldsters concluded a lower diabetes risk among people taking AA or calcium supplements whereas no beneficial correlation was observed for any other multivitamin (Song et al., 2011). Antioxidants such as AA have found useful in diabetic retinopathy due to scavenging the ROS, produced in the retinal cells as a result of insulin therapy (Wu et al., 2012). AA has also found to improve cell survival in diabetic patients by reducing cytotoxicity (Franke et al., 2013).

Another clinical study has recommended the use of oral supplementation of AA with metformin in patients with type 2 diabetes. The combined therapy resulted in better therapeutic outcome as compared to metformin alone in maintaining good glycemic condition (Dakhale et al., 2011).

On the contrary, the use of AA in diabetes mellitus has been discouraged by some workers as no beneficial outcome was observed in their studies (Cuerda et al., 2011; Golbidi et al., 2011; Kataja-Tuomola et al., 2011).

2.8. Asthma

During an acute attack of asthma, an increased amount of ROS is formed due to the oxidative stress (Al-Abdulla et al., 2010). Lower levels of AA were reported to be associated with increased frequency of asthmatic attacks (Kalayci et al., 2000; Kongerud et al., 2003; Harik-Khan et al., 2004; Rubin et al., 2004; Allen et al., 2009). Due to this property, the use of AA in the treatment and prevention of asthma has gained some popularity (Shidfar et al., 2005; Patel et al., 2006; Riccioni et al., 2007).

It has also proved to be effective in the treatment of patients with exercise-induced bronchoconstriction, cough and wheezing (Omenaas et al., 2003; Tecklenburg et al., 2007; Allen et al., 2009). However, more clinical trials should be undertaken to further confirm the protective role of this vitamin in the treatment of asthma and associated conditions (Kaur et al., 2001, 2009; Ram et al., 2004).

2.9. Pregnancy

During pregnancy an appropriate amount of minerals and vitamins is extremely important for consumption for both mother and the child. Like all other vitamins, AA deficiency is associated with some severe complications in pregnancy including eclampsia, pre-eclampsia, premature rupture of membranes, abortion, preterm birth, increased risk of infections, etc. (Dror and Allen, 2012; Kiondo et al., 2011; Osaikhuwuomwan et al., 2011; Ikpen et al., 2012). Although AA is excreted in the milk and is also known to be actively transported to the fetus, it is still considered safe because no maternal toxicity or teratogenic effects have been reported (Dror and Allen, 2012).

2.10. Wound Healing

AA has also been found to be effective in the healing of wounds. Wound healing is a complex procedure that involves a number of steps including collagen deposition and formation of ROS by the inflammatory cells at the wound site.

Various studies involving animal models such as rats and mice have reported effective recovery of the wounds when treated with AA thus showing the potential of this vitamin in healing and reducing inflammation (Collins, 2009; Lima et al., 2009; Ekci et al., 2011; Jewo et al., 2012; Konerding et al., 2012; Lee et al., 2012).

2.11. Gout

AA has also demonstrated some potential in lowering of serum uric acid level, hence, a supplementation of this vitamin may reduce the symptoms of gout. Further trials can establish the usefulness of this vitamin in lowering hyperuricemia and preventing gout (Suresh and Das, 2012; Huang et al., 2005; Gao et al., 2008; Choi et al., 2009; Juraschek et al., 2011).

2.12. Cataracts and Glaucoma

Oxidative stress and formation of ROS are considered to be the major reasons behind the development and progression of age related cataracts. Humans and other diurnal animals contain 20–70 times higher concentrations of AA in ocular tissues as compared to its plasma concentration. High concentration of AA in aqueous humor is known to protect the lens of the eye from the penetration of UV light, thus preventing photo as well as oxidative damage of the eye tissue (Kisic et al., 2012). A strong and inverse correlation has been observed between AA concentration and development of cataracts. Various studies have reported lower levels of the vitamin in elderly patients as compared to normal individuals (Rodríguez-Rodríguez et al., 2006; Yoshida et al., 2007; Linetsky et al., 2008; Nourmohammadi et al., 2008; Jalal et al., 2009; Leite et al., 2009; Ravindran et al., 2011; Kisic et al., 2012). Similarly in the other study, diabetic patients were characterized by lower level of AA radical in cataract lenses as compared to patients without diabetes (Goslawski et al., 2008). In spite of these findings, some workers on the basis of their results have opposed this concept and the use of vitamins in age related cataracts (Christen et al., 2010; Mathew et al., 2012).

Not much work has been carried out regarding the use of AA in the prevention or treatment of glaucoma. However, few studies have reported a reduction of AA level in patients with glaucoma indicating a potential role of this vitamin in the prevention of this disease (Aleksidze et al., 1989; Leite et al., 2009; Yuki et al., 2010).

2.13. Depression

ROS species were reported to play a role in the progression of depression (Moretti et al., 2012). Anxiety and depression are the most common stress-induced psychiatric disorders. A comparative study between anxiety, depression and healthy volunteers was carried out with an aim to establish any correlation in blood serum levels of vitamin A, C and E. Antioxidant therapy as an adjuvant was found useful in the stress-induced psychiatric patients (Gautam et al., 2012) and is suggested for the used in the management of depression (Moretti et al., 2012). In another study, performed on mice, AA produced effects similar to antidepressants (Binfare et al., 2009). Some studies have also reported development of scurvy in patients suffering from depression (Nguyen et al., 2003; Chang et al., 2007).

2.14. Parkinsonism

Oxidative stress is suggested to be one of the factors involved in the etiology and progression of Parkinson's disease (PD) (Paraskevas et al., 2003; Jomova et al., 2010; Sutachan et al., 2012). A new finding based on AA and zinc deficiency-associated Parkinsonism has been recently reported in an 83 years old man (Noble et al., 2013). Intravenous administration of AA and zinc in Parkinsonism or other movement disorders has also been suggested by Shavit and Brown (2013). Paraskevas et al. (2003) measured the levels of vitamin A, E and AA in patients with PD, vascular Parkinsonism (VP) and other syndromes of Parkinsonism, and noted decreased levels of AA and vitamin E in patients of VP only.

However, their findings were opposed by Iwasaki et al. (2004) as no difference in the vitamins level was observed by them in various PD and VP patients. Similarly, Zhang et al. (2002) has reported insignificant correlation between the use of AA with the risk of PD. AA has also been shown to improve the pharmacokinetics of levodopa in patients with PD, which is the most effective drug against this disease (Nagayama et al., 2004).

2.15. Schizophrenia

Schizophrenia is a mental disorder, which is associated with the formation of ROS in response to the use of antipsychotic drugs. Addition of vitamins, especially AA, has been reported to improve the symptoms of schizophrenia as well as in reducing the side effects of the antipsychotic drugs (Hoffer, 2008; Michael et al., 2002; Arvindakshan et al., 2003; Dakhale et al., 2004, 2005; Sivrioglu et al., 2007; Heiser et al., 2010).

Reduced levels of leucocyte AA have been observed in schizophrenic patients. This reduction indicates the depletion of AA body stores with advancing age and hence worsening of the diseased condition (Dadheech et al., 2006).

2.16. Alzheimer Disease

Oxidative stress can induce protein and DNA damage in Alzheimer disease (AD) patients and is therefore related to its pathophysiology (Bowman, 2012; Gackowski et al., 2008; Jomova et al., 2010; Murakami et al., 2011). The concentration of AA is 3–4 times higher in cerebrospinal fluid and about 200 times higher in the neurons as compared to plasma (Bowman, 2012).

Some studies have shown protective activity of AA in the treatment of AD (Bowman, 2012; Harrison, 2012; Bowman et al., 2009; Murakami et al., 2011) while others have discourage the use of this vitamin on the basis of their results or inconsistent data (Landmark, 2006; Boothby and Doering, 2005; Fillenbaum et al., 2005; Galasko et al., 2012).

2.17. Urinary Tract Infections

AA may also be used in the treatment and prevention of urinary tract infections (UTI). Low levels of plasma AA have been observed in patients with UTI (Ciftci et al., 2008). Dietary and endogenous nitrates are excreted in urine, which are reduced to nitrites by nitrate-reducing bacteria such as *E. coli*, *Pseudomonas aeruginosa* and *Staphylococcus aureus*. The acidification of urine by AA converts this nitrite into a variety of nitrogen oxides which are toxic to a variety of microorganisms (Carlsson et al., 2001, 2003). Daily oral administration of 100 mg AA has also been found to reduce the chances of UTI development in pregnant women (Ochoa-Brust et al., 2007).

3. ADVERSE EFFECTS AND CONTRAINDICATIONS

Not much adverse effects or toxicities are associated with the use of AA (Combs, 2008). However, some adverse events associated with its consumption in large doses are as follows:

3.1. Kidney Stones

The use of AA is associated with the formation of kidney stones due to its enzymatic conversion into oxalate. Various workers have reported the formation of stones in individuals consuming AA (Allison, 2013; Combs, 2008; Sweetman, 2009; Baxmann et al., 2003; Traxer et al., 2003; Taylor et al., 2004; Massey et al., 2005; Moyad et al., 2009). Formation of kidney stone has also been reported in a cancer patient treated with intravenous AA who was initially diagnosed with reduced plasma AA levels (Riordan et al., 2005).

3.2. Other Complications

High dose usage of AA may cause diarrhea and other gastrointestinal disturbances. Large doses may also result in disturbed water and electrolyte balance, increased red cell lysis, rebound scurvy and renal calcification (Dollery, 1991; Combs, 2008; Sweetman, 2009). Hemolysis in patients with G-6-PD deficiency following large doses of AA either intravenously or in soft drinks has also been reported (Reynolds, 1993; Sweetman, 2009). Dental enamel erosion has been observed in patients as a consequence of AA consumption (Giunta 1983; Sweetman, 2009; Beyer et al., 2011).

3.3. Contraindications

AA is contraindicated in patients with hyperoxaluria and G-6-PD deficiency (Dollery, 1991; Sweetman, 2009) hemochromatosis or other forms of excess iron accumulation (Combs, 2008).

CONCLUSION

On the basis of the findings of a number of studies, it is now proved that the clinical use of ascorbic acid is not only limited to the treatment of scurvy. This antioxidant has demonstrated a tremendous potential in the prevention and curing of various pathological cases. Its use is associated with very few toxicities or adverse events, which further enhances its medical importance. However, due to some contradictory data, it is necessary to further evaluate the effectiveness of ascorbic acid especially against some devastating disease conditions such as hypertension, various heart diseases, cancers, etc. Future investigations on the vitamin may prove its therapeutic efficacy in a number of diseases and it may be used as a safe supplement for currently available drugs.

ACKNOWLEDGMENTS

The present chapter has been reviewed by:

- Prof. Syed Riaz Baquar (PhD, DSc), Institute of Pharmaceutical Sciences, Baqai Medical University, Karachi, Pakistan.
- Prof. Maxim P. Evstigneev (PhD, DrSci), Sevastopol National Technical University, Sevastopol, Ukraine.

REFERENCES

Ahmad, I.; Sheraz, M. A.; Shaikh, R. H.; Ahmed, S., and Vaid, F. H. M. (2010). Photostability of ascorbic acid in aqueous and organic solvents. *J. Pharm. Res.,* 3, 1237–1239.

Ahmad, I.; Sheraz, M. A.; Ahmed, S.; Bano, R., and Vaid, F. H. M. (2012a). Photochemical interaction of ascorbic acid with riboflavin, nicotinamide and alpha-tocopherol in cream formulations. *Int. J. Cosm. Sci.*, 34, 123–131.

Ahmad, I.; Sheraz, M. A.; Ahmed, S.; Shad, Z., and Vaid, F. H. M. (2012b). Photostabilization of ascorbic acid with citric acid, tartaric acid and boric acid in cream formulations. *Int. J. Cosm. Sci.,* 34, 240–245.

Ahmad, I.; Sheraz, M. A.; Ahmed, S.; Shaikh, R. H.; Vaid, F. H. M.; Khattak, S. U. R., and Ansari, S. A. (2011). Photostability and interaction of ascorbic acid in cream formulations. *AAPS PharmSciTech*, 12, 917–923.

Al-Abdulla, N. O.; Al Naama, L. M. and Hassan, M. K. (2010). Antioxidant status in acute asthmatic attack in children. *J. Pak. Med. Assoc.,* 60, 1023–1027.

Aleksidze, A. T.; Beradze, I. N. and Golovachev, O. G. (1989). Effect of the ascorbic acid of the aqueous humor on the lipid peroxidation process in the eye in primary open-angle glaucoma. *Oftalmol. Zh.,* 2, 114–116.

Allen, S.; Britton, J. R. and Leonardi-Bee, J. A. (2009). Association between antioxidant vitamins and asthma outcome measures: systematic review and meta-analysis. *Thorax,* 64, 610–619.

Allison, S. J. (2013). Stones: Ascorbic acid and risk of kidney stones. *Nat. Rev. Nephrol.,* 9, 187.

Arvindakshan, M.; Ghate, M.; Ranjekar, P. K.; Evans, D. R., and Mahadik, S. P. (2003). Supplementation with a combination of omega-3 fatty acids and antioxidants (vitamins E and C) improves the outcome of schizophrenia. *Schizophr. Res.,* 62, 195–204.

Audera, C.; Patulny, R. V.; Sander, B. H., and Douglas, R. M. (2001). Mega-dose vitamin C in treatment of the common cold: a randomised controlled trial. *Med. J. Aust.,* 175, 359–362.

Baxmann, A. C.; De, O. G.; Mendonça, C., and Heilberg, I. P. (2003). Effect of vitamin C supplements on urinary oxalate and pH in calcium stone-forming patients. *Kidney Int.,* 63, 1066–1071.

Beyer, M.; Reichert, J.; Bossert, J.; Sigusch, B. W.; Watts, D. C., and Jandt, K. D. (2011). Acids with an equivalent taste lead to different erosion of human dental enamel. *Dent. Mater.,* 27, 1017–1023.

Binfare, R. W.; Rosa, A. O.; Lobato, K. R.; Santos, A. R., and Rodrigues, A. L. (2009). Ascorbic acid administration produces an antidepressant-like effect: evidence for the involvement of monoaminergic neurotransmission. *Prog. Neuropsychopharmacol. Biol. Psychiatry,* 33, 530–540.

Bjordahl, P. M.; Helmer, S. D.; Gosnell, D. J.; Wemmer, G. E.; O' Hara, W. W., and Milfeld, D. J. (2012). Perioperative supplementation with ascorbic acid does not prevent atrial fibrillation in coronary artery bypass graft patients. *Am. J. Surg.,* 204, 862–867.

Block, G.; Norkus, E.; Hudes, M.; Mandel, S., and Helzlsouer, K. (2001). Which plasma antioxidants are most related to fruit and vegetable consumption? *Am. J. Epidemiol.,* 154, 1113–1118.

Boothby, L. A. and Doering, P. L. (2005). Vitamin C and vitamin E for Alzheimer's disease. *Ann. Pharmacother.,* 39, 2073–2080.

Bowman, G. L. (2012). Ascorbic acid, cognitive function, and Alzheimer's disease: a current review and future direction. *Biofactors,* 38, 114–122.

Bowman, G. L.; Dodge, H.; Frei, B.; Calabrese, C.; Oken, B. S.; Kaye, J. A., and Quinn, J. F. (2009). Ascorbic acid and rates of cognitive decline in Alzheimer's disease. *J. Alzheimers Dis.,* 16, 93–98.

British National Formulary (BNF) 61. (2011). *British National Formulary* (61st edition, p. 617). London, UK: BMJ Group and RPS Publishing.

Canter, P. H.; Wider, B. and Ernst, E. (2007). The antioxidant vitamins A, C, E and selenium in the treatment of arthritis: a systematic review of randomized clinical trials. *Rheumatology,* 46, 1223–1233.

Carlsson, S.; Wiklund, N. P.; Engstrand, L.; Weitzberg, E., and Lundberg, J. O. (2001). Effects of pH, nitrite, and ascorbic acid on nonenzymatic nitric oxide generation and bacterial growth in urine. *Nitric Oxide,* 5, 580–586.

Carlsson, S.; Govoni, M.; Wiklund, N. P.; Weitzberg, E., and Lundberg, J. O. (2003). In vitro evaluation of a new treatment for urinary tract infections caused by nitrate-reducing bacteria. *Antimicrob Agents Chemother.,* 47, 3713–3718.

Cha, J.; Roomi, M. W.; Ivanov, V.; Kalinovsky, T.; Niedzwiecki, A., and Rath, M. (2013). Ascorbatesupplementation inhibits growth and metastasis of B16FO melanoma and 4T1 breast cancer cells in vitamin C-deficient mice. *Int. J. Oncol.,* 42, 55–64.

Chang, C. W.; Chen, M. J.; Wang, T. E.; Chang, W. H.; Lin, C. C., and Liu, C. Y. (2007). Scurvy in a patient with depression. *Dig. Dis. Sci.,* 52, 1259–1261.

Choi, H. K.; Gao, X. and Curhan, G. (2009). Vitamin C intake and the risk of gout in men: A prospective study. *Arch. Intern. Med.,* 169, 502–507.

Christen, W. G.; Glynn, R. J.; Sesso, H. D.; Kurth, T.; MacFadyen, J.; Bubes, V.; Buring, J. E.; Manson, J. E., and Gaziano, J. M. (2010). Age-related cataract in a randomized trial of vitamins E and C in men. *Arch. Ophthalmol.,* 128, 1397–1405.

Ciftci, H.; Verit, A.; Yeni, E., and Savas, M. (2008). Decreased oxidative stress index of urine in patients with urinary tract infection. *Urol. Int.,* 81, 312–315.

Collins, N. (2009). The facts about vitamin C and wound healing. *Ostomy Wound Manage,* 55, 8–9.

Combs, G. F. (2008). *The Vitamins: Fundamental Aspects in Nutrition and Health* (3rd edition, pp. 235–263) Burlington, MA, US: Elsevier Academic Press.

Crott, J. W. and Fenech, M. (1999). Effect of vitamin C supplementation on chromosome damage, apoptosis and necrosis ex vivo. *Carcinogenesis,* 20, 1035–1041.

Cuerda, C.; Luengo, L. M.; Valero, M. A.; Vidal, A.; Burgos, R.; Calvo, F. L., and Martínez, C. (2011). Antioxidants and diabetes mellitus: review of the evidence. *Nutr. Hosp.,* 26, 68–78.

Cullen, J. J. (2010). Ascorbate induces autophagy in pancreatic cancer. *Autophagy,* 6, 421–422.

Dadheech, G.; Mishra, S.; Gautam, S., and Sharma, P. (2006). Oxidative stress, α-tocopherol, ascorbic acid and reduced glutathione status in schizophrenics. *Indian J. Clin. Biochem.,* 21, 34–38.

Dakhale, G. N.; Chaudhari, H. V. and Shrivastava, M. (2011). Supplementation of vitamin C reduces blood glucose and improves glycosylated hemoglobin in type 2 diabetes mellitus: a randomized, double-blind study. *Adv. Pharmacol. Sci.,* 2011, 195271.

Dakhale, G. N.; Khanzode, S. D.; Khanzode, S. S., and Saoji, A. (2005). Supplementation of vitamin C with atypical antipsychotics reduces oxidative stress and improves the outcome of schizophrenia. *Psychopharmacology (Berl.),* 182, 494–498.

Dakhale, G.; Khanzode, S.; Khanzode, S.; Saoji, A.; Khobragade, L., and Turankar, A. (2004). Oxidative damage and schizophrenia: the potential benefit by atypical antipsychotics. *Neuropsychobiology,* 49, 205–209.

Dollery, C. (1991) *Therapeutic Drugs* (Volume 1, A181–A185) London, UK: Churchill Livingstone.

Donpunha, W.; Kukongviriyapan, U.; Sompamit, K.; Pakdeechote, P.; Kukongviriyapan, V., and Pannangpetch, P. (2011). Protective effect of ascorbic acid on cadmium-induced hypertension and vascular dysfunction in mice. *Biometals,* 24, 105–115.

Douglas, R. M.; Chalker, E. B. and Treacy, B. (2007). Vitamin C for preventing and treating the common cold. *Cochrane Database Syst. Rev.,* 2, CD000980.

Douglas, R. M.; Hemila, H.; D'Souza, R.; Chalker, E. B., and Treacy, B. (2004). Vitamin C for preventing and treating the common cold. *Cochrane Database Syst. Rev.,* 4, CD000 980.

Dror, D. K. and Allen, L. H. (2012). Interventions with vitamins B6, B12 and C in pregnancy. *Paediatr. Perinat. Epidemiol.,* 26, 55–74.

Du, J.; Cullen, J. J. and Buettner, G. R. (2012). Ascorbic acid: chemistry, biology and the treatment of cancer. *Biochim. Biophys. Acta,* 1826, 443–457.

Ekci, B.; Karabicak, I.; Atukeren, P.; Altinlio, E.; Tomaoglu, K., and Tasci, I. (2011). The effect of omega-3 fatty acid and ascorbic acid on healing of ischemic colon anastomoses. *Ann. Ital. Chir.*, 82, 475–479.

Fernandes, P. R.; Lira, F. A.; Borba, V. V.; Costa, M. J.; Trombeta, I. C.; Santos Mdo, S., and Santos Ada, C. (2011). Vitamin C restores blood pressure and vasodilator response during mental stress in obese children. *Arq. Bras. Cardiol.*, 96, 490–497.

Fillenbaum, G. G.; Kuchibhatla, M. N.; Hanlon, J. T.; Artz, M. B.; Pieper, C. F.; Schmader, K. E.; Dysken, M. W., and Gray, S. L. (2005). Dementia and Alzheimer's disease in community-dwelling elders taking vitamin C and/or vitamin E. *Ann. Pharmacother.*, 39, 2009–2014.

Ford, E. S. and Mokdad, A. H. (2001). Fruit and vegetable consumption and diabetes mellitus incidence among US adults. *Prev. Med.*, 32, 33–39.

Franke, S. I. R.; Muller, L. L.; Santos, M. C.; Fishborn, A.; Hermes, L.; Molz, P.; Pereira, C. S.; Wichmann, F. M. A.; Horta, J. A.; Maluf, S. W., and Pra, D. (2013). Vitamin C intake reduces the cytotoxicity associated with hyperglycemia in prediabetes and type 2 diabetes. *BioMed Res. Int.*, 2013, 896536.

Frech, T. M. and Clegg, D. O. (2007). The utility of nutraceuticals in the treatment of osteoarthritis. *Curr. Rheumatol. Rep.*, 9, 25–30.

Gackowski, D.; Rozalski, R.; Siomek, A.; Dziaman, T.; Nicpon, K.; Klimarczyk, M.; Araszkiewicz, A., and Olinski, R. (2008). Oxidative stress and oxidative DNA damage is characteristic for mixed Alzheimer disease/vascular dementia. *J. Neurol. Sci.*, 266, 57–62.

Galasko, D. R.; Peskind, E.; Clark, C. M.; Quinn, J. F.; Ringman, J. M.; Jicha, G. A.; Cotman, C.; Cottrell, B.; Montine, T. J.; Thomas, R. G., and Aisen, P. (2012). Alzheimer's disease cooperative study. Antioxidants for Alzheimer disease: a randomized clinical trial with cerebrospinal fluid biomarker measures. *Arch. Neurol.*, 69, 836–841.

Gao, X.; Curhan, G.; Forman, J. P.; Ascherio, A., and Choi, H. K. (2008). Vitamin C intake and serum uric acid concentration in men. *J. Rheumatol.*, 35, 1853–1858.

Gautam, M.; Agrawal, M.; Gautam, M.; Sharma, P.; Gautam, A. S., and Gautam, S. (2012). Role of antioxidants in generalised anxiety disorder and depression. *Indian J. Psychiatry*, 54, 244–247.

Giunta, J. L. (1983). Dental erosion resulting from chewable vitamin C tablets. *J. Am. Dent. Assoc.*, 107, 253–256.

Golbidi, S.; Ebadi, S. A. and Laher, I. (2011). Antioxidants in the treatment of diabetes. *Curr. Diabetes Rev.*, 7, 106–125.

Gomes, M. E.; El Messaoudi, S.; Lenders, J. W.; Bellersen, L.; Verheugt, F. W.; Smits, P., and Tack, C. J. (2011). High dose ascorbic acid does not reverse central sympathetic over activity in chronic heart failure. *J. Clin. Pharm. Ther.*, 36, 546–552.

Goslawski, W.; Mozolewska-Piotrowska, K.; Gonet, B., and Karczewicz, D. (2008). In vitro level of L-ascorbic acid radical in lenses of patients with senile or diabetic cataract-preliminary study. *Ann. Acad. Med. Stetin*, 54, 65–69.

Grober, U. (2009) Vitamin C in complementary oncology-update 2009. *Med. Monatsschr. Pharm.*, 32, 263–267.

Harding, A. H.; Wareham, N. J.; Bingham, S. A.; Khaw, K.; Luben, R.; Welch, A., and Forouhi, N. G. (2008). Plasma vitamin C level, fruit and vegetable consumption, and the risk of new-onset type 2 diabetes mellitus: the European prospective investigation of cancer-Norfolk prospective study. *Arch. Intern. Med.,* 168, 1493–1499.

Harik-Khan, R. I.; Muller, D. C. and Wise, R. A. (2004). Serum vitamin levels and the risk of asthma in children. *Am. J. Epidemiol.,* 159, 351–357.

Harrison, F. E. (2012). A critical review of vitamin C for the prevention of age-related cognitive decline and Alzheimer's disease. *J. Alzheimers Dis.,* 29, 711–726.

Heiser, P.; Sommer, O.; Schmidt, A. J.; Clement, H. W.; Hoinkes, A.; Hopt, U. T.; Schulz, E.; Krieg, J. C., and Dobschütz, E. (2010). Effects of antipsychotics and vitamin C on the formation of reactive oxygen species. *J. Psychopharmacol.,* 24, 1499–1504.

Hemila, H. and Chalker, E. (2013). Vitamin C for preventing and treating the common cold. *Cochrane Database Syst. Rev.,* 1, CD000980.

Hoffer, L. J. (2008). Vitamin therapy in schizophrenia. *Isr. J. Psychiatry Relat. Sci.,* 45, 3–10.

Hoffer, L. J.; Levine, M.; Assouline, S.; Melnychuk, D.; Padayatty, S. J.; Rosadiuk, K.; Rousseau, C.; Robitaille, L., and Miller, W. H. Jr. (2008). Phase I clinical trial of i.v. ascorbic acid in advanced malignancy. *Ann. Oncol.,* 19, 1969–1974.

Huang, H. Y.; Appel, L. J.; Choi, M. J.; Gelber, A. C.; Charleston, J.; Norkus, E. P., and Miller, E. R. (2005). The effects of vitamin C supplementation on serum concentrations of uric acid: results of a randomized controlled trial. *Arthritis Rheum.,* 52, 1843–1847.

Ikpen, M. A.; Eigbefoh, J.; Eifediyi, R. A.; Isabu, P. A.; Okogbenin, S.; Okogbo, F. O.; Momoh, M., and Ekwedigwe, K. C. (2012). Determination of antioxidant status of pre-eclamptic and normotensive sub-rural Nigerian pregnant women at the Irrua Specialist Teaching Hospital, Irrua, Edo State. *J. Matern. Fetal. Neonatal. Med.,* 25, 2046–2050.

Iwasaki, Y.; Igarashi, O.; Ichikawa, Y.; Kawabe, K., and Ikeda, K. (2004). Vitamins A, C and E in vascular parkinsonism. *J. Neurol. Sci.,* 227, 149.

Jalal, D.; Koorosh, F. and Fereidoun, H. (2009). Comparative study of plasma ascorbic acid levels in senile cataract patients and in normal individuals. *Curr. Eye Res.,* 34, 118–122.

Jewo, P. I.; Duru, F. I.; Fadeyibi, I. O.; Saalu, L. C., and Noronha, C. C. (2012). The protective role of ascorbic acid in burn-induced testicular damage in rats. *Burns,* 38, 113–119.

Jomova, K.; Vondrakova, D.; Lawson, M., and Valko, M. (2010). Metals, oxidative stress and neurodegenerative disorders. *Mol. Cell Biochem.,* 345, 91–104.

Juraschek, S. P.; Miller, E. R. and Gelber, A. C. (2011). Effect of oral vitamin C supplementation on serum uric acid: a meta-analysis of randomized controlled trials. *Arthritis Care Res. (Hoboken),* 63, 1295–1306.

Juraschek, S. P.; Guallar, E.; Appel, L. J., and Miller, E. R. (2012). Effects of vitamin C supplementation on blood pressure: a meta-analysis of randomized controlled trials. *Am. J. Clin. Nutr.,* 95, 1079–1088.

Kalayci, O.; Besler, T.; Kilinç, K.; Sekerel, B. E., and Saraçlar, Y. (2000). Serum levels of antioxidant vitamins (alpha tocopherol, beta carotene, and ascorbic acid) in children with bronchial asthma. *Turk. J. Pediatr.,* 42, 17–21.

Kataja-Tuomola, M. K.; Kontto, J. P.; Männistö, S.; Albanes, D., and Virtamo, J. (2011). Intake of antioxidants and risk of type 2 diabetes in a cohort of male smokers. *Eur. J. Clin. Nutr.,* 65, 590–597.

Kato, K.; Fukuma, N.; Kimura-Kato, Y.; Aisu, N.; Tuchida, T.; Mabuchi, K., and Takano, T. (2006). Improvement of sympathetic response to exercise by oral administration of ascorbic acid in patients after myocardial infarction. *Int. J. Cardiol.,* 111, 240–246.

Kaur, B.; Rowe, B. H. and Ram, F. S. (2001). Vitamin C supplementation for asthma. *Cochrane Database Syst. Rev.*, 4, CD000993.

Kaur, B.; Rowe, B. H. and Arnold, E. (2009) Vitamin C supplementation for asthma. *Cochrane Database Syst. Rev.,* 1, CD000993.

Kim, J.; Lee, S. D.; Chang, B.; Jin, D. H.; Jung, S. I.; Park, M. Y.; Han, Y.; Yang, Y.; Il Kim, K.; Lim, J. S.; Kang, Y. S., and Lee, M. S. (2012). Enhanced antitumor activity of vitamin C via p53 in cancer cells. *Free Radic. Biol. Med.,* 53, 1607–1615.

Kiondo, P.; Welishe, G.; Wandabwa, J.; Wamuyu-Maina, G.; Bimenya, G. S., and Okong, P. (2011). Plasma vitamin C concentration in pregnant women with pre-eclampsia in Mulago hospital, Kampala, Uganda. *Afr. Health Sci.,* 11, 566–572.

Kisic, B.; Miric, D.; Zoric, L.; Ilic, A., and Dragojevic, I. (2012). Antioxidant capacity of lenses with age-related cataract. *Oxid. Med. Cell Longev.,* 2012, 467130.

Konerding, M. A.; Ziebart, T.; Wolloscheck, T.; Wellmann, A., and Ackermann, M. (2012). Impact of single-dose application of TGF-β, copper peptide, stanozolol and ascorbic acid in hydrogel on midline laparatomy wound healing in a diabetic mouse model. *Int. J. Mol. Med.,* 30, 271–276.

Kongerud, J.; Crissman, K.; Hatch, G., and Alexis, N. (2003). Ascorbic acid is decreased in induced sputum of mild asthmatics. *Inhal. Toxicol.,* 15, 101–109.

Kumar, P. and Clark, M. (2009). *Kumar and Clark's Clinical Medicine* (7th edition, p. 223). Spain: Saunders Elsevier Limited.

Kurotani, K.; Nanri, A.; Goto, A.; Mizoue, T.; Noda, M.; Kato, M.; Inoue, M.; Tsugane, S., and the Japan Public Health Center-based Prospective Study Group. (2013). Vegetable and fruit intake and risk of type 2 diabetes: Japan Public Health Center-based Prospective Study. *Br. J. Nutr.*, 109, 709–717.

Landmark, K. (2006). Could intake of vitamins C and E inhibit development of Alzheimer dementia? *Tidsskr Nor Laegeforen,* 126, 159–161.

Lee, J. Y.; Kim, C. J. and Chung, M. Y. (2010). Effect of high-dose vitamin C on oxygen free radical production and myocardial enzyme after tourniquet ischaemia-reperfusion injury during bilateral total knee replacement. *J. Int. Med. Res.,* 38, 1519–1529.

Lee, Y. H.; Chang, J. J.; Chien, C. T.; Yang, M. C., and Chien, H. F. (2012). Antioxidant sol-gel improves cutaneous wound healing in streptozotocin-induced diabetic rats. *Exp. Diabetes Res.*, 2012, 504693.

Leite, M. T.; Prata, T. S.; Kera, C. Z.; Miranda, D. V.; de Moraes Barros, S. B., and Melo, L. A. Jr. (2009). Ascorbic acid concentration is reduced in the secondary aqueous humour of glaucomatous patients. *Clin. Experiment Ophthalmol.*, 37, 402–406.

Lima, C. C.; Pereira, A. P.; Silva, J. R.; Oliveira, L. S.; Resck, M. C.; Grechi, C. O.; Bernardes, M. T.; Olímpio, F. M.; Santos, A. M.; Incerpi, E. K., and Garcia, J. A. (2009). Ascorbic acid for the healing of skin wounds in rats. *Braz. J. Biol.,* 69, 1195–1201.

Linetsky, M.; Shipova, E.; Cheng, R., and Ortwerth, B. J. (2008). Glycation by ascorbic acid oxidation products leads to the aggregation of lens proteins. *Biochim. Biophys. Acta,* 1782, 22–34.

Liu, S.; Serdula, M.; Janket, S. J.; Cook, N. R.; Sesso, H. D.; Willett, W. C.; Manson, J. E., and Buring, J. E. (2004). A prospective study of fruit and vegetable intake and the risk of type 2 diabetes in women. *Diabetes Care,* 27, 2993–2996.

Lukic, M.; Segec, A.; Segec, I.; Pinotić, L.; Pinotić, K.; Atalić, B.; Solić, K., and Vcev, A. (2012). The impact of the vitamins A, C and E in the prevention of gastroesophageal reflux disease, Barrett's oesophagus and oesophageal adenocarcinoma. *Coll Antropol.,* 36, 867–872.

Maggini, S.; Beveridge, S. and Suter, M. (2012). A combination of high-dose vitamin C plus zinc for the common cold. *J. Int. Med. Res.,* 40, 28–42.

Mamede, A. N.; Tavares, S. D.; Abrantes, A. M.; Trindade, J.; Maia, J. M., and Botelho, M. F. (2011). The role of vitamins in cancer: a review. *Nutrition and Cancer,* 63, 479–494.

Mamede, A. C.; Pires, A. S.; Abrantes, A. M.; Tavares, S. D.; Gonçalves, A. C.; Casalta-Lopes, J. E.; Sarmento-Ribeiro, A. B.; Maia, J. M., and Botelho, M. F. (2012). Cytotoxicity of ascorbic acid in a human colorectal adenocarcinoma cell line (WiDr): in vitro and in vivo studies. *Nutr. Cancer,* 64, 1049–1057.

Massey, L. K.; Liebman, M. and Kynast-Gales, S. A. (2005). Ascorbate increases human oxaluria and kidney stone risk. *J. Nutr.,* 135, 1673–1677.

Mathew, M. C.; Ervin, A. M.; Tao, J., and Davis, R. M. (2012). Antioxidant vitamin supplementation for preventing and slowing the progression of age-related cataract. *Cochrane Database Syst. Rev.,* 6, CD004567.

Mazloom, Z.; Hejazi, N.; Dabbaghmanesh, M. H.; Tabatabaei, H. R.; Ahmadi, A., and Ansar, H. (2011). Effect of vitamin C supplementation on postprandial oxidative stress and lipid profile in type 2 diabetic patients. *Pak. J. Biol. Sci.,* 14, 900–904.

Michael, N.; Sourgens, H.; Arolt, V., and Erfurth, A. (2002). Severe tardive dyskinesia in affective disorders: treatment with vitamin E and C. *Neuropsychobiology,* 46, 28–30.

Michels, K. B.; Welch, A. A.; Luben, R.; Bingham, S. A., and Day, N. E. (2005). Measurement of fruit and vegetable consumption with diet questionnaires and implications for analyses and interpretation. *Am. J. Epidemiol.,* 161, 987–994.

Mikirova, N.; Casciari, J.; Rogers, A., and Taylor, P. (2012). Effect of high-dose intravenous vitamin C on inflammation in cancer patients. *J. Transl. Med.,* 10, 189.

Moffat, A. C.; Osselton, M. D. and Widdop, B. (2004). *Clarke's Analysis of Drugs and Poisons* (3rd edition, pp. 649–650). London, UK: Pharmaceutical Press.

Mohammad, A.; Ali, N.; Reza, B., and Ali, K. (2010). Effect of ascorbic acid supplementation on nitric oxide metabolites and systolic blood pressure in rats exposed to lead. *Indian J. Pharmacol.,* 42, 78–81.

Moretti, M.; Colla, A.; de Oliveira Balen, G.; dos Santos, D. B.; Budni, J.; de Freitas, A. E.; Farina, M., and Severo Rodrigues, A. L. (2012). Ascorbic acid treatment, similarly to fluoxetine, reverses depressive-like behavior and brain oxidative damage induced by chronic unpredictable stress. *J. Psychiatr. Res.,* 46, 331–340.

Moyad, M. A.; Combs, M. A.; Crowley, D. C.; Baisley, J. E.; Sharma, P.; Vrablic, A. S., and Evans, M. (2009). Vitamin C with metabolites reduce oxalate levels compared to ascorbic acid: a preliminary and novel clinical urologic finding. *Urol. Nurs.,* 29, 95–102.

Murakami, K.; Murata, N.; Ozawa, Y.; Kinoshita, N.; Irie, K.; Shirasawa, T., and Shimizu, T. (2011). Vitamin C restores behavioral deficits and amyloid-β oligo.merization without affecting plaque formation in a mouse model of Alzheimer's disease. *J. Alzheimers Dis.,* 26, 7–18.

Myint, P. K.; Luben, R. N.; Wareham, N. J., and Khaw, K. T. (2011). Association between plasma vitamin C concentrations and blood pressure in the European prospective investigation into cancer-Norfolk population-based study. *Hypertension,* 58, 372–379.

Nagappan, A.; Park, K. I.; Park, H. S.; Kim, J. A.; Hong, G. E.; Kang, S. R.; Lee do, H.; Kim, E. H.; Lee, W. S.; Won, C. K., and Kim, G. S. (2012). Vitamin C induces apoptosis in

AGS cells by down-regulation of 14-3-3σ via a mitochondrial dependent pathway. *Food Chem.,* 135, 1920–1928.

Nagayama, H.; Hamamoto, M.; Ueda, M.; Nito, C.; Yamaguchi, H., and Katayama, Y. (2004). The effect of ascorbic acid on the pharmacokinetics of levodopa in elderly patients with Parkinson disease. *Clin. Neuropharmacol.,* 27, 270–273.

Nahas, R. and Balla, A. (2011). Complementary and alternative medicine for prevention and treatment of the common cold. *Can. Fam. Physician,* 57, 31–36.

Nguyen, R. T. D.; Cowley, D. M. and Muir, J. B. (2003). Scurvy: a cutaneous clinical diagnosis. *Aust. J. Dermatol.,* 44, 48–51.

Nishikimi, M.; Fukuyama, R.; Minoshima, S.; Shimizu, N., and Yagi, K. (1994). Cloning and chromosomal mapping of the human nonfunctional gene for L-gulono-gamma-lactone oxidase, the enzyme for L-ascorbic acid biosynthesis missing in man. *J. Biol. Chem.,* 269, 13685–13688.

Noble, M.; Healey, C. S.; McDougal-Chukwumah, L. D., and Brown, T. M. (2013). Old disease, new look? A first report of Parkinsonism due to scurvy, and of refeeding-induced worsening of scurvy. *Psychosomatics,* 54, 277–283.

Nourmohammadi, I.; Modarress, M.; Khanaki, K., and Shaabani, M. (2008). Association of serum alpha-tocopherol, retinol and ascorbic acid with the risk of cataract development. *Ann. Nutr. Metab.,* 52, 296–298.

O' Neil, M. J. (2013). *The Merck Index* (15th edition, Electronic version). White House Station, NJ, US: Royal Society of Chemistry, Merck and Co., Inc.

Ochoa-Brust, G. J.; Fernández, A. R.; Villanueva-Ruiz, G. J.; Velasco, R.; Trujillo-Hernández, B., and Vásquez, C. (2007). Daily intake of 100 mg ascorbic acid as urinary tract infection prophylactic agent during pregnancy. *Acta Obstet. Gynecol. Scand.,* 86, 783–787.

Odum, E. P.; Ejilemele, A. A. and Wakwe, V. C. (2012). Antioxidant status of type 2 diabetic patients in Port Harcourt, Nigeria. *Niger. J. Clin. Pract.,* 15, 55–58.

Ohno, S.; Ohno, Y.; Suzuki, N.; Soma, G., and Inoue, M. (2009). High-dose vitamin C (ascorbic acid) therapy in the treatment of patients with advanced cancer. *Anticancer Res.,* 29, 809–815.

Omenaas, E.; Fluge, O.; Buist, A. S.; Vollmer, W. M., and Gulsvik, A. (2003). Dietary vitamin C intake is inversely related to cough and wheeze in young smokers. *Respir. Med.,* 97, 134–142.

Osaikhuwuomwan, J. A.; Okpere, E. E.; Okonkwo, C. A.; Ande, A. B., and Idogun, E. S. (2011). Plasma vitamin C levels and risk of preterm prelabour rupture of membranes. *Arch. Gynecol. Obstet.,* 284, 593–597.

Padayatty, S. J.; Riordan, H. D.; Hewitt, S. M.; Katz, A.; Hoffer, L. J., and Levine, M. (2006). Intravenously administered vitamin C as cancer therapy: three cases. *CMAJ,* 174, 937–942.

Paraskevas, G. P.; Kapaki, E.; Petropoulou, O.; Anagnostouli, M.; Vagenas, V., and Papageorgiou, C. (2003). Plasma levels of antioxidant vitamins C and E are decreased in vascular parkinsonism. *J. Neurol. Sci.,* 215, 51–55.

Patel, B. D.; Welch, A. A.; Bingham, S. A.; Luben, R. N.; Day, N. E.; Khaw, K. T.; Lomas, D. A., and Wareham, N. J. (2006). Dietary antioxidants and asthma in adults. *Thorax,* 61, 388–393.

Peregoy, J. and Wilder, F. V. (2011). The effects of vitamin C supplementation on incident and progressive knee osteoarthritis: a longitudinal study. *Public Health Nutr.*, 14, 709–715.

Pfister, R.; Sharp, S. J.; Luben, R.; Wareham, N. J., and Khaw, K. T. (2011). Plasma vitamin C predicts incident heart failure in men and women in European Prospective Investigation into Cancer and Nutrition-Norfolk prospective study. *Am. Heart. J.*, 162, 246–253.

Porter, R. S. (2011). *The Merck Manual of Diagnosis and Therapy* (19th edition, Electronic version) Whitehouse Station, NJ, US: Merck and Co., Inc.

Putchala, M. C.; Ramani, P.; Sherlin, H. J.; Premkumar, P., and Natesan, A. (2013). Ascorbic acid and its pro-oxidant activity as a therapy for tumours of oral cavity – A systematic review. *Arch. Oral Biol.*, 58, 563–574.

Ram, F. S.; Rowe, B. H. and Kaur, B. (2004). Vitamin C supplementation for asthma. *Cochrane Database Syst. Rev.*, 3, CD000993.

Ravindran, R. D.; Vashist, P.; Gupta, S. K.; Young, I. S.; Maraini, G.; Camparini, M.; Jayanthi, R.; John, N.; Fitzpatrick, K. E.; Chakravarthy, U.; Ravilla, T. D., and Fletcher, A. E. (2011). Inverse association of vitamin C with cataract in older people in India. *Ophthalmology*, 118, 1958–1965.

Riccioni, G.; Barbara, M.; Bucciarelli, T.; di Ilio, C.m and D' Orazio, N. (2007). Antioxidant vitamin supplementation in asthma. *Ann. Clin. Lab. Sci.*, 37, 96–101.

Riccioni, G.; Frigiola, A.; Pasquale, S.; Massimo de, G., and D' Orazio, N. (2012). Vitamin C and E consumption and coronary heart disease in men. *Front Biosci. (Elite Ed.)*, 4, 373–380.

Riordan, H. D.; Casciari, J. J.; González, M. J.; Riordan, N. H.; Miranda-Massari, J. R.; Taylor, P., and Jackson, J. A. (2005). A pilot clinical study of continuous intravenous ascorbate in terminal cancer patients. *P R Health Sci. J.*, 24, 269–276.

Rodriguez-Rodríguez, E.; Ortega, R. M.; López-Sobaler, A. M.; Aparicio, A.; Bermejo, L. M., and Marín-Arias, L. I. (2006). The relationship between antioxidant nutrient intake and cataracts in older people. *Int. J. Vitam. Nutr. Res.*, 76, 359–366.

Rosenbaum, C. C.; O' Mathúna, D. P.; Chavez, M., and Shields, K. (2010). Antioxidants and antiinflammatory dietary supplements for osteoarthritis and rheumatoid arthritis. *Altern. Ther. Health Med.*, 16, 32–40.

Rowe, R. C.; Sheskey, P. J. and Quinn, M. E. (2009). *Handbook of Pharmaceutical Excipients* (4th edition, pp. 43–46). London, UK: Pharmaceutical Press.

Rubin, R. N.; Navon, L. and Cassano, P. A. (2004). Relationship of serum antioxidants to asthma prevalence in youth. *Am. J. Respir. Crit. Care Med.*, 169, 393–398.

Shavit, I. and Brown, T. M. (2013). Simultaneous scurvy and wernicke's encephalopathy in a patient with an ascorbate-responsive dyskinesia. *Psychosomatics*, 54, 181–186.

Sheraz, M. A.; Ahmed, S.; Ahmad, I.; Vaid, F. H. M., and Iqbal, K. (2011). Formulation and stability of ascorbic acid in topical preparations. *Syst. Rev. Pharm.*, 2, 86–90.

Shidfar, F.; Baghai, N.; Keshavarz, A.; Ameri, A., and Shidfar, S. (2005). Comparison of plasma and leukocyte vitamin C status between asthmatic and healthy subjects. *East Mediterr. Health J.*, 11, 87–95.

Shim, J. E.; Paik, H. Y.; Shin, C. S.; Park, K. S., and Lee, H. K. (2010). Vitamin C nurtiure in newly diagnosed diabetes. *J. Nutr. Sci. Vitaminol. (Tokyo)*, 56, 217–221.

Simon, J. A. and Hudes, E. S. (1999). Serum ascorbic acid and cardiovascular disease prevalence in US adults: The Third National Health and Nutrition Examination Survey (NHANES III). *Ann. Epidemiol.,* 9, 358–365.

Sivrioglu, E. Y.; Kirli, S.; Sipahioglu, D.; Gursoy, B., and Sarandöl, E. (2007). The impact of omega-3 fatty acids, vitamins E and C supplementation on treatment outcome and side effects in schizophrenia patients treated with haloperidol: an open-label pilot study. *Prog. Neuropsychopharmacol. Biol. Psychiatry,* 31, 1493–1499.

Song, Y.; Xu, Q.; Park, Y.; Hollenbeck, A.; Schatzkin, A., and Chen, H. (2011). Multivitamins, individual vitamin and mineral supplements, and risk of diabetes among older US adults. *Diabetes Care,* 34, 108–114.

Suresh, E. and Das, P. (2012). Recent advances in management of gout. *QJM,* 105, 407–417.

Sutachan, J. J.; Casas, Z.; Albarracin, S. L.; Stab, B. R.; Samudio, I.; Gonzalez, J.; Morales, L., and Barreto, G. E. (2012). Cellular and molecular mechanisms of antioxidants in Parkinson's disease. *Nutr. Neurosci.,* 15, 120–126.

Sweetman, S. C. (2009). *Martindale: The Complete Drug Reference* (36th edition, pp. 1983–1985). London, UK: Pharmaceutical Press.

Taylor, E. N.; Stampfer, M. J. and Curhan, G. C. (2004). Dietary factors and the risk of incident kidney stones in men: new insights after 14 years of follow-up. *J. Am. Soc. Nephrol.,* 15, 3225–3232.

Tecklenburg, S. L.; Mickleborough, T. D.; Fly, A. D.; Bai, Y., and Stager, J. M. (2007). Ascorbic acid supplementation attenuates exercise-induced bronchoconstriction in patients with asthma. *Respir. Med.,* 101, 1770–1778.

Traxer, O.; Pearle, M. S.; Gattegno, B., and Thibault, P. (2003). Vitamin C and stone risk. Review of the literature. *Prog. Urol.,* 13, 1290–1294.

Uchide, N. and Toyoda, H. (2011). Antioxidant therapy as a potential approach to severe influenza-associated complications. *Molecules,* 16, 2032–2052.

Ullah, M. F.; Bhat, S. H.; Hussain, E.; Abu-Duhier, F.; Ahmad, A., and Hadi, S. M. (2012). Ascorbic acid in cancer chemoprevention: translational perspectives and efficacy. *Curr. Drug Targets,* 13, 1757–1771.

Wu, H.; Xu, G.; Liao, Y.; Ren, H.; Fan, J.; Sun, Z., and Zhang, M. (2012). Supplementation with antioxidants attenuates transient worsening of retinopathy in diabetes caused by acute intensive insulin therapy. *Graefes Arch. Clin. Exp. Ophthalmol.,* 250, 1453–1458.

Yoshida, M.; Takashima, Y.; Inoue, M.; Iwasaki, M.; Otani, T.; Sasaki, S., and Tsugane, S. (2007). JPHC Study Group. Prospective study showing that dietary vitamin C reduced the risk of age-related cataracts in a middle-aged Japanese population. *Eur. J. Nutr.,* 46, 118–124.

Yuki, K.; Murat, D.; Kimura, I.; Ohtake, Y., and Tsubota, K. (2010). Reduced-serum vitamin C and increased uric acid levels in normal-tension glaucoma. *Graefes Arch. Clin. Exp. Ophthalmol.,* 248, 243–248.

Zhang, S. M.; Hernán, M. A.; Chen, H.; Spiegelman, D.; Willett, W. C., and Ascherio, A. (2002). Intakes of vitamins E and C, carotenoids, vitamin supplements, and PD risk. *Neurology,* 59, 1161–1169.

In: Vitamin C
Editor: Raquel Guiné

ISBN: 978-1-62948-154-8
© 2013 Nova Science Publishers, Inc.

Chapter 11

CONTRADICTIONS AND AMBIVALENCES OF VITAMIN C CONSUMPTION ON HUMAN HEALTH: A REVIEW OF THE LITERATURE

Vanessa A. Ferreira[1],*, Ivy S. C. Pires[1],† and Milton C. Ribeiro[2],‡
[1]Departamento de Nutrição, Faculdade de Ciências Biológicas e da Saúde,
Universidade Federal dos Vales do Jequitinhonha e Mucuri, Diamantina,
Minas Gerais, Brasil
[2]Pós Graduação Profissional em Ensino e Saúde, Faculdade de Ciências Biológicas
e da Saúde, Universidade Federal dos Vales do Jequitinhonha e Mucuri, Diamantina,
Minas Gerais, Brasil

ABSTRACT

Vitamin C (ascorbic acid) has numerous physicochemical properties that are fundamental to the proper functioning of the human body; it promotes collagen production, carnitine, biosynthesis of neurotransmitters, among many other functions. Different from others living things, we humans are incapable of synthesize vitamin C, due to the absence of the enzyme that promotes their conversion (gulonolactone oxidase). A deficiency of this vitamin can lead to severe clinical manifestations being the most well documented scurvy. Therefore, the daily intake of vitamin C is essential for the proper maintenance of human life. In this sense, the consumption of dietary sources of vitamin C should be present in our daily diet including citrus fruits and vegetables. The Recommended Dietary Allowance (RDA) for vitamin C (ascorbic acid) is 100-120 mg/day for adults. However, it is important to highlight that there is controversy about the benefits of ascorbic acid consumption on human health. The literature points, especially that the antioxidant properties may contribute on the neutralize free radicals, delaying the premature aging, the protective effect against viral infections, property anti-atherogenesis and anti-carcinogenesis of vitamin and also the immunomodulatory. Taking into consideration the functional importance of vitamin C as a component of the

* E-mail: vanessa.nutr@ig.com.br.
† E-mail: ivycazelli@gmail.com.
‡ E-mail: miltoncribeiro@gmail.com.

human food to the promotion of health and prevention of disease, it has beene noted the growth of a variety of food products fortified with ascorbic acid which are available to world population. Moreover, the excessive intake of this vitamin can lead to clinical condition, such as diarrhea, indigestion and the development of kidney stones. We acknowledge that a detailed study on the adverse effects of vitamin C on the health of populations is an important, current and relevant theme. In this perspective, the objective of this chapter is to review the main evidence on the benefits of vitamin C in human health, and to highlight the adverse effects most commonly observed in the excessive consumption of this vitamin A in populations. The purpose is to present the ambivalences and contradictions of the theme on a contemporary basis, contigent on a review of a consistent literature.

1. INTRODUCTION

Vitamin C, also called ascorbic acid is widely recognized in the scientific field, for performing different physiological functions in the human body and for being used as a preservative in the food industry. Like other water-soluble vitamins, it must be derived from exogenous sources, since they cannot be synthesized by the body. The main dietary sources of this vitamin are citrus fruits, and some vegetables.

The extensive disclosure regarding the consumption of vitamin C in health promotion and disease prevention,generates great interest at society, researchers, food (Abassa et al., 2011) and pharmaceutical industry that may lead to increase production, acquisition and or consumption of foods rich in such vitamin.

In healthy adult humans, the reserve of ascorbic acid is approximately 1500 mg with an average daily intake 45-75 mg. When there isn't the intake of the vitamin, about 3% of the reserves are diminished daily and clinical symptoms of scurvy is presented in about 30 to 45 days when the organic reserve reach below 300 mg (Guilland and Lequeu, 1995). Thus, there has been a longtime recognition that the lack of vitamin C leads to scurvy, a disease that manifests through a variety of clinical symptoms including petechiae, ecchymosis, hyperkeratosis, purpura, gum disease, tooth loss, anemia, muscle degeneration, cardiac hypertrophy, arthritis, swelling, and alopecia. In this situation, the mere treatment with ascorbic acid solves the manifestations of the disease (Olmedo et al., 2006).

Recent work has been attributed to vitamin C many benefits, such as protection against viral infections, antiatherogenic effect (Aguirre et al., 2008; Lee et al., 2004; Osganian et al., 2003; Neumann et al., 2006; Sesso et al., 2008; Who et al., 2002; Who et al., 2001; Wilcoxet et al., 2008; Ye et al., 2008), anticancer (Hutchinson et al., 2012, Yang et al., 2009), and Immunomodulation (Yang et al., 2009). There are reports of vitamin C has been involved in the protection of the vascular endothelium in situations of oxidative stress (Dias et al., 2012; Weinstein et al., 2001), collagen biosynthesis and optimization of iron absorption in humans (Day et al., 2012; Chen et al., 2003). Studies also report that oxidation of lipids in our body causes the production of free radicals and that such action could result in tissue damage and toxic production or harmful compounds, a process known as oxidative stress. In this context the antioxidant compounds are considered very important because they act in order to prevent oxidative stress (Cerqueira et al., 2007, Dias et al., 2012; Frei and Lawson et al., 2008; Yang et al., 2009) or inflammatory processes triggered by exercise (Silva et al., 2012). In contrast, if they are consumed in excess, they can cause vitamin C to produce pro-oxidative effect

(Cerqueira et al., 2007; Green et al., 1994; Halliwell et al., 1999, Lenita et al., 2006; Podoaro et al., 1998, Rover Junior et al., 2001, Welch et al., 1999) and can be involved in the development of kidney stones (Rivas et al. and Yang et al., 2008, 2009).

The science clash about the therapeutic effect of vitamin C is still persistent and often paradoxical because of the contradictions and ambiguities on the consumption of this vitamin. Therefore, this chapter will present the actions and benefits of the micronutrient for human health, based on scientific evidence and epidemiological studies which has recently been the most published.

2. BENEFICIAL EFFECTS OF VITAMIN C IN HUMAN HEALTH

Some studies have associated the consumption of fruits and vegetables rich in vitamin C to prevent the development of cancers of the esophagus, stomach, oral cavity and pancreas, although the mechanisms are still controversial and poorly understood (González et al., 2005; Ramos et al., 2009), It is worth noting that most of these studies are restricted to animal testing.

Several epidemiological evidence suggests that high doses of ascorbate can act as a pro-oxidant in order to reduce the development of cancer cells, while other studies using this and other supplemental antioxidant vitamins (A, C, E and β-carotene) administered alone or in combination, showed no protective effects against carcinomas (Du et al., 2012).

According to a review by Sampaio and Almeida (2009), vitamin C ensures a protective effect on cancer of the cervix, due not only for being an antioxidant, but because of its essential roles in maintaining the integrity and regeneration of the epidermis. These authors also report that it can increase immunity against infections caused by human papillomavirus (HPV). Other studies, however, depict inconsistent investigations as a prevention mechanism. Furthermore, according to Gold et al. (2003) and Halliwell et al. (2001) showed that vitamin C stimulates the immune system, inhibits the formation of nitrosamines and blocks the metabolic activation of carcinogens. However, tumor cells appear to require ascorbic acid and compete with healthy cells of this nutrient.

The relationship among the vitamin C in the prevention and control of chronic diseases has also been discussed in the scientific field. A prospective study that followed European adults for 12 years showed a strong inverse association between serum concentrations of vitamin C and the risk of type 2 diabetes mellitus (Harding et al., 2008). In the same study, the authors found that the consumption of fruits and vegetables were also associated with a lower risk of type 2 DM. It is known that patients with metabolic syndrome or type 2 diabetes have reduced serum concentration of vitamin C supplementation but high doses (800 mg daily) were not able to completely restore the serum concentrations of vitamin C, or to improve the dysfunction Endothelial and insulin resistance in these individuals (Chen et al., 2006).

Observational epidemiologic studies conducted by Catania, et al. (2009) suggest that the high intake of antioxidants from the diet, and especially those diets rich in fruits and vegetables reduce the risk of cardiovascular disease. Moreover, the same authors show that when investing in a micronutrient supplementation with specific antioxidant, such as vitamin C to reduce the incidence of cardiovascular disease, the impact is non –existent or sometimes negative. Regarding mortality, in a study conducted in Sweden, with approximately 40 .000 men aged 45 to 79 years, who were followed for about eight years, there were no associations between vitamin C intake and cardiovascular mortality (Messerer et al., 2008). However,in this same study, men who reported improper diet and use of multivitamin supplements, showed a significant reduction of cardiovascular mortality.

In the neurological, more specifically in Alzheimer's disease, the benefit of vitamin C and other antioxidants has been controversial. In a large observational study showed a reduction in the prevalence and incidence of the disease after three years of supplementation with 500 mg / day. Another similar study found no difference in the incidence of dementia, after monitoring for four years.

For these individuals although the risks of moderate doses of vitamin C are relatively low, a lack of consistent evidence of the efficacy of the vitamin discourages its use in the prevention of disease (Boothby and Doering, 2005).

Vitamin C appears to be involved with strengthening of the immune system. In the systematic review by Douglaset al., (2006) which analyzed the doses of vitamin C in reducing the duration or severity of symptoms of common cold (both prophylaxis and continued after onset of symptoms) revealed the reduction in duration of clinical 8% of adults and 13.5% of the children who were studied. In 15 comparative studies, the severity of respiratory episodes under different measures decreased with intake of vitamin C. The authors also demonstrated that the duration of symptoms showed no significant difference when vitamin C was compared with placebo. Other studies show that despite the significant reduction in the frequency of disease, severity and duration of cold are not affected (Sasazuki et al., 2006).

Several studies report the action of vitamin C as an antioxidant essential for humans. This action is only possible due to its ability to provide electrons, becoming in ascorbic acid (reduced form) or *acid dehydroascorbic,* its oxidized form (Cerqueira et al., 2007, Dias et al., 2012; Frei and Lawson et al., 2008), can neutralize free radicals (Costa, 2004, Dias et al., 2012; Frei and Lawson et al., 2008). According Cerqueira et al., (2007), oxidative stress is characterized by an imbalance in the relationship between the oxidant system and the body's antioxidant defenses, noting a increased with the first one. Oxidative stress is produced by free radicals, ie, molecules that contain one or more unpaired electrons. Due to this feature, free radicals are very unstable and reactive, and pilfer electrons from other molecules in order to pair their electrons. After losing their electrons, those molecules whose electrons are transferred, become unstable and turn into free radicals.

Several authors have reported that the antioxidant defenses of the body become insufficient against oxidative stress acute and chronic oxidative stress, there is a predisposition for the development of a number of degenerative diseases, such as atherosclerosis and diabetes (Lankin et al., 2005), ischemic injury (Saito et al., 2005), cancer (Valko et al., 2006), neurological disorders (Parkinson's disease, amyotrophic lateral sclerosis, Down's syndrome, Alzheimer's disease (Bondy et al., 1995), Hypertension (de la Fuente et al., 2005), eye diseases, including age-related macular degeneration and cataracts (Santosa et al., 2005), among lung diseases such as asthma and chronic obstructive pulmonary disease (Ramhman et al., 2002) and inflammatory diseases such as rheumatoid arthritis (Tak et al., 2000), ulcerative colitis (Prauda et al., 2005) and pancreatitis (Andican et al., 2005). Besides the fact that the chronic effects of free radicals are considered key players in the aging process (Droge et al., 2003; Halliwell et al., 1999).

According Auguto et al. (2006) and Rover Junior et al. (2001) the main substances capable of generating free radicals are oxygen in the ground state (O2) and nitric oxide (NO). The molecules whose electrons are focused on free O2 and nitrogen receive designations of reactive oxygen species (ROS) and nitrogen (ERN), respectively. The main examples of free radicals are super-oxide (O2 • -), the hydroxyl (OH •), thiol (RS •), the trichloromethyl (CHCl3 •) and nitric oxide (NO •). According Chauhan and Chauhan (2006), low concentrations of free radicals, ERROR and RNA are important for the maintenance of cellular redox state for the proper functioning of the immune system and appropriate cell signaling. However, if they are not neutralized, they often react with proteins, lipids and acids, nucleic causing damage to cellular functions. According Cerqueira et al. (2007) Oxidative damage to biomolecules can lead to enzyme inactivation, mutation, membrane rupture, increase in the atherogenicity of low density lipoproteins and cell death.

The authors Chauhan and Chauhan (2006) and Zhu et al. (2007) reported that the central nervous system is particularly vulnerable to damage caused by lipid peroxidation due to its high oxygen consumption, large amounts of polyunsaturated fatty acids and decreased level of antioxidant enzymes compared to other tissues, contributing much to neurodegenerative disorders such as Alzheimer's disease (Bains and Shaw, 1997; Bourdel-Marchasson et al. 2001).

Castro and Freeman (2001), Cui et al. (2004) and Brenneisen et al. (2005) have described the actions for combating cytotoxic ROS cells are equipped with a variety of antioxidant defenses, which include enzymes such as super-oxide dismutase (SOD), catalase and glutationaperoxidase (GPx). Although endogenous antioxidant defenses are effective and not infallible, there is a continuously forming reactive species of oxygen and nitrogen (ROS / RNS) that interact at different levels with the cellular environment prior to disposal, which, at first glance, it may seem an evolutionary failure (Burdon et al., 1996).

Other authors (Apleton et al., 2009; Dauchet et al., 2006; Dias et al., 2012; Hardling et al., 2008, Holt et al., 2009; Lampe et al., 1999) describes the context which is reported as indisputable health benefits associated with the consumption of fruits and vegetables and their antioxidant vitamins. Castro and Freeman (2001) and Mas et al. (2006) reported that vitamins C and E after neutralizing free radicals can be regenerated by the antioxidant system. They work in a synergistic way, so the vitamin E and form the tocoferoxil compound and in order to be regenerated they need electrons provided by vitamin C.

Other authors (Cuddihy et al., 2008; Dias et al., 2012; Foyer and Frei et al., 2011; Halpner et al., 1998; Jacob, 1998; Lawson et al., 2008; Valero et al., 2009) reported on their studies that the most important indirect functions of vitamin C is its ability to regenerate other biologically important antioxidants such as vitamin E and glutathione in its reduced state.

3. ACTION OF VITAMIN C AS A PRO-OXIDANT

Despite the great efficiency of antioxidants, vitamin C also acts, paradoxically, as a pro-oxidant "*in vitro*" (Yang et al., 2009). This is very reactive when consumed in high doses, and it can cause the pro-oxidant effect (Cerqueira et al., 2007; Green et al., 1994; Halliwell et al., 1999; Lenita et al., 2006; Podoaro et al., 1998; Rover Junior et al., 2001; Welch et al., 1999).

This oxidizing effect of vitamin C, inclusive, has been used for decades to induce oxidative modification of lipids, proteins and DNA. Another example of vitamin C act as a pro-oxidant is the Fenton reaction, reduction of hydrogen peroxide by $Cu1+$ or $Fe 2+$ to hydroxyl radical, when it is favored in the presence of vitamin C can reduce the transition metals, making them suitable for this reaction. *In vivo*, metals are found complexed in protein thus unavailable (Halliwell et al., 1999).

Many intervention studies in humans relate to supplementation with vitamin C and oxidative lesions in DNA, including injury and nitrogenous bases of DNA strand breaks. The results are contradictory. It has already occurred a decrease (Green et al., 1994) and a increase (Podoaro et al., 1998) of injuries and in some cases the effects were null (Welch et al., 1999). Despite conflicting data, these authors reiterate the importance of vitamin C as an antioxidant considering the recommended doses, which is usually achieved through food. Halliwell (2000) reported that micronutrients are coenzymes for many enzymes involved in DNA synthesis and repair and apoptosis.

In cell culture studies demonstrate that vitamin C can alter the expression of genes involved in inflammatory response (Berneti et al., 2003), apoptosis (Catani et al., 2002), and cell differentiation (Alcain et al., 1994). The mechanism which this occurs is still unknown, but it is assumed that it acts indirectly by altering the gene expression of endogenous antioxidants or directly modulating the binding of some transcription factors to the core (Lee et al., 2003).

4. THE HYPERVITAMINOSIS C

Excessive consumption of Vitamin C has been reported in some studies. The most common symptom of hypervitaminosis C is diarrhea, probably determined by carrying of large amounts of water into the intestine. Other clinical symptoms also seem to be present such as nausea, vomiting, increased iron absorption and renal damage and the bladder, due to the increase of their excretions, because ascorbic acid is partially converted into oxalic acid, and this may induce lithiasis oxalic (Guilland, 1992).

5. CONSIDERATIONS ON THE EFFECTS OF VITAMIN C, ITS CONSUMPTION AND THE ESTABLISHMENT OF NUTRITIONAL RECOMMENDATIONS FOR POPULATIONS

Despite all the benefits that described Vitamin C as an antioxidant, it can be too reactive when consumed in high doses, causing the pro-oxidant effect (Cerqueira et al., 2007; Green et al., 1994; Halliwell et al., 1999; Lenita et al., 2006; Podoaro et al., 1998; Rover Junior et al., 2001, Welch et al., 1999). Faced with these contradictions and ambivalences of the subject, it is up to the researchers in the nutrition, epidemiology and statistics fields to institute an organized reference in health, assessing the benefits and risks of excessive consumption, mediating information and publishing secure recommendations.

In this sense, even in response to the proven benefits, dietary doses of vitamin C recommended by the "Recommended Dietary Allowance-RDA" (1989) were higher in 2000 at 15 mg for women over 19 years and 30 mg and for men of the same age.

The U. S. daily recommendation for vitamin C intake in 1989 was 60 mg and it was increased to 75 mg for women and 90 mg for men in the international level by publication of "Dietary Reference Intakes" IOM / FNB (2000). Taking into consideration that this recommendation does not correspond either the tenth fraction of 2 g proposed by Pauling in 1970 as the ideal for maintaining health and or below the amount consumed daily by our Paleolithic ancestors (Key et al., 1996). Including 2000 mg which was considered as the maximum level of intake for individuals with more than 19 years old.

For children 1-3 years is 15mg/day, increasing the doses as the age advances 75 mg / day for male adolescents 14-18 years (IOM / FNB, 2000e RDA, 1989). For women the recommendation increases slightly during pregnancy and lactation 80 and 115 mg / day, respectively. For minors below 18 years of age is 85 and 120 mg /day and for adults over 19 respectively (IOM/ FNB, 2000).

Despite the increase recommendation of vitamin C in 2000, international studies show that the consumption of vitamin C remains inadequate in many places. Researchers add that the insufficient intake of micronutrients is among the ten leading risk factors of the global total disease burden worldwide and it is considered the third risk factor for preventable diseases and non-communicable diseases (Leo and Santos, 2012.)

When Canoy et al. (2005) was evaluating the nutritional status DE19, thousand Englishmen between 45-79 years reported that they had low plasma concentrations of ascorbic acid. Other European prospective study, lasting 12 years, found a high prevalence of low serum concentrations of vitamin C (Harding et al., 2008). Moreover, Appleton et al. also found inadequate consumption of fruits and vegetables among older adults in Great Britain (England, Wales and Scotland) and those living in socially deprived areas in 2009. After selecting 426 individuals, the authors observed an average of 4 and 4.1 of fruits and vegetables which were served and consumed on weekdays and weekends, respectively. The same author reports that the amount of fruits and vegetables reported in this study is slightly higher than reported in population from elderly people in Britain.

Ma et al. (2009) studied, in great detail, the data consumption of more than 24 000 Chinese adults between 50 and 79 years by 24 h recalls of the "Health and Nutrition Survey" conducted in 1991, 1993, 1997, 2000, 2004, 2006 and 2009 in nine provinces. These authors observed that the consumption of vitamin C of the population of the rural area decreased between the years 1991 and 2009, an average of 12.1 mg and 11.8 mg for men and women, respectively. Moreover, they observed that the intake of vitamin C, increased by 8.7 and 10.2 mg, respectively, among men and women who lived in the cities. It was reported yet that the intake of vitamin C, from dark green vegetables, decreased 15.1 mg in males and 13.9 mg females from rural areas. The adjustments were found for this vitamin from 19.8% to 30.4% for men in urban, 31.1% to 43.9% for men living in rural areas and in the range of 15.9% to 24, 9% and 26.4% to 38.1% for women in urban and rural areas, respectively. Furthermore, the amount of vitamin C intake by the population of rural and urban is getting closer to the consumption of vegetables and fruits, They are still insufficient.

Su et al. (2012) on the other hand is interested in comparing the eating habits of Chinese born in 1960 and 1980. It was observed that the data of micronutrient intakes were significantly lower in Chinese born in the 60s. Griep et al., for their part in 2013, when they compared the consumption of fruit in the U.S. and in China found that the average consumption in the first country was 52-65 kcal gm/1000 while the second is 68-70 g / 1000 kcal. Azadbakhtet al. (2007) in the district of Tehran, Iran, have identified low vitamin C intake when assessing 926 women.

Particularly in Brazil, for example, there is almost the same consumption profile in several states. Analyzing the data on Brazilian states with higher purchasing power were found inadequate intake of antioxidant nutrients (food sources of vitamin C, A, E, beta carotene, zinc and selenium). Silva et al. (2012) observed that a high percentage of women who engage in regular physical activity in São Paulo, had antioxidant intake below recommended levels (52% compared to the consumption of Vitamin C, 57% relative to Vitamin E consumption, 52% consumption compared to Vitamin A, 52% in simultaneously, ie, the best public awareness about healthy eating and at the same time improving their purchasing power may occur excessive vitamin C intake by this population. Abassa et al. (2011) reports that the scientific evidence on health promotion and consumption of vitamin C has encouraged the emergence of research on food fortification.

In the study by Dias et al. (2012) the authors reported that approximately 90% of vitamin C in the typical human diet comes from vegetables and fruits, such as citrus fruits (lemon, orange), green leafy vegetables (Yang et al., 2009), chilies, papayas, kiwi and tomatoes. According to Liu et al. (2009) Vitamin C can be obtained by daily consumption of fruits, vegetables and supplements. Lenita et al. (2006), however, disagree with the authors mentioned above and reports that ascorbic acid comes from the intake of various food, especially citrus fruits, strawberries, green vegetables and tomatoes, and the evidence on the benefit from vitamin C does not establish its supplementation indiscriminately.

In the work of Key et al. (1996) the authors reported that the bioavailability of vitamin C consumed from fruits and vegetables is approximately 100%. He also reports that the bioavailability is impaired only if this consumption is above 200 mg / day, due to saturation of tissue with consequent lower absorption, or due to processing effects or the presence of flavonoids or other compounds or the effects in processing it Szeto et al. (2004) and Choi et al. (2004) reported that vitamin C is very well absorbed in the gastrointestinal tract. Yang et al. (2009) reported that plasma levels may be increased in response to a diet rich in fruits and vegetables for long periods of time or in cases of supplementation and the vitamin C in these, it is only reduced during the storing and processing. Dias et al. (2012) reported that water soluble vitamin is highly sensitive to water and air temperature and about 25% may be lost by bleaching (boiling or steaming the food for a few minutes). This same degree of loss occurs in freezing vegetables.Cooking for long periods of time (10-20 minutes) may result in a loss of more than 50% of the total content of vitamin C.

For these reasons, the best way to maximize the consumption of vitamin C is to ingest raw vegetables. In this sense, to encourage consumption of healthy foods and optimize the nutritional value of foods, contributes to increase the level of this vitamin in most plant foods. The content of Vitamin C may also be increased by increasing expression of the enzyme responsible for recycling ascorbate (Chen et al., 2003).

Other studies are reflections on the use of supplements containing vitamin C. Dias et al. (2012) reported that high doses of vitamin C may interfere with copper metabolism. Lenita (2006) reports that the widespread use of vitamin C, alone or in combination with other nutrients, a priori cannot be recommended until new and more robust evidence is found. The explanation is that many biochemical functions occurring in different tissues of the body are related to vitamin C and the evidence points to contemporary benefit with few indications, ie in scurvy and age-related macular degeneration. Predominating the lack of efficacy in many others, such as the common cold, preeclampsia, atherosclerosis, hypertension, cataracts, pain and changes in muscle function after exercise, Alzheimer's disease, bronchial asthma and hemodialysis.

Results jobs Osganian et al. (2003) suggest that the intake of vitamin C supplements have a negative association with early atherosclerosis, while vitamin C from foods has a protective association. The results also suggest that adverse reactions of vitamin C supplements may be relatively higher among individuals with elevated cholesterol levels.

Studies report that while diets rich in fruits and vegetables are associated with a reduction in cardiovascular disease (Dauchet et al., 2008, Li et al., 2007, Willcox et al., 2008; Ye et al., 2008) antioxidants from vitamin supplements containing vitamin C, failed to reduce cardiovascular events in randomized controlled trials (Augusto et al., 2006; Cook et al., 2007; Dauchet et al., 2008; Halliwell et al., 2000, Li et al., 2007; Knoops et al., 2004; Sesso et al., 2008; Willcox et al., 2008; Ye et al., 2008). Lee et al. (2004) and Muntwyler et al., (2002) reported, however that the mechanisms for this differential impact between fruits and supplements have not been fully understood.

Halliwell et al. (2000) tried to list some explanations for this dichotomy. When analyzing supplements containing beta-carotene he noted that this is the only one of 600 identified carotenoids,and it may not be the most active. Gray et al. (2008) also described this fact, reporting that while supplements have only one of the existing forms of vitamin, foods rich in these vitamins have combinations among different forms of vitamin. Recent publications suggest that antioxidants are effective in the prevention of chronic diseases associated with oxidative stress when administered to groups that have inadequate plasma concentrations of these micronutrients. The study called SUVIMAX (The Supplémentationen Vitamines et MinérauxAntioxydants) that followed for 7.5 years thousands of French people receiving daily doses of ascorbic acid, alpha-tocopherol and beta carotene found that the reduction of cancer incidence and mortality was observed among males. These were defective in plasma levels of antioxidants administered prior to the study (Hercberg et al., 2004). These authors report that there is no evidence that consumption of foods rich in antioxidants will bring harmful effects throughout the life –cycle. On the contrary, there is strong epidemiological evidence that it is associated with healthy aging and functional longevity.

Other authors explain that maybe the intake of fruits and vegetables will prove more effective than consuming supplements, because they contain components and photochemical that interact, potentialized beneficial effects in the body (Cannella, 2007; Cerqueira et al., 2007; Dai et al., 2006; Halliwell, 2000; Levine et al. 1996). Due the above mentioned, it is believed that supplementation is little recommended because the literature is still inconclusive. It is unable to establish safe and effective dosages. Thus, it is suggested that prospective studies in this area need a longer follow-up (Cardoso et al., 2009).

CONCLUSION

Reviewing this literature we conclude that the role of ascorbic acid on human health is still controversial.More researches and discussions on the mechanisms of action are necessary.Such as "*in vivo*""(experimentation using a whole, living organism as opposed to a partial or dead organism, or an *in vitro* ("within the glass", i.e., in a test tube or petri dish) to understand and elucidate the properties and benefits of ascorbic acid to population health.

REFERENCES

Abassa, S., Weia, C., Hayatb, K. Xiaominga, Z. (2011). Ascorbic Acid: microencapsulation techniques and trends: a review. *Food Reviews international, 28*, 343-374.

Aguirre, R. & May, J. M. (2008). Inflammation in the vascular bed: importance of vitamin C. *Pharmacol Ther., 119,* 96–103.

Alcain, F. J. & Buron, M. I. (1994). Ascorbate is regenerated by HL-60 cells through the transplasmalemma redox system. *J. Bioenerg.Biomembr.,* 26, 8, 393-410.

Andican, G., Gelisgen, R., Unal, E. Tortum, O. B., Dervisoglu, S., Karahasanoglu, T., Burcak, G. (2005). Antioxidants in cardiovascular health and disease. *World J. Gastroenterol, 11, 9,* 23-40.

Appleton, K. M., McGill, R. & Woodside, J. V. (2009). Fruit and vegetable consumption in older individuals in Northern Ireland: levels and patterns. *British Journal of Nutrition,* 102, 949–53.

Augusto, O. (2006) *Radicais Livres: bons, maus e naturais.* São Paulo: Oficina de Textos.

Azadbakht, L., & Esmaillzadeh, A. (2007). Dietary and non-dietary determinants of central adiposity among Tehrani women. *Public Health Nutrition, 1, 5,* 528–34.

Bains, J. S. & Shaw, C. A. (1997). Neurodegenerative disorders in humans: the role of gluthatione in oxidative stress-mediated neuronal death. *Brain Res. Rev., 25, 3,* 335-58.

Bernotti, S., Seidman, E., Sinnett, D., Brunet, S., Dionne, S., Delvim, E. & Levy, E. (2003). Prevention of chronic diseases. *Am. J. Physiol. Gastrointest. Liver Physiol., 285, 6,* 898– 912.

Bondy, S. C. (1995). The relation of oxidative stress and hyperexcitation to neurological disease. *Proc. Soc. Exp. Biol. Med., 208, 6,* 337-44.

Boothby, L. A. & Doering, P. L. (2005). Vitamin C and vitamin E for Alzheimer's disease. *Ann Pharmacother, 39, 12,* 2073- 80.

Bourdel-Marchsson, I., Delmasbeauvieux, M. C., Peuchant, E., Richardhartson, S., Decanps, A., Reignier, B., Emeriau, J. P. & Rainfray, M. (2001). Antioxidant defences and oxidative stress markers in erythrocytes and plasma from normally nourished eldery Alzheimer patients. *Age Ageing, 30, 3,* 235-51.

Brenneisen, P., Steinbrenner, H. & Sies, H. (2005). Selenium, oxidative stress, and health aspects. *Mol. Aspects Med., 26, 4,* 256-67.

Burdon, R. H., Gill, V. & Alliangana, D. (1996). Lipid peroxidation in liver and plasma of ODS rats supplemented with alpha-tocopherol and ascorbic acid. *Free Radical. Res., 24, 4,* 81-96.

Canoy, D., Wareham, N. & Welch, A. (2005). Plasma ascorbic acid concentrations and fat distribution in 19.068 British men and women in the European Prospective Investigation into Cancer and Nutrition Norfolk cohort study. *Am J. Sem. Nutr., 82, 3,* 1203–09.

Cardoso, B. R. & Cozzolino, S. M. F. (2009). Estresse oxidativo na Doença de Alzheimer: o papel das vitaminas C e E. Nutrire: *Rev. Soc. Bras. Alim. Nutr., 34, 3,* 249-59.

Castro, L. & Freeman, B. A. (2011). Reactive oxygen species in human health and disease. *Nutrition, 17, 2,* 161-65.

Catani, M. V., Constanzo, A., Savini, I., Leviero, M., de Laurenzi, V., Wang, J. Y. J., Melino, G. & Avigilian, O. L. (2002). Ascorbate up-regulates MLH1 (Mut L homologue-1) and p73: implications for the cellular response to DNA damage. *Biochem. J. 364, 6,* 441-47.

Catania, S. A., Barros, C. R., Ferreira, S. R. G. (2009). Vitaminas e minerais com propriedades antioxidantes e risco cardiometabólico: controvérsias e perspectivas. *Arq. Bras. Endocrinol. Metab., 53, 5,* 550 – 59.

Cerqueira, F. M., Medeiros, M. H. G. & Ohara, A. (2007). Antioxidantes Dietéticos: controvérsias e perspectivas. *Quim. Nova, 30, 2,* 441-9.

Chauhan, V. & Chauhan, A. (2006). Oxidative stress in alzheimer's disease. *Pathophysiology, 13, 3,* 195-208.

Chen, H., Karne, R. J., Hall, G., Campia, U., Panza, J. A. & Cannon, R. O. (2003). High-dose oral vitamin C partially replenishes vitamin C levels in patients with type 2 diabetes and low vitamin C levels but does not improve endothelial dysfunction or insulin resistance. *Am. J. Physiol. Heart Circ. Physiol., 290, 1,* 137-45.

Choi, S. W., Benzie, I. F.; Collins, A. R.; Hannigan, B. M.; Strain, J. (2004). Vitamins C and E: acute interactive effects on biomarkers of antioxidant defense and oxidative stress. *Mutation Res, 551, 7,* 109-17.

Cook, N. R.; Albert, C. M. & Gaziano, J. M. (2007). A randomized factorial trial of vitamins C and E and beta carotene in the secondary prevention of cardiovascular events in women: results from the Women's Antioxidant Cardiovascular Study. *Arch. Intern. Med., 167,* 1610–618.

Costa, N. M. B. (2004). Biotecnologia aplicada ao valor nutricional dos alimentos. *Biotecnologia, Ciência e Desenvolvimento, 32, 2,* 47-54.

Cuddihy, S. L., Parker, A., Harwood, D. T., Vissers, M. C. & Winterbourn, C. C. (2008). Ascorbate interacts with reduced glutathione to scavenge phenoxyl radicals in HL60 cells. *Free Radic. Biol. Med., 44, 8,* 1637-44.

Cui, K.; Luo, X., Xu, K. & Ven Murthy, M. R. (2004). Role of oxidative stress in neurodegeneration: recent developments in assay methods for oxidative stress and nutraceutical antioxidants. *Prog. Neuropsychopharmacol. Biol. Psychiatry, 28, 5,* 771-99.

Dai, Q., Borenstein, A. R., Wu, Y., Jackson, J. C. & Larson, E. B. (2006). Fruit and Vegetable Juices and Alzheimer's Disease: The Kame Project. *Am. J. Med., 119, 9,* 751-59.

Dauchet, L., Amouyel, P., Hercberg, S. & Dallongeville, J. (2008). Fruit and vegetable consumption and risk of coronary heart disease: a meta-analysis of cohort studies. *J. Nutr., 136,* 2588–93.

Day, R. & Lal, S. S. (2012). Supplementation Effects of Vitamin C and Vitamin E on Oxidative Stress in Post Menopausal Diabetic Women. *Int J Cur Biomed Phar Res, 2*(2), 269-271.

de la Fuente, M.; Hanz, A. & Vallejo, M. C. (2005). Daily requirements, dietary sources and adverse effects vitamin C. *Antiox. Redox Signaling, 7, 3,* 1356-69.

Dias, J. S. (2012). Major Classes of Phytonutriceuticals in Vegetables and Health Benefits. *Journal of Nutritional Therapeutics, 1, 1,* 245-65.

Douglas, R. M., Hemila, H., Chalker, E. & D'Souza, R. R. D. (2006). Treacy B. Vitamin C forpreventing and treating the common cold (Cochrane Review). In: *The Cochrane Library*. Oxford: Update Software.

Droge, W. (2003). Fruit and vegetable consumption and risk of coronary heart disease: a meta-analysis. *Adv. Exp. Med. Biol. 543, 3,* 191-213.

Du, J., Cullen, J. J. & Buettner, G. R. (2012). Ascorbic acid: Chemistry, biology and the treatment of cancer. *Biochimica et Biophysica Acta, 1826, 2, 443-457.*

Frei, B. & Lawson, S. (2008). Vitamin C and cancer revisited. *Proc. Natl. Acad. Sci.,* 105, 32, 1, 1037-38.

Gold, M. D. (2003). Does vitamin C act as a pro-oxidant under physiological conditions? *Integr. Cancer Ther., 2, 3,* 151-68.

González, M. L., Miranda-Massari, J. R., Mora, E. M., Guzmán, A., Riordan, N. R., Riordan, H. D., Casciari, J. J., Jackson, J. A. & Roman-Franco, A. (2005). Orthomolecular oncology review: ascorbic acid and 25 years later. *Integrative Cancer Therapies,* 4, 1, 32 – 44.

Gray, S. L., Anderson, M. L., Crane, P. K., Breitner, J. C. S., Mccormick, W., Bowen, J. D., Teri, L. & Larson, E. (2008). Antioxidant Vitamin Supplement Use and Risk of Dementia or Alzheimer's Disease in Older Adults. *J. Am. Geriatr. Soc., 56, 2,* 251-95.

Green, M. H. L., Lowe, J. E., Waugh, A. P. W., Aldridge, K. E., Cole, J. & Arlett, C. F. (1994) *Mutat. Res., 316, 2,* 91-110.

Griep, L. M., Stamler, J., Chan, Q., van Horn, L., Steffen, L. M., Miura, K., Ueshima, H., Okuda, N., Zhao, L., Daviglus M. L., Elliott, P. (2013). Association of raw fruit and fruit juice consumption with blood pressure: the INTERMAP Study. *Am J Clin Nutr,* volume 97, 1083–1091.

Guilland, J. C. & Lequeu, B. (1995). *As vitaminas do nutriente ao medicamento*. São Paulo: Santos.

Guilland, J. C. (1992). Vieillissementet vitamines. *La Revue de Gériatrie, 17, 10,* 545-53.

Halliwell, B. (1999) Vitamin C: poison, prophylactic our panacea? *Trends Biochem. Sci.,* 24, 7, 255- 259.

Halliwell, B. (2001) Vitamin C and genomic stability. *Mutat. Res.* 475, 6, 29-35.

Halpner, A. D., Handelman, G. J., Belmont, C. A., Harris, J. M. & Blumberg, J. B. (1998). Protection by vitamin C of oxidant-induced loss of vitamin of vitamin E in rat hepatocytes. *J. Nutr. Biochem., 9,* 355-59.

Hardling, A., Wareham, N. J., Bingham, S. A., Khaw, K., Luben, R. & Welch, A. (2008). Plasma vitamin C level, fruit and vegetable consumption, and the risk of new-onset type 2 diabetes mellitus. The European Prospective Investigation of Cancer-Norfolk Prospective Study. *Arch Intern Med, 168, 14,* 1493-9.

Hercberg, S., Galan, P., Preziosi, P., Bertrais, S., Mennen, L., Malvy, D., Roussel, A. F., Serge, A. B. (2004). The SU.VI.MAX Study: a randomized, placebo-controlled trial of the health effects of antioxidant vitamins and minerals. *Arch. Intern. Med.,* 164 (21), 2335-2342.

Holt, E. M., Steffen, L. M., Moran, A., Basu, S., Steinberger, J. & Ross, J. A. (2009). Fruit and vegetable consumption and its relation to markers of inflammation and oxidative stress in adolescents. *J. Am. Diet Assoc., 109, 3,* 414-21.

Hutchinson, M. A. H., Lentjes, D. C., Greenwood, V. J., Burley, J. E., Cade, C. L., Cleghorn, D. E., Threapleton, T. J., Key, B. J., Cairns, R. H.; Keogh, C. C., Dahm, E. J., Brunner,

M. J., Shipley, D., Kuh, G., Mishra, A. M., Stephen, A. & Bhaniani, G. (2012). Vitamin C intake from diary recordings and risk of breast cancer in the UK Dietary Cohort Consortium. *European Journal of Clinical Nutrition, 66,* 561-68.

Institute of Medicine. National Research Council. Dietary (2002). *Reference intakes for vitamin C, vitamin E, selenium, and carotenoids.* Washington, DC: National Academy Press; 2002.

Institute of Medicine. National Research Council. Dietary (2000). *Reference intakes for vitamin C, vitamin E, selenium, and carotenoids.* Washington, DC: National Academy Press.

Jacob, R. A. (1998). The integrated antioxidant system. *Nutr Res*, volume 15, 3, 755-66.

Key, T., Oakes, S., Davey, G., Moore, J., Edmond, L. M.; Mc Loone, U. J. & Thurnham, D. I. (1996). Focused on aldehyde dehydrogenase 2 (ALDH2), the enzyme for elimination of acetaldehyde *Cancer Epidemiol., 5, 2,* 811-23.

Knoops, K. T., de Groot, L. C., Kromhout, D., Perrin, A. E., Moreiras-Varela, O., Menotti, A. & van Staveren, W. A. (2004). Mediterranean diet, lifestyle factors and 10 year mortality in elderly European men and women: The hale project. J. *Am. Med. Assoc., 292, 5,* 1433-43.

Lampe, J. W. (1999). The association between HIGH intake of vegetables and fruits and LOW risk of chronic disease. *Am. J. Clin. Nutr., 70, 3,* 475-90.

Lankin, V. Z., Lisina, M. O., Arzamastseva, N. E., Konovalova, G. G., Nedosugova, V. V., Kaminnyi, A. K., Tikhase, A. K., Aglev, F. T., Kukharchuk, V. V. & Belenkov, Y. N.; (2005). Oxidatite stress in atherosclerosis and Diabetes. *Bull. Exp. Biol. Med., 140, 1,* 41-3.

Lee, D. H., Folsom, A. R., Harnack, L., Halliwell, B. & Jacobs, D. R. (2004). Does supplemental vitamin C increase cardiovascular disease risk in women with diabetes? *Am. J. Clin. Nutr., 80,* 1194–200.

Lee, K. W., Lee, H. J., Surh, Y. J. & Lee, C.Y. (2003). Vitamin C and cancer chemoprevention: reappraisal, *Am. J. Clin. Nutr., 78, 3,* 1074-1078.

Levine, M., Conrycantilena, C., Wang, Y. H., Welch, R. W., Washko, P. W., Dhariwal, K. R., Park, J. B., Lazarev, A., Graumlich, J. F., King, J. & Cantilena, L. R. (1996). *Proc. Natl. Acad. Sci. U. S. A., 93, 3,* 704-9.

Li Y. & Schellhorn, H. E. (2007). New developments and novel therapeutic perspectives for vitamin C. *J Nutr., 137,* 2171–84.

Ma, Y. X., Zhang, B., Wang, H. J., Du, W.W., Su, C., Zhang, J. G., Zhang, J., Zhaif, Y. & Zhonghua, M. (2012). Trend on vitamin C intake among Chinese population aged 50 - 79 years in 9 provinces, from 1991 to 2009. *Zhonghua Liu Xing Bing XueZaZhi, 33, 5,* 496-500.

Mas, E., Dupuy, A. M., Sylvaine, A., Portet, F., Cristol, J. P., Ritchie, K. & Touchon, J. (2006). Functional Vitamin E Deficiency in ApoE4 Patients with Alzheimer's Disease. *Dement Geriatr. Cogn. Disord., 21, 3,* 198-204.

Muntwyler, J., Hennekens, C. H., Manson, J. E., Buring, J. E. & Gaziano, J. M. (2002). Vitamin supplement use in a low-risk population of US male physicians and subsequent cardiovascular mortality. *Arch. Intern Med., 162,* 1472–6.

Neumann, A. I. C. P., Shirassu, M. M. & Fisberg, R. M. (2006). Consumo de alimentos de risco e proteção para doenças cardiovasculares entre funcionários públicos. *Rev Nutr, 19, 1,* 19-28.

Olmedo, J. M., Yiannias, J. A., Windgassen, E. B. & Gornet, M. K. (2006). Scurvy: a disease almostforgotten. *Int. J. Dermatol., 45, 8,* 909-13.

Osganian, S. K., Stampfer, M. J. & Rimm, E. (2003). Vitamin C and risk of coronary heart disease in women. *J. Am. Coll. Cardiol., 42,* 246–52.

Podoaro, I. D., Griffiths, H. R., Herbert, K. E., Mistry, N., Mistry, P., Lunec, J. (1998) Vitamin C exhibits pro-oxidant properties. *Nature*, 392, 3, 558-559.

Prauda, J. (2005). Terapeutic perpectives for vitamim C. *Wrold Gastroenteol, 11, 7,* 2371-85. Consumption of dietary antioxidants in overweight and obese individuals, users of the health promotion center. *Clin Nutr, 23, 4,* 1005-6.

Ramhman, I. (2002). Vitamin and inflame. Curr. Drug TargetsInflam. *Allergy*,1, 1, 291-311.

Ramos, A. C., Araujo, M. R., Lopes, L. R. & Andreollo, N. A. (2009). Role of the vitamin C indiethylnitrosamine-induced esophageal cancer in Wistar. *Acta Cirúrgica Brasileira, 24, 3,* 183-8.

Rivas, F. A., Zúñiga, A., Salas-Burgos, L., Mardones, V. & Ormazabal, J. C. (2008). Vitamin C transporters. *Journal of Physiology and Biochemistry, 64,* 357-75.

Rover Júnior, l., Höehr, N. F. & Vellasco, A. P. (2001). Sistema antioxidante envolvendo o ciclo metabólico da glutationa associado a métodos eletroanalíticos na avaliação do estresse oxidativo. *Quim. Nova, 24, 1,* 112-9.

Saito, A., Maier, C. M., Narasimham, P., Nishi, T., Song, Y. S., Yu, F., Liu, J., Lee, Y. S., Neto, C., Kamada, H., Doda, R. L., Hseeh, L. B., Hassid, B., Kim, E. E., Gonzalez, M. & Chan, P. H. (2005). Oxidative stress and neuronal death/ survival signaling cerebral ischemia *Mol. Neurobiol., 31, 3,* 105-16.

Sampaio, L. C. & Almeida, C. F. (2009). O papel dos alimentos funcionais na prevenção e controle do câncer de colo uterino. *Revista Brasileira de Cancerologia, 55, 3,* 251-60.

Santosa, S. & Jones, P. J. H. (2005). Efects of vitamin C. CMAJ, *Can. Med. Assoc. J., 173, 3,* 861-74.

Sasazuki, S., Sasaki, S., Tsubono, Y., Okubo, S., Hayashi, M. & Tsugane, S. (2006). Effect of vitamin C on common cold: randomized controlled trial. *Eur. J. Clin. Nutr., 60, 1,* 9-17.

Sesso, H. D., Buring, J. E., Christen, W. G. (2008). Vitamins E and C in the prevention of cardiovascular disease in men: the Physicians' Health Study II randomized controlled trial. *Jama, 300,* 2123–33.

Silva, J. V. F. P., Moreira, L. de N., Oliveira, D. C., Santos, T. R. dos; Padilha, H. G., Stulbach, T. & Crispim, C. A. (2012). Avaliação do consumo de nutrientes antioxidantes por mulheres fisicamente ativas. *Brazilian Journal of Sports Nutrition, 1, 1,* 30–6.

Su, C., Wang, H., Zhang, J., Du, W., Wang, Z., Zhang, J., Zhai, F. & Zhang, B. (2012). Free radicals and antioxidants. *Journal of Hygiene Research, 41, 3,* 357-62.

Szeto, Y. T., Kwork, T. C. Y. & Benzie, I. F. (2004). Effect of long term vegetarian diet on biomarks of antioxidant status and cardiovascular. *Nutrition, 20, 3,* 863-66.

Tak, P. P., Zvaifler, N. J., Green, P. R. & Forestein, G. S. (2000). Rheumatoid arthirit is and p53: how oxidative stress might alter of the course of inflammatory diseases. *Immunol. Today, 21,5,* 78-82.

Valero, E., Gonzalez-Sanchez, M. I., Macia, H. & Garcia-Carmona, F. (2009). Computer simulation of the dynamic behavior of the glutathione-ascorbate redox cycle in chloroplasts. *Plant Physiol, 149, 4,* 1958-69.

Valko, M., Rhodes, C. J., Moncol, J., Izakovic, M. & Mazur, M. (2006). Free radicals, metals and antioxidants in oxidative stress-induced cancer. *Chem. Biol. Interact., 160, 1,* 40-52.

Wannmache, L. (2006). *Vitamina C: seis problemas em busca de uma solução*. Brasília. Ministério da Saúde.

Weinstein, M., Babyn, P. & Zlotkin, S. (2001). An Orange a Day Keeps the Doctor Away: Scurvy in the Year 2000. *Pediatrics, 108, 3,* 528-34.

Welch, R. W., Turley, E., Sweetman, S. F., Kennedy, G., Collins, A. R., Dunne, A., Livingstone, M. B. E., Mckenna, P. G., Mckelvey-Martin, V. J. & Strain, J. (1999). Vitamin C and cancer. *Nutr. Cancer, 34*, 167-75.

Willcox, B. J., Curb, J. D. & Rodriguez, B. L. (2008). Antioxidants in cardiovascular health and disease: key lessons from epidemiologic studies. *Am. J. Cardiol., 101*, 75–86.

World Health Organization. (2002). *Diet, nutrition and prevention of chronic diseases: report of a joint.* WHO/FAO expert consultation. Geneva: WHO.

World Health Report (2001). *Reducing risks, promoting healthy life.* Geneva: World Health Organization.

Yang, J., Liu, J. R., Parry, J., Frito-Lay, R., Texas, U. S. A.; Kucharski, H. & Zajac, J. (2009). *Handbook of vitamin C research: daily requirements, dietary sources and adverse effects*. Nutrition and Diet Research Progress Series.

Ye, Z. & Song, H. (2008). Antioxidant vitamins intake and the risk of coronary heart disease: meta-analysis of cohort studies. *Eur. J. Cardiovasc. Prev. Rehabil., 15*, 26–34.

Zhu, X., Lee, H., Perry, G., Smith, M. A. (2007). Alzheimer disease, the two-hit hypothesis: An update. *Biochim. Biophys. Acta,* volume 4, 5, p. 494-502.

In: Vitamin C
Editor: Raquel Guiné

ISBN: 978-1-62948-154-8
© 2013 Nova Science Publishers, Inc.

Chapter 12

VITAMIN C ROLE IN HUMAN HEALTH, DISEASE AND SPORT

Goreti Botelho[1,*] and Marco Aguiar[2]

[1]Food Science and Technology Department, CERNAS Research Unit, Coimbra College of Agriculture, Polytechnic Institute of Coimbra, Bencanta, Coimbra, Portugal
[2]Sport Sciences, Exercise and Health Department, University of Trás-os-Montes e Alto Douro, Quinta de Prados, Vila Real, Portugal

ABSTRACT

Vitamin C (chemical names: ascorbic acid and ascorbate) is a six-carbon lactone which is synthesized from glucose by many animals. Vitamin C is synthesized in the liver of some mammals and in the kidney of birds and reptiles. However, several species, including humans, non-human primates and guinea pigs are unable to synthesize vitamin C. It is one of the important water soluble vitamins for human health. Vitamin C is needed for many physiological functions in our body, such as, for collagen, carnitine and neurotransmitters biosynthesis. These physiological functions are largely dependent on the oxido-reduction properties of this vitamin.

The most widely known health beneficial effect of vitamin C is in the the prevention or relief of common cold. However, the role of oral vitamin C in the prevention and treatment of colds remains controversial despite many controlled trials.

Vitamin C plays a critical role in wound repair and in the healing/regeneration process by stimulating collagen synthesis. It also protects against oxidation of isolated low density lipoproteins by different types of oxidative stress, including metal ion dependent and independent processes, some implicated in development of atherosclerosis. Some scientific findings also refer to the positive role of Vitamin C in cancer treatment.

In sport, some recent studies indicate important effects of Vitamin C in reducing inflammation secondary related to exercise and improving recovery.

The present chapter provides an up-to-date overview of the different Vitamin C roles in promoting human health, preventing disease and sport performance.

---

* Email: goreti@esac.pt

1. INTRODUCTION

Vitamin C, also known as ascorbate or ascorbic acid, is synthesized by all animals except humans, monkeys, guinea pigs, bats, and several bird species (Linster et al., 2007). L-ascorbic acid ($C_6H_8O_6$) is the trivial name of vitamin C and the chemical name is 2-oxo-L-threo-hexono-1,4-lactone-2,3-enediol. L-ascorbic and dehydroascorbic acid are the major dietary forms of vitamin C (Moser & Bendich, 1990). In this chapter the terms vitamin C and ascorbic acid will be used synonymously.

During recent decades, in clinical and experimental research, attention is paid to the role of antioxidant defense systems in the prevention of human diseases such as cancer, diabetes mellitus, and cardiovascular pathologies (Cross et al., 1987; Sabuncu et al., 2001; Vural et al., 2000; Vural et al., 2001). During the progression of these diseases, oxidative stress events occur, and free radicals and reactive oxygen species (ROS) are generated from the molecular oxygen to form superoxide radical, hydrogen peroxide, hypocloride, hydroxyl, and peroxyl radicals.

These free radicals and ROS are thought to contribute to lipid peroxidation (LPO) (Hochstein & Ernster, 1963), DNA damage (Kasai et al., 1986), and protein degradation (Dreher & Junod, 1996). Host survival depends upon the ability of cells and tissues to adapt to or resist the stress and repair or remove damaged molecules and cells. Multiple enzymatic and nonenzymatic antioxidant defense systems present in cells inactivate those free radicals and reduce the amount of cellular oxidative damage they cause.

These antioxidants include free radical scavengers; exogenous vitamins A, C, E and endogenous like glutathione (GSH) and enzymatic systems; and superoxide dismutase (SOD), catalase (CAT) and glutathione peroxidase (GSH-Px), uric acid, bilirubin, and albumin. The beneficial effects of the antioxidant supplements have been assessed in many degenerative diseases that are recognized as being a consequence of oxidative stress and free radical damage (Abe et al., 1994; Cross et al., 1987; Montilla et al., 1998; Rosenblat & Aviram, 2002; Sabuncu et al., 2001; Vural et al., 2000; Vural et al., 2001).

Vitamin C can limit the formation of carcinogens, such as nitrosamines (Carr & Frei, 1999; Hecht, 1997), *in vivo*; modulate immune response (Carr & Frei, 1999; Jacob & Sotoudeh, 2002); and, through its antioxidant function, possibly attenuate oxidative damage that can lead to cancer (Li & Schellhorn, 2007).

Several scientific studies have been undertaken on how the vitamin C is involved in the delay or prevention of the onset or progression of the diseases and their complications. By this, the relationship between vitamin C and disease/health condition will be the focus of the first section on the present chapter.

The second section describes the effects of vitamin C intake on human physiologic function during exercise and physical performance.

2. VITAMIN C IN HUMAN HEALTH AND DISEASE

Ascorbic acid is one of the most important water soluble vitamins present in foods and is readily available and easily absorbed by active transport in the intestine (Sauberlich, 1985).

Most of it (80–90 %) will be absorbed when the intake is up to 100 mg/day, whereas at higher levels of intake (500 mg/day) the efficiency of absorption of ascorbic acid rapidly declines.

As ascorbic acid is a water soluble compound, it is easily absorbed but it is not stored in the body. The average adult has a body pool of 1.2–2.0 g of ascorbic acid that may be maintained with 75 mg/day of ascorbic acid. About 140 mg/day of ascorbic acid will saturate the total body pool of vitamin C (Sauberlich, 1990). The average half life of ascorbic acid in adult human is about 10–20 days, with a turnover of 1 mg/kg body and a body pool of 22 mg/kg at plasma ascorbate concentration of 50 μmol/L (Hellman & Burns, 1958; Kallner et al., 1982). Hence ascorbic acid has to be regularly supplemented through diet or tablets to maintain ascorbic acid pool in the body.

Deruelle & Baron (2008), from the current literature, advise healthy people to consume five servings of fruits and vegetables daily, added to 1 g of vitamin C supplementation divided in two or three doses during the day, in order to ensure an optimal allowance in vitamin C.The recommended dietary allowance (RDA) for vitamin C was set at 75 mg daily for adult females and 90 mg daily for adult males, an increase of 25 % for women and 50% for men, over the previous recommendation (FNB, 2000). Gram doses (1–2 g/day) of vitamin C are well tolerated by most individuals. A number of studies suggest that optimal health benefits are achieved at intakes of 100–200 mg/day. Supported by clinical trial evidence from several studies, Hathcock et al. (2005), concluded that vitamin C supplements of ≤ 2000 mg/day are safe for most adults. The Food and Nutrition Board's panel on Dietary Antioxidant and Related Compounds of the NAS (National Academy of Sciences) has defined an antioxidant as ''any substance that, when present at low concentrations compared to those of an oxidizable substrate (e.g., proteins, lipids, carbohydrates, and nucleic acids), significantly delays or prevents oxidation of that substrate'' (FNB, 1998).

Table 1. Tissue concentrations of ascorbic acid in rat and human body (adapted from Banhegyi et al., 1998, with permission).

Tissue	Rat (mg/100 g)	Human (mg/100 g)
Adrenal glands	280-400	30-40
Pituitary gland	100-130	40-50
Liver	25-40	10-16
Spleen	40-50	10-15
Lungs	20-40	7
Kidneys	15-20	5-15
Testes	25-30	3
Thyroid	22	2
Thymus	40	
Brain	35-50	13-15
Pancreas	10-16	
Eye lens	8-10	25-31
Skeletal muscle	5	3-4
Heart muscle	5-10	5-15
Bone marrow	12	
Plasma	1.6	0.4-1.0
Saliva	0.07-0.09	

Many cells accumulate ascorbic acid against a concentration gradient. Intracellular concentrations of ascorbic acid are up to 40-fold higher than plasma concentrations (Banhegyi et al., 1998, Table 1).

When activated, neutrophils accumulate ascorbate with intracellular ascorbic acid levels ranging from 2 mM to as much as 10 mM. Although simple diffusion accounts for some of this movement, ascorbic acid transport is primarily carrier-mediated (Goldenberg & Schweinzer, 1994; McCormick & Rose et al., 1998; Rumsey et al., 1997; Zhang, 1993).

Ascorbic acid enters cells on a sodium- and energy-dependent transporter, and with the exception of the intestine, simple diffusion is of minor importance. Most of the intracellular ascorbate, however, is derived from rapid conversion of dehydroascorbic acid (Behrens & Madere, 1994; Rumsey & Levine, 1998). Dehydroascorbic acid enters cells on GLUT 1, 2, or 4 transporters, and this transport is inhibited by glucose in vitro.

Oxidative stress is now known to be implicated in the pathogenesis of a wide variety of health disorders, including coronary heart diseases, cerebrovascular diseases, emphysema, bronchitis, chronic obstructive lung disease, some forms of cancer, diabetes, skeletal muscular dystrophy, infertility, cataractogenesis, dermatitis, rheumatoid arthritis, AIDS-related dysfunctions, and Alzheimer's and Parkinson's diseases (Davies & Ursini 1995; Sen & Hanninen 1994). In addition, reactive oxygen species are thought to critically contribute to ageing and age-related disorders (Levine & Stadtman 1996).

Ascorbic acid readily scavenges reactive oxygen and nitrogen species, such as superoxide and hydroperoxyl radicals, aqueous peroxyl radicals, singlet oxygen, ozone, peroxynitrite, nitrogen, dioxide, nitroxide radicals and hypochlorous acid. Moreover, ascorbic acid supplementation has been associated with reduced lipid, DNA, and protein oxidation in experimental systems (Bors & Buettner, 1997; Halliwell &Whiteman, 1997).

Due to its function as an antioxidant and its role in immune function, vitamin C has been promoted as a means to help prevent and/or treat numerous health conditions. This chapter' section focuses on diseases and unhealthy habits in which vitamin C might play a role: diabetes, cancer, cardiovascular disease, age-related macular degeneration and cataracts, virus-induced respiratory infections, and tobacco usage. The health risks from excessive intake of vitamin C will also be discussed.

2.1. Vitamin C and Diabetes

It was reported that 194 million people representing a global prevalence exceeding 3 % of the world population were diabetic and is expected to reach 6.3 % by the year 2025, with the type 2 diabetes mellitus representing the major part (85-90 %) (Boutayeb et al., 2004).

The chronic intake of high-heat-treated foods was shown to accelerate cardiovascular complications in animals and humans with diabetes (Lin et al., 2003; Vlassara et al., 2002) and to help type 1 and 2 diabetes development in mice (Peppa et al., 2003; Sandu et al., 2005). It was shown that a typical Western diet characterized by a significantly higher consumption of processed foods (processed meat, pizza, or snacks) is associated with an increased risk of insulin resistance and metabolic syndrome when compared with a healthier diet (higher intake of vegetables and significantly reduced amounts of processed foods) (Esmaillzadeh et al., 2007). In addition, more recently, in a randomized, crossover, intervention trial, it was found that a diet that is based on high-heat-treated foods increases markers associated with an enhanced risk of type 2 diabetes and cardiovascular diseases in healthy people. Replacing high-heat-treatment techniques by mild cooking techniques may help to positively modulate biomarkers associated with an increased risk of diabetes mellitus and cardiovascular diseases (Birlouez-Aragon et al., 2010).

On the other hand, several nutraceuticals used in clinical practice have been shown to target the pathogenesis of diabetes mellitus, metabolic syndrome and their complications and to favourably modulate a number of biochemical and clinical endpoints. These compounds include antioxidant vitamins, such as vitamins C and E, flavonoids, vitamin D, conjugated linoleic acid, omega-3 fatty acids, minerals such as chromium and magnesium, α-lipoic acid, phytoestrogens and dietary fibers (Davì et al., 2010).

Most of the intracellular ascorbate is derived from rapid conversion of dehydroascorbic acid (Behrens & Madere, 1994, Rumsey & Levine, 1998), and the transfer of dehydroascorbic acid to cells is made through GLUT 1, 2, or 4 transporters, a process that is inhibited by glucose *in vitro*. Of clinical significance, it has been postulated that diabetic patients may have compromised ascorbic status due in part to the inference made by glucose on dehydroascorbic acid uptake (Rumsey et al., 1997; Rumsey & Levine, 1998).

Knowledge that oxidative changes may actually trigger deterioration in cell function has led to investigations for identifying agents that may have possible therapeutic value.

Vitamin C (ascorbic acid) is a powerful water-soluble antioxidant present in the cytosolic compartment of the cell that serves as an electron donor to vitamin E radicals generated in the cell membrane during oxidative stress. The major store of membranebound vitamin E is in the inner mitochondrial membrane, the site of the electron transport system. Vitamin E neutralizes free radicals, preventing the chain reaction that contributes to oxidative damage (Murase et al., 1998; Sun et al., 1999; Tavan et al., 1997). In animals, vitamin C reduces diabetes-induced sorbitol accumulation and lipid peroxides in erythrocytes (Riccioni et al., 2007). Vitamin C (800 mg/day) partially replenishes vitamin C levels in patients with type 2 diabetes and low vitamin C levels but does not improve endothelial dysfunction or insulin resistance (Chen et al., 2006).

Observational epidemiologic studies have shown significant inverse correlations between antioxidant concentrations and several biomarkers of insulin resistance or glucose intolerance in healthy individuals (Sargeant et al., 2000). Concentrations of antioxidants in the blood, such as vitamins C (Sargeant et al., 2000; Sinclair et al., 1994; Will et al., 1999) and E (Abahusain et al., 1999; Polidori et al., 2000) and β-carotene (Abahusain et al., 1999; Ford et al., 1999; Polidori et al., 2000) were also significantly lower in individuals with type 2 diabetes than in nondiabetic control subjects.

Oxidative stress due to hyperglycemia and dyslipidemia in diabetes is known to initiate and promote either of micro and macro vascular complications (Maritim et al., 2003). The authors Aksoy et al., (2005) conducted a study to describe the effects of these vitamins on the oxidative-antioxidative system in diabetic rats. Diabetes in rats increased oxidative stress in erythrocytes and the supplementation of vitamins C and E significantly reduced LPO levels and increased GSH, GSH-Px, and SOD activities. These results indicate that combined ingestion of vitamins C and E exerted beneficial effects of antioxidative defense systems against that imposed by diabetes mellitus. More recently, in addition to hyperglycemia, it was reported that dyslipidemia may also contribute to excess free radical generation leading to oxidative stress (Suchitra et al., 2011).

Diabetes increases the cardiovascular risk leading to high morbidity and mortality in diabetic patients (Fox et al., 2007). Moreover, in diabetes, dyslipidemia in the form of increased levels of total cholesterol, triglycerides, low density lipoprotein cholesterol, very low density lipoprotein cholesterol and reduced high density lipoprotein cholesterol may substantially contribute to the excess cardiovascular risk in diabetes (Garg & Grundy, 1990). A randomized trial study showed no significant overall effects of vitamin C, vitamin E and β-carotene on risk of developing type 2 diabetes in women at high risk of cardiovascular disease (Song et al., 2009).

A very recent study showed that vitamin C supplementation (1 g/day) for four week duration among 30 patients, in addition to regular management of diabetic patients (with type 2 diabetes mellitus) was effective in improving hyperglycemia and hyperlipidemia as a therapeutic measure preventing associated complications (Vaksh et al., 2013). However, as the authors recognized, the low sample size and short duration of vitamin C supplementation should be regarded as limitations of the study.

2.2. Vitamin C and Cancer

Cancer is the second leading cause of death in the U.S.A. and in most high-income countries (Heron, 2011). Cancer is responsible for 44 % of all deaths in Japan, 35 % in Australia, 33 % in Spain and in United Kingdom, 30 % in Poland, 29 % in the U.S.A. and in Germany, 22 % in China, 20 % in South Africa and in Brazil, 18 % in Mexico, 15 % in India, and 9 % in Egypt (WCRF/AICR, 2007).

In epidemiologic studies, diets rich in fruits and vegetables are consistently related to decreased risk for cancers (Carr & Frei, 1999; Gandini et al., 2000; Levi et al., 1999; Mosby et al., 2012; Steinmaus et al., 2000; Voorrips et al., 2000; WCRF/AICR, 2007). Phytochemicals, the bioactive nonnutrient plant compounds in fruit, vegetables, grains, and other plant foods, have been linked to reductions in the risk of major chronic diseases. It is estimated that more than 5000 phytochemicals have been identified, but a large percentage still remain unknown (Shahidi & Naczk, 1995) and need to be identified before their health benefits are fully understood. Phytochemical extracts from fruit have strong antioxidant and antiproliferative effects and the combination of phytochemicals in fruit and vegetables is critical to powerful antioxidant and anticancer activity (Chu et al., 2002; Ederhardt et al., 2000; Liu, 2003; Sun et al., 2002).

For example, the total antioxidant activity of phytochemicals in 1 g of apples with skin is equivalent to 83.3 μmol vitamin C equivalents, that is, the antioxidant value of 100 g of apples is equivalent to 1500 mg of vitamin C. This is much higher than the total antioxidant activity of 0.057 mg of vitamin C (the amount of vitamin C in 1 g of apples with skin). In other words, vitamin C in apples contributed only < 0.4 % of total antioxidant activity (Ederhardt et al., 2000). By this, vitamin C may simply be a marker for fruit and vegetable consumption (Drewnowski et al., 1997).

On the other hand, cancer incidence and deaths appear inversely related to regular use of vitamin C supplements (Carr & Frei, 1999). But, although it is likely that ascorbic acid may have some limited effect given the complexity of protective mechanism(s), the relative importance of ascorbic acid in various cancers has yet to be resolved.

The great majority of case-control studies have found an inverse association between dietary vitamin C intake and cancers of the lung, breast, colon or rectum, stomach, oral cavity, larynx or pharynx, and esophagus (Carr & Frei, 1999; Jacob & Sotoudeh, 2002). Nevertheless, evidence from prospective cohort studies is inconsistent, possibly due to varying intakes of vitamin C among studies.

In a cohort of 82,234 women aged 33–60 years from the Nurses' Health Study, consumption of an average of 205 mg/day of vitamin C from food (highest quintile of intake) compared with an average of 70 mg/day (lowest quintile of intake) was associated with a 63 % lower risk of breast cancer among premenopausal women with a family history of breast cancer (Zhang et al., 1999). In opposition, a significantly lower risk of breast cancer among postmenopausal women consuming at least 198 mg/day (highest quintile of intake) of vitamin C from food compared with those consuming less than 87 mg/day (lowest quintile of intake) was not found (Kushi et al., 1996). Currently, millions of postmenopausal women use multivitamins, often believing that supplements prevent chronic diseases such as cancer and cardiovascular disease. After a median follow-up of 8.0 and 7.9 years in the clinical trial and observational study cohorts, respectively, the Women's Health Initiative study provided convincing evidence that multivitamin (including vitamin C) use has little or no influence on the risk of common cancers, cardiovascular disease, or total mortality in postmenopausal women (Neuhouser et al., 2009).

There are several studies that suggest that an intake of 90-100 mg vitamin C/day is required for optimum reduction of chronic disease risk (including significantly lower cancer risk) in nonsmoking men and women (Carr & Frei, 1999; Levine et al., 1996; Levine et al., 2001).

Experimental studies have demonstrated that vitamin C inhibits the growth of androgen-independent and androgen-dependent prostate cancer cells in vitro (Maramag et al., 1997) and decreases the production of reactive oxygen species in androgen-treated prostate cancer cells (Ripple et al., 1997).

In addition, plasma vitamin C has been shown to be inversely correlated with biomarkers of oxidative stress even after adjusting for other antioxidants (Block et al., 2002), suggesting that vitamin C may decrease oxidative stress. Prospective studies examining blood levels (Eichholzer et al., 1999; Huang et al., 2003) or dietary intake (Daviglus et al., 1996; Giovannucci et al., 1995; Shibata et al., 1992; Schuurman et al., 2002) of vitamin C and prostate cancer risk have not observed a significant protective association. However, two retrospective case-control studies found that higher dietary intake of vitamin C was associated with a decreased risk of prostate cancer (Deneo-Pellegrini et al., 1999; Ramon et al., 2000). More recently, a prospective study conducted by Berndt et al. (2005), found that higher plasma vitamin C concentrations within the normal physiologic range are not associated with a lower risk of prostate cancer in well-nourished men.

A 2008 review of vitamin C and other antioxidant supplements for the prevention of gastrointestinal cancers found no convincing evidence that vitamin C (or beta-carotene, vitamin A, or vitamin E) prevents gastrointestinal cancers (Bjelakovic et al., 2008). A similar review revealed that vitamin C supplementation, in combination with vitamin E, had no significant effect on death risk due to cancer in healthy individuals (Coulter et al., 2003).

Research in mice suggests that pharmacologic doses of vitamin C by intravenous (IV) administration may be promising in treating otherwise difficult-to-treat tumors (Chen et al., 2008). A high concentration of vitamin C may act as a pro-oxidant and generate hydrogen peroxide that has selective toxicity toward cancer cells (Chen et al., 2005; Chen et al., 2007; Chen et al., 2008). Based on these findings and a few case reports of patients with advanced cancers who had remarkably long survival times following administration of high-dose IV vitamin C, some researchers support reassessment of the use of high-dose IV vitamin C as a drug to treat cancer (Chen et al., 2008; Frei et al., 1989; Levine et al., 2009; Padayatty et al., 2006).

A significant limitation in interpreting many of these studies is that the measurement of plasmatic or tissue vitamin C concentrations before or after supplementation are not performed. Additionally, at daily intakes of 100 mg or higher, cells appear to be saturated and at intakes of at least 200 mg, plasma concentrations increase only marginally (Carr & Frei, 1999; Kushi et al., 1996; Levine et al., 1996; Padayatty et al., 2004; Taylor et al., 1994). If subjects' vitamin C levels were already close to saturation at study entry, supplementation would be expected to have made little or no difference on measured outcomes (Levine et al., 1996; Levine et al., 1999; Padayatty & Levine, 2006, 2009).

In conclusion, the evidence is inconsistent on whether dietary vitamin C intake affects cancer risk. Results from most clinical trials suggest that modest vitamin C supplementation alone or with other nutrients offers no benefit in the prevention of cancer.

2.3. Vitamin C and Cardiovascular Disease

Epidemiologic studies have shown that high intakes of fruits and vegetables are associated with a reduced risk of cardiovascular disease (Li & Schellhorn, 2007; Ye & Song, 2008; Willcox et al., 2008). This association might be partly attributable to the antioxidant content of these foods because oxidative damage, including oxidative modification of low-density lipoproteins, is a major cause of cardiovascular disease (Jacob & Sotoudeh, 2002; Li & Schellhorn, 2007; Willcox et al., 2008).

Some studies revealed that death due to cardiovascular disease is inversely related to regular use of vitamin C supplements (Carr & Frei, 1999; Ernstrom et al., 1992). Males with vitamin C deficiency (plasma vitamin C 0.2 mg/dL) were at significantly increased risk of myocardial infarction after controlling for potentially confounding variables (Ernstrom et al., 1992).

In addition to its antioxidant properties, vitamin C has been shown to reduce monocyte adherence to the endothelium, improve endothelium-dependent nitric oxide production and vasodilation, and reduce vascular smooth-muscle-cell apoptosis, thus preventing plaque instability in atherosclerosis (Carr & Frei, 1999; Honarbakhsh & Schachter, 2008).

The oxidation of low-density lipoproteins has been implicated in the etiology of atherosclerosis and serum lipid peroxides were significantly reduced in patients hospitalized with acute myocardial infarction after consuming diets rich in vitamin C (Singh et al., 1995).

Results from prospective studies focused on associations between vitamin C intake and cardiovascular disease risk are contradictory (Willcox et al., 2008). In the Nurses' Health Study, a 16-year prospective study involving 85,118 female nurses, total intake of vitamin C from both dietary and supplemental sources was inversely associated with coronary heart disease risk (Osganian et al., 2003). However, intake of vitamin C from diet alone showed no significant associations, suggesting that vitamin C supplement users might be at lower risk of coronary heart disease.

A prospective study in 20,649 British adults found that those in the top quartile of baseline plasma vitamin C concentrations had a 42 % lower risk of stroke than those in the bottom quartile (Myint et al., 2008). In male physicians participating in the Physicians' Health Study, use of vitamin C supplements for a mean of 5.5 years was not associated with a significant decrease in total cardiovascular disease mortality or coronary heart disease mortality (Muntwyler et al., 2002).

A collective analysis of nine prospective studies that included 293,172 subjects free of coronary heart disease at baseline found that people who took ≥700 mg/day of supplemental vitamin C had a 25 % lower risk of coronary heart disease incidence than those who took no supplemental vitamin C (Knekt et al., 2004). The authors of a meta-analysis of prospective cohort studies, including 14 studies reporting on vitamin C for a median follow-up of 10 years, concluded that dietary, but not supplemental, intake of vitamin C is inversely associated with coronary heart disease risk (Ye & Song, 2008).

Follow-up data from the Linxian trial, a population nutrition intervention trial conducted in China shows that daily vitamin C supplements (120 mg) plus molybdenum (30 mcg) for 5–6 years significantly reduced the risk of cerebrovascular deaths by 8 % during 10 years of follow-up after the end of the active intervention (Qiao et al., 2009).

Contradicting the "positive effect" evidence, a study indicated that postmenopausal women with diabetes who took at least 300 mg/day vitamin C supplements had increased cardiovascular disease mortality (Lee et al., 2004).

Results from other clinical intervention trials have failed to show a beneficial effect of vitamin C supplementation on the primary or secondary prevention of cardiovascular disease. For example, in the Women's Antioxidant Cardiovascular Study, a secondary prevention trial involving 8,171 women aged 40 years or older with a history of cardiovascular disease, supplementation with 500 mg/day vitamin C for a mean of 9.4 years showed no overall effect on cardiovascular events (Cook et al., 2007). Similarly, vitamin C supplementation (500 mg/day) for a mean follow-up of 8 years had no effect on major cardiovascular events in male physicians enrolled in the Physicians' Health Study II (Sesso et al., 2008).

The authors of a 2006 meta-analysis of randomized controlled trials concluded that antioxidant supplements (vitamins C and E and beta-carotene or selenium) do not affect the progression of atherosclerosis (Bleys et al., 2006). Similarly, a systematic review of vitamin C's effects on the prevention and treatment of cardiovascular disease found that vitamin C did not have favorable effects on cardiovascular disease prevention (Shekelle et al., 2003).

Several studies reported that dialysis patients had an impaired antioxidant system, including antioxidant status (Clermont et al., 2000; Ha et al., 1996; Hultqvist et al., 1997; Jackson et al., 1995), antioxidant enzyme activities (Durak et al., 1994; Canestrari et al., 1995; Chen et al., 1997; Mohora et al., 1995; Paul et al., 1993; Shurtz-Swirski et al., 1995; Toborek et al., 1992), and reduced antioxidant defense against lipid peroxidation (Canestrari et al., 1995; Fiorillo et al., 1998; Galli et al., 2001; Mohora et al., 1995; Paul et al., 1993; Peuchant et al., 1997; Toborek et al., 1992). Due to hemobioincompatibility of the dialysis system, the formation of free oxygen radical species and trace amounts of endotoxins were induced during the inflammatory state in hemodialysis patients (Morena et al., 2000). Both the abnormalities in the antioxidant defense system and the increased oxidative stress may increase their susceptibility to lipid peroxidation in low density lipoprotein (LDL), which may lead to the subsequent development of atherosclerotic cardiovascular disesase in hemodialysis patients (Clermont et al., 2000; Galli et al., 2001; Morena et al., 2000).

According to Chao et al. (2002), vitamin C and E supplements improve the impaired antioxidant status and decrease plasma lipid peroxides in hemodialysis patients.

Although the results from several studies, like the Linxian trial data, suggest a possible benefit, overall, the findings from most intervention trials do not provide conclusive evidence that vitamin C supplements provide protection against cardiovascular disease or reduce its morbidity or mortality. However, clinical trial data for vitamin C are limited by the fact that plasma and tissue concentrations of vitamin C are tightly controlled in humans. Ascorbic acid is also necessary for the transformation of cholesterol to bile acids as it modulates the microsomal 7-α-hydroxylation, the rate limiting reaction of cholesterol catabolism in liver. In ascorbic acid deficiency, this reaction becomes slowed down, thus, resulting in an accumulation of cholesterol in liver, hypercholesterolemia, formation of cholesterol gall stones, among others (Ginter et al., 1982). Moreover, Harats et al., (1998) reported that 2 months of supplementation with 500 mg vitamin C/day slightly increased plasma cholesterol (this was offset by reduced *in vitro* LDL susceptibility to oxidation).

2.4. Vitamin C and Age-Related Macular Degeneration and Cataracts

Age-related macular degeneration (AMD) and cataracts are two of the leading causes of vision loss in older individuals. Oxidative stress might contribute to the etiology of both conditions. Therefore, researchers have hypothesized that vitamin C and other antioxidants play a role in the development and/or treatment of these diseases.

High dietary intakes of vitamin C and higher plasma ascorbate concentrations have been associated with a lower risk of cataract formation in some studies (Carr & Frei, 1999; Jacob & Sotoudeh, 2002). In a 5-year prospective cohort study conducted in Japan, higher dietary vitamin C intake was associated with a reduced risk of developing cataracts in a cohort of more than 30,000 adults aged 45–64 years (Yoshida et al., 2007). Furthermore, results from two case-control studies indicate that vitamin C intakes greater than 300 mg/day reduce the risk of cataract formation by 70 %–75 % (Carr & Frei, 1999; Jacob & Sotoudeh, 2002).

A population-based cohort study in the Netherlands found that adults aged 55 years or older who had high dietary intakes of vitamin C as well as beta-carotene, zinc, and vitamin E had a reduced risk of AMD (van Leeuwen et al., 2005).

Epidemiologic studies have also shown that the risk of cataract, particularly posterior subcapsular cataract, is significantly higher in individuals with moderate to low blood concentrations of vitamin C (odds ratio, 3.3 to 11.3 after adjustment for age, gender, race, and diabetes) (Jacques & Chylack, 1991; Jacques et al., 1997). After controlling for potentially confounding variables, including diabetes, smoking, sunlight exposure and regular aspirin use, taking vitamin C supplements for 10 years was associated with reduced risk for early (odds ratio, 0.23; 95 % CI, 0.99-0.60) and moderate (odds ratio, 0.17; 95 % CI, 0.03-0.87) age-related lens opacities in women (Jacques et al., 1997). When consumed for less than 10 years little or no association to cataract formation has been observed.

However, most prospective studies do not support those findings (Evans, 2007). The authors of a systematic review and meta-analysis of prospective cohort studies and randomized clinical trials concluded that the current evidence does not support a role for vitamin C and other antioxidants, including antioxidant supplements, in the primary prevention of early AMD (Chong et al., 2007).

Although research has not shown that antioxidants play a role in AMD development, some evidence suggests that they might help slow AMD progression (Evans, 2006). The Age-Related Eye Disease Study (AREDS), a large, randomized, placebo-controlled clinical trial, evaluated the effect of high doses of selected antioxidants (500 mg vitamin C, 400 IU vitamin E, 15 mg beta-carotene, 80 mg zinc, and 2 mg copper) on the development of advanced AMD in 3,597 older individuals with varying degrees of AMD (AREDSRG, 2001a,b). After an average follow-up period of 6.3 years, participants with intermediate AMD who received antioxidant supplements had a 28 % lower risk of progression to advanced AMD than participants who received a placebo.

2.5. Vitamin C and Immune Function

The most prominent link of vitamin C to immune system seems to be its suggested preventive role on virus-induced respiratory infections.

There are many synonyms or acronyms for cold and flu. Most generally, flu refers to constitutional symptoms of fever and aching with occasional gastrointestinal upset. Cold generally refers to symptoms in the upper respiratory tract. The two may or may not accompany each other and both are largely viral infections.

In the 1970s, Nobel laureate Linus Pauling suggested that vitamin C could successfully treat and/or prevent the common cold (Pauling, 1971). Results of subsequent controlled studies have been inconsistent, resulting in confusion and controversy, although public interest in the subject remains high (Douglas & Hemilä, 2005; Douglas et al., 2007).

The search for the unequivocal demonstration of the effectiveness of vitamin C in preventing and relieving the symptoms of virus-induced respiratory infections such as colds and influenza has been the target of a few research works. One of the obstacles has been the assumption that as a water-soluble vitamin, excess vitamin C is passed off in the urine, and therefore the application of megadoses is ineffective.

Positive results in treating the symptoms of virus-induced respiratory infections by the application of moderate-to-large doses of vitamin C (300 mg and 2000 mg) have been reported (Bernasconi & Massera, 1985; Bucca et al., 1990; Hemilia, 1994; Hunt et al., 1994; Peters et al., 1993). In 1999, during a prospective, clinically controlled study, Gorton & Jarvis, reported that vitamin C in megadoses (1000 mg each), administered before or after the appearance of cold and flu symptoms relieved and prevented the symptoms (85 % less symptoms) in the test population compared with the control group.

More recently, a 2007 Cochrane review examined placebo-controlled trials involving the use of at least 200 mg/day vitamin C taken either continuously as a prophylactic treatment or after the onset of cold symptoms (Douglas et al., 2007). Prophylactic use of vitamin C did not significantly reduce the risk of developing a cold in the general population. However, in trials involving marathon runners, skiers, and soldiers exposed to extreme physical exercise and/or cold environments, prophylactic use of vitamin C in doses ranging from 250 mg/day to 1 g/day reduced cold incidence by 50 %. In the general population, use of prophylactic vitamin C modestly reduced cold duration by 8 % in adults and 14 % in children. When taken after the onset of cold symptoms, vitamin C did not affect cold duration or symptom severity.

Overall, the evidence to date suggests that regular intakes of vitamin C at doses of at least 200 mg/day do not reduce the incidence of the common cold in the general population, but such intakes might be helpful in people exposed to extreme physical exercise or cold environments and those with marginal vitamin C status, such as the elderly and chronic smokers (Douglas et al., 2007; Hemilä, 2007; Wintergerst et al., 2006). A study with hospitalized elderly patients, diagnosed with acute respiratory infections, receiving 200 mg of vitamin C daily fared better than patients receiving a placebo (Hunt et al., 1994).

The mechanisms by which vitamin C reduces the severity of upper respiratory tract infections are not well established, but must be related to any number of redox sensitive signals and sites associated with enzymes and receptors. Further, reducing agents and proton donors are needed to drive the activation of phagocytes. Vitamin C can also accelerate the destruction of histamine, a mediator of allergy and cold symptoms in vitro (Bucca et al., 1990; Johnston et al., 1992; Johnston et al., 1996). Vitamin C supplementation consistently reduces blood histamine concentrations 30 % to 40 % in adult subjects (Johnston et al., 1992; Johnston et al., 1996). An acute dose of vitamin C (e.g., 2 g) can also reduce bronchial responsiveness to inhaled histamine in patients with allergy (Bucca et al., 1990). Thus, the antihistamine effect of vitamin C may attenuate the severity of symptoms associated with respiratory tract infections.

The use of vitamin C supplements might shorten the duration of the common cold and ameliorate symptom severity in the general population (Douglas & Hemilä, 2005; Hemilä, 2007), possibly due to the anti-histamine effect of high-dose vitamin C (Johnston, 1996).

2.6. Vitamin C and Tobacco Usage

Smoking is known to increase the metabolic turnover of ascorbic acid due to its oxidation by free radicals and reactive oxygen species generated by cigarette smoking (Frei et al., 1981). It has been suggested that a daily intake of at least 140 mg/day is required for smokers to maintain a total body pool similar to that of non-smokers consuming 100 mg/day (Kallner et al., 1981).

Supplementation of 100 mg vitamin C/day for 20 weeks to both smokers and non-smokers resulted in a significant decrease in oxidative base damage to lymphocyte DNA as measured by a modified comet assay. In addition the lymphocytes showed an increased resistance to H_2O_2 induced oxidative damage in vitro (Duthie et al., 1996).

In smokers, acute smoking (5–7 cigarettes in 90 min) increased LDL lipid peroxidation twofold; vitamin C supplementation (1.5 g daily) reversed LDL lipid smoking-induced peroxidation (Harats et al., 1990).

Vitamin C intake is positively associated with bone mineral density (Hall & Greendale, 1998; Leveille et al., 1997; Melhus et al., 1999; Weber, 1999). This association is independent of other nutrients correlated with dietary vitamin C, including vitamin A and β-carotene. The relationship is particularly strong at high calcium intakes in postmenopausal women (Hall & Greendale, 1998; Melhus et al., 1999). Among persons with low vitamin E intake (6 mg per day) and those with modest vitamin C intake (70 mg per day or less), the odds of sustaining a fracture were 2–4 times greater for current smokers than for women who never smoked. Among persons with low intakes of both vitamins, the odds of fracture were nearly five times greater among current smokers than among women who never smoked. Compared with those who have never smoked, the odds of fracture were not increased among smokers who also had high intakes of vitamin E and/or vitamin C, e.g., 200 mg/day (Hall & Greendale, 1998; Melhus et al., 1999; Weber, 1999).

According to the FNB (2000) recommendations, the RDA of vitamin C for smokers must be increased in more 35 mg in both genders.

2.7. Health Risks from Excessive Vitamin C Intake

It has been recommended that the RDA for ascorbic acid should be 100–120 mg/day to maintain cellular saturation and optimum risk reduction of heart disease, stroke and cancer in healthy individuals (Carr & Frei, 1999). There is no scientific evidence to show that even very large doses of vitamin C are toxic or exert serious adverse health effects (Bendich, 1997; FNB, 2000; Johnson, 1999).

Furthermore, the panel on dietary antioxidants and related compounds suggested that *in vivo* data do not clearly show a relationship between excess vitamin C intake and kidney stone formation, pro-oxidant effects, excess iron absorption (FNB, 2000). The most common complaints are diarrhea, nausea, abdominal cramps, and other gastrointestinal disturbances due to the osmotic effect of unabsorbed vitamin C in the gastrointestinal tract (FNB, 2000; Jacob & Sotoudeh, 2002).

Plasma vitamin C concentrations in people who regularly consume vitamin C supplements are 60–70 % higher than those who do not take supplements (75–80 and 45–50 μmol/L, respectively (Byerley & Kirksey, 1985; Dickinson et al., 1994; Moss, 1989; Subar & Block, 1990). A daily intake of 500–1000 mg is necessary to maintain plasma vitamin C concentrations at 75–80 μmol/L. The recently revised RDA for vitamin C, 75 mg daily for adult females and 90 mg daily for adult males, represents a 25–50 % increase over the 1989 RDA, 60 mg (FNB, 2000). Exclusively breastfed infants ingest approximately 10 mg vitamin C/kg body weight (Byerley & Kirksey, 1985).

Approximately 70 % of a 500 mg dose is absorbed. However, much of the absorbed dose (50 %) is excreted unmetabolized in urine. With a dose of 1250 mg, only 50 % of the dose is absorbed and nearly all (85 %) of the absorbed dose is excreted (Johnson, 1999).

About 75 % of kidney stones contain calcium oxalate; another 5–10 % is composed of uric acid. High doses of vitamin C have been shown to increase urinary excretion of both oxalic acid and uric acid; and thus, theoretically promote the formation of kidney stones (Berger & Gerson, 1977; Curhan et al., 1996; FNB, 2000; Goldfarb, 1994; Levine et al., 1996; Nahata et al., 1977; Schrauzer & Rhead, 1973; Stein et al., 1976; Wandzilak et al., 1994). Chronic daily ingestion of 1000 mg vitamin C increased urinary uric acid by 30% (Stein et al., 1976). However, studies evaluating the effects on urinary oxalate excretion of vitamin C intakes ranging from 30 mg to 10 g/day have had conflicting results, so it is not clear whether vitamin C actually plays a role in the development of kidney stones (Curhan et al., 1996, Curhan et al., 1999; FNB, 2000; Taylor et al., 2004). The best evidence that vitamin C contributes to kidney stone formation was found in patients with pre-existing hyperoxaluria (Levine et al., 1999).

In their review, Levine et al. (1999), concluded that the safe upper limit for vitamin C should be 1 g/day. At higher dosages of vitamin C patients with pre-existing hyperoxaluria may increase the risk of nephrolithiasis and in some healthy people there is an increase in oxalate excretion, although the consequences of this increase are unclear.

Epidemiologic data do not support an association between vitamin C supplementation and kidney stones. In the Harvard Prospective Health Professional Follow-Up Study involving over 45,000 men from 40–75 years of age, 751 incident cases of kidney stones were documented over a six-year period (Curhan et al., 1996). The age-adjusted relative risk for men consuming 1500 mg or more vitamin C/day was 0.78, when compared with those consuming less than 251 mg/day (95 % confidence interval, 0.54–1.11).

Another matter of concern is the influence of vitamin C over iron absorption. Due to the enhancement of nonheme iron absorption by vitamin C, a theoretical concern is that high vitamin C intakes might cause excess iron absorption. In healthy individuals, this does not appear to be a concern (FNB, 2000). However, in individuals with hereditary hemochromatosis, chronic consumption of high doses of vitamin C could exacerbate iron overload and result in tissue damage (FNB, 2000; Jacob & Sotoudeh, 2002).

Vitamin C is a redox active compound and can not only act as an antioxidant but also as a pro-oxidant in the presence of redox active transition metal ions. Reduction of metal ions e.g. copper and iron, by vitamin C in vitro can result in formation of highly reactive hydroxyl radicals via reaction of the reduced metal ion with hydrogen peroxide by the Fenton reaction (Carr & Frei, 1999). In fact, under specific conditions, vitamin C can act as a pro-oxidant, potentially contributing to oxidative damage (FNB, 2000). It was reported that vitamin C can cause oxidative damage to erythrocytes (Ballin et al., 1988).

A few studies in vitro have suggested that by acting as a pro-oxidant, supplemental oral vitamin C could cause chromosomal and/or DNA damage and possibly contribute to the development of cancer (Lee et al., 2001; Podmore et al., 1998).

Doses of 500 mg vitamin C per day given to volunteers (16 females and 14 males aged between 17 and 49) exhibited a pro-oxidative effect. The levels of the potentially mutagenic lesions, 8-oxoadenine and 8-oxoguanine, markers for DNA damage mediated by oxygen radicals, were measured. Supplementation of diets with 500 mg vitamin C for 6 weeks gave a statistically significant increase in 8-oxoadenine levels in DNA harvested from lymphocytes. No significant increase was observed in those subjects receiving placebo. In the 6 week period following treatment 8-oxoadenine levels returned to those observed at baseline or during placebo. In contrast, 8-oxoguanine levels were significantly reduced (Podmore et al., 1998).

However, other studies have not shown increased oxidative damage or increased cancer risk with high intakes of vitamin C (Carr & Frei, 1999; FNB, 2000).

The diet of most athletes usually contains vitamins in their naturally occurring state, or when the foods are enriched (e.g. breakfast cereals). Unfortunately, many athletes regularly consume megadoses of vitamins (between 10 to 1000 times RDA) as an ergogenic aid in the belief that, 'if a little is good, more must be better' (Bishop et al., 1999). However, supplementation studies in athletes eating well-balanced diets do not support this practice (van der Beek, 1992), and ingestion of megadoses of vitamins is likely to do more harm than good. By this, athletes are advised to be supervised by a qualified sports nutritionist to assess their nutritional status and needs before taking large amounts of unnecessary vitaminic supplements, such as vitamin C, in particular.

3. VITAMIN C AND SPORTS

The detrimental outcomes associated with unregulated and excessive production of free radicals remains a physiological concern that has implications to health, medicine and performance. Available evidence suggests that physiological adaptations to exercise training can enhance the body's ability to quench free radicals and circumstantial evidence exists to suggest that key vitamins and nutrients may provide additional support to mitigate the untoward effects associated with increased free radical production. However, controversy has risen regarding the potential outcomes associated with vitamin C.

3.1. Vitamine C as Ergogenic Aid in Sport

An ergogenic aid is defined as any training technique, mechanical device, nutritional practice, pharmacological method, or psychological technique that can improve exercise performance capacity and/or enhance training adaptations (Kreider et al., 2009; Leutholtz & Kreider, 2001; Williams, 1999). This includes aids that may help prepare an individual to exercise, improve the efficiency of exercise, and/or enhance recovery from exercise. Ergogenic aids may also allow an individual to tolerate heavy training to a greater degree by helping them recover faster or help them stay injury-free and/or healthy during intense training.

According to Kreider et al., who published in 2010 an extensive review focused on research and recommendations about exercise and sport nutrition, individuals who better adapt to high levels of training usually experience greater gains from training over time which can lead to improved performance. Consequently, employing nutritional practices that help prepare individuals to perform and/or enhance recovery from exercise should also be viewed as ergogenic.

Changes in nutrient intake may induce homeostatic adaptations in absorption and metabolic use that redistribute nutrients without any effect on performance. Failure to assess biochemical indicators of nutritional status also limits any conclusions about influence of intake on biological function. Lukaski (2004) presented a model that includes these key components and emphasisis feedback regulation among these components (Figure 1).

According to Lukaski (2004), the use of this model will enable rigorous research designs to test hypothesis relating nutrient intake, nutritional status, and human performance.

The metabolic functions of vitamins required in sports are mainly those needed for production of energy and for neuromuscular functions (skills). Physical performance involves several metabolic pathways, all including several biochemical reactions. The relation between vitamin supply and functional capacity is S-shaped or 'bell-shaped', depending on whether the examination is extended to megadoses (Figure 2). The core in the above relation is that the output (functional capacity) is not improved after the 'minimal requirement for maximal output' is reached (Brubacher, 1989). In contrast, overvitaminosis may in some cases reduce the output below the maximal level.

Although research has demonstrated that specific vitamins may possess some health benefit (for instance, vitamin E, vitamin C, and folic acid), few have been reported to directly provide ergogenic value for athletes.

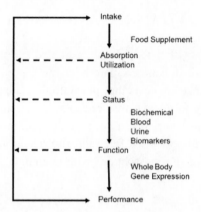

Figure 1. Model to assess the interactions among nutrient intake, status, function, and performance (adapted from Lukaski, 2004, with permission).

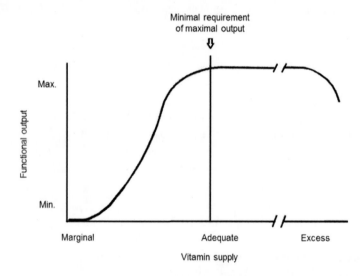

Figure 2. The association between vitamin supply and functional output (adapted from Fogelholm, 2000, with permission).

However, some vitamins may help athletes tolerate training to a greater degree by reducing oxidative damage (vitamin E, C) and/or help to maintain a healthy immune system during heavy training (vitamin C). Theoretically, this may help athletes tolerate heavy training leading to improved performance (Kreider et al., 2010).

Vitamin supplements frequently used by athletes include B-complex vitamins, vitamin E and, especially, vitamin C (Sobal & Marquart, 1994). The common motivation for vitamin supplementation is to improve sports performance and enhance recovery (Williams, 1986).

Vitamin C is involved in a number of metabolic processes in the human body, including those that may be important for the optimal functioning of the oxygen energy system. The reductant properties of vitamin C help to absorb dietary iron, which is needed for the formation of haemoglobin in the red blood cell.

**Table 2. Functions of vitamin C associated with specific enzymes
(adapted from Johnston et al., 2001, with permission)**

Function	Associated enzyme(s)	Associated mechanism and features
Extracellular matrix maturation (Collagen biosynthesis)	Prolyl-3-hydroxylase Prolyl-4-hydroxylase Lysyl hydroxylase	Dioxygenase; Fe^{+2}
Cq1 complement synthesis Carnitine biosynthesis	Prolyl-3-hydroxylase 6-N-Trimethyl-L-lysine hydroxylase γ-Butyrobetaine hydroxylase	Dioxygenase; Fe^{+2} Dioxygenase; Fe^{+2}
Pyridine metabolism	Pyrimidine deoxyribonucleoside Hydroxylase (fungi)	Dioxygenase; Fe^{+2}
Cephalosporin synthesis	Deacetoxycephalosporin C synthetase	Dioxygenase; Fe^{+2}
Tyrosine metabolism	Tyrosine-4-hydroxyphenylpyruvate hydrolase	Dioxygenase; Fe^{+2}
Norepinephrine biosynthesis	Dopamine-β-monooxygenase or hydrolase	Monooxygenase; Cu^{+1}
Peptidylglycine-α-amidation in the activation of hormones	Peptidylglycine-α-amidating monooxygenase	Monooxygenase; Cu^{+1}

Most of all, it is a powerful antioxidant, helping prevent cellular damage and impairment of the immune system from free radicals generated during intense aerobic exercise (Evans, 2000).

Ascorbic acid is distributed in varying concentrations throughout the body and is involved in a variety of metabolic reactions related to exercise, such as, the synthesis and activation of neuropeptides, collagen, carnitine and protection against the harmful effects of reactive oxidant species (Table 2). Athletes who increased dietary vitamin C requirements and intake may have important effects on aerobic capacity, antioxidant status and immunity (Peake, 2003). Vitamin C is a required cofactor for the biosynthesis of muscle carnitine (β-hydroxy butyric acid), a fatty acid transport molecule that facilitates fat oxidation during exercise. Vitamin C depletion is associated with decreased tissue carnitine, a consequence that is believed to contribute to fatigue and decreased fat oxidation during exercise (Hughes et al., 1980; Johnston et al., 2006). Vitamin C is required for norepinephrine synthesis, a neurotransmitter with roles in mood states, exercise performance, and heart rate recovery after exertion (Carlezon et al., 2009; Zouhal et al., 2008). Although conflicting data exist, the preponderance of available information suggests that physical exercise promotes an increase in free-radical generation. There are few studies that were focused on the effects of vitamin C intake in the oxidative stress parameters of professional athetes during submaximal and/or maximal exercise. Cholewa et al. (2008), conducted a study with well-trained basketball players and found that supplementation in vitamin C (240 mg/d for 21 days) does not change the blood antioxidant status, both at rest and after maximal exercise. It also has no effect on maximal oxygen uptake, thus, does not increase aerobic capacity.

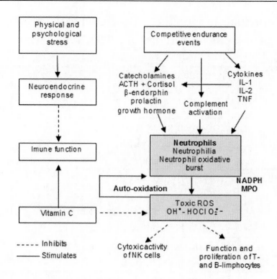

Figure 3. Ascorbic acid (vitamin C) and immunosuppression in runners. A hypothetical model of prophylactic mechanisms of action (adapted from Peters, 1997, with permission). ACTH= adrenocorticotrophic hormone; IL = interleukin; MPO = myeloperoxidase; NADPH = nicotinamide adenine dinucleotide phosphate (reduced form); NK = natural killer; ROS = reactive oxygen species; TNF = tumour necrosis factor.

Vasankari et al. (1998) found no improvement in exercise induced oxidative stress in Finnish runners who were supplemented with vitamin C. Although Bryant et al. (2003) reported diminished membrane damage with 400 IU/day of vitamin E in trained cyclists (22.3 ± 2 years old, who participated in four separate supplementation trials—placebo, 1 g/day of vitamin C, 400 IU/day of vitamin E, or 1 g/day of vitamin C plus 200 IU/day of vitamin E), 1 g/day of vitamin C promoted cellular damage. Neither vitamin E nor vitamin C (alone or taken together) improved exercise performance.

Vitamin C may enhance immune function. In fact, a number of reports suggest ascorbic acid supplementation lowers the incidence of upper respiratory tract infection in individuals under heavy physical stress (Peters et al., 1993; Peters et al., 1996). Ascorbic acid acts as a free radical scavenger, neutralising the ROS that are produced by neutrophils during exercise-induced phagocytosis and degranulation. This is hypothesised to reduce the auto-oxidative effect on neutrophil function and the apparent post-event immunosuppression (Figure 3).

Male runners consuming 500 mg/day of vitamin C received 600 mg of vitamin C or placebo for 21 days and then ran in a marathon race (Peters et al., 1993). During the 14 days after the race, the runners supplemented with vitamin C had fewer upper respiratory tract infections than did men receiving the placebo (33 % against 68 %).

3.2. Potential Action of Vitamine C in Sports Injuries and Muscle Recovery

The regulation of inflammation is an active area of research. Anti-inflammatory cytokines provide endogenous protection against proinflammatory cytokines.

The anterior crutiate ligament (ACL) is one of four major ligaments in the knee that provides stability and strength to the knee joint. Immediate (1 week post-ACL surgery) and persistent (months to years) leg muscle atrophy commonly follows an ACL injury and surgery (Arangio et al., 1997; Arvidsson et al., 1986; Elmqvist et al., 1989; Risberg et al., 1999; Rosenberg et al., 1992). Synovial fluid proinflammatory cytocines (Zysk et al., 2004) have been observed following ACL surgery and they induce oxidative and nitrative stress (Adams et al., 2002; Hardin et al., 2008) and mediate muscle atrophy or proteolysis (Dehoux et al., 2007; Goodman, 1991, 1994; Li et al., 1998). In a randomized, double-blind, placebo-controlled trial in men undergoing ACL surgery, conduted by Barker et al., (2009), it was found that vitamin E and C supplementation prior to ACL surgery attenuated the increase in IL-10 (an anti-inflammatory cytocine) in patients at 90 min and 72 h postsurgery.

Thompson et al. (2003) investigated the effects of 200 mg vitamin C supplementation following an intense shuttle-running test. These investigators did not observe improved indices of muscle damage, muscle function, or muscle soreness compared to a placebo group. Similar results were reported in a study by Close et al. (2006). In this study, supplementation with ascorbic acid after downhill running exercise decreased indices of oxidative muscle damage compared to placebo but did not attenuate delayed-onset muscle soreness. In fact, at least two studies have reported that postexercise vitamin C supplementation may delay the recovery process, especially following prolonged eccentric exercise (Childs et al., 2001; Thompson et al., 2003). Thus, although preexercise vitamin C supplementation has been clearly demonstrated to play a protective role in muscle (Bryer & Goldfarb, 2006; Goldfarb et al., 2005; Thompson et al., 2001), its application to postexercise recovery is less clear.

Vitamin C does appear to control ROS formed during exercise. If not controlled, these species have the ability to react with cell membranes and damage them. In 1992, Kaminski & Boal examined the relation between vitamin C (given to 19 subjects for 3 days before exercise and 7 days afterward) and the muscle damage induced by two bouts of eccentric exercise. The authors concluded that vitamin C reduced muscle damage.

Brites et al., (1999) found that football players participating in regular training demonstrated higher levels of oxidative stress damage, despite an increase in endogenous antioxidant capacity.

More recently, the effects of vitamin C and E supplementation on markers of oxidative stress, muscle damage and performance of elite football players, under regular training during their pre-competitive season, was studied (Zoppi, 2006). This study demonstrated that these vitamins may reduce lipid peroxidation and muscle damage during high intensity efforts, but did not enhance performance.

CONCLUSION

Vitamin C is one of the most important and essential vitamins for human health. It is needed for many physiological functions in human biology.

Ongoing research is examining whether vitamin C, by limiting the damaging effects of free radicals through its antioxidant activity, might help prevent or delay the development of certain cancers, diabetes mellitus, cardiovascular disease, and other diseases in which oxidative stress plays a causal role. Nevertheless, evidence from most randomized clinical trials suggests that vitamin C supplementation, usually in combination with other micronutrients, does not affect cancer risk.

The effect of vitamin C supplementation on physical performance has been investigated intermittently over the past 50 years, but the results of these studies have been contradictory. The possible benefits of vitamin C supplementation on exercise-induced muscle damage remain doubtful and further research is requested. In fact, clear evidence of a benefit of vitamin C supplementation on physical performance is lacking. Vitamin C, however, may exert permissive effects on physiologic fuctions (such as, antioxidant, imunocompetence, and collagen repair) that facilitate recovery from intense training and, thus, promote performance.

In summary, though vitamin C was discovered in 17th century, the exact role of this vitamin in human biology and health is still a mystery in view of the many beneficial claims and controversies.

ACKNOWLEDGMENTS/REVISION

The present chapter has been reviewed by:

- Cecília Morais (PhD), Faculty of Nutrition and Food Sciences, University of Porto. R. Dr. Roberto Frias, 4200-465 Porto, Portugal. E-mail: ceciliamorais@fcna.up.pt
- Jorge Lameiras (MSc), Nutrition Sciences Department, ISEIT-Viseu, Institute Piaget. Alto do Gaio - Galifonge, 3515-776 Lordosa (Viseu), Portugal. E-mail: jlameiras@ipiaget.org
- The authors thank Angela Carvalho (Jersey City, NJ, USA) for her proofreading of the English manuscript.

REFERENCES

Abahusain, M. A.; Wright, J.; Dickerson, J. W. & de Vol E. B. (1999). Retinol, alphatocopherol and carotenoids in diabetes. *Eur. J. Clin. Nutr.*, 53, 630-5.

Abe, M.; Reiter, R. J.; Orhii, P. B.; Hara, M. & Poeggeler, B. (1994). Inhibitory effect of melatonin on cataract formation in newborn rats: evidence for an antioxidative role for melatonin. *J. Pineal Res.*, 17, 94- 100.

Adams, V.; Nehrhoff, B.; Spate, U.; Linke, A.; Schulze, P. C.; Baur, A.; Gielen, S.; Hambrecht, R. & Schuler, G. (2002). Induction of iNOS expression in skeletal muscle by IL- 1beta and NFkappaB activation: an in vitro and in vivo study. *Cardiovasc. Res.*, 54, 95–104.

Age-Related Eye Disease Study Research Group. (2001a). A randomized, placebo-controlled, clinical trial of high-dose supplementation with vitamins C and E, beta carotene, and zinc for age-related macular degeneration and vision loss: AREDS report no. 8. *Arch. Ophthalmol.*, 119(10), 1417-1436.

Age-Related Eye Disease Study Research Group. (2001b). A randomized, placebo-controlled, clinical trial of high-dose supplementation with vitamins C and E, beta carotene, and zinc for age-related macular degeneration and vision loss: AREDS report no. 9. *Arch. Ophthalmol.*, 119(10), 1439-1452.

Aksoy, N.; Vurala, H.; Sabuncu, T.; Arslan, O. & Aksoy, S. (2005). Beneficial effects of vitamins C and E against oxidative stress in diabetic rats. *Nutrition Research*, 25, 625–630.

Arangio, G. A.; Chen, C.; Kalady, M. & Reed, J. F. (1997). Thigh muscle size and strength after anterior cruciate ligament reconstruction and rehabilitation. *JOSPT*, 26, 238–243.

Arvidsson, I.; Arvidsson, H.; Eriksson, E. & Jansson, E. (1986). Prevention of quadriceps wasting after immobilization: an evaluation of the effect of electrical stimulation. *Orthopedics*, 9, 1519–1528.

Ballin, A.; Brown, E. J.; Koren, G. & Zipursky, A. (1988). Vitamin C induced erythrocyte damage in premature infants. *J. Pediatr.*, 113, 114-20.

Banhegyi, G.; Marcolongo, P.; Puskas, F.; Fulceri.; R.; Mandl, J. & Benedetti, A. (1998). Dehydroascorbate and ascorbate transport in rat liver microsomal vesicles. *J .Biol. Chem.*, 273, 2758–2762.

Barker, T.; Leonard, S. W.; Trawick, R. H.; Martins, T. B.; Kjeldsberg, C. R.; Hill, H. R. & Traber, M. G. (2009). Modulation of inflammation by vitamin E and C supplementation prior to anterior cruciate ligament surgery. *Free Radical Biology & Medicine*, 46, 599–606.

Behrens, W. A. & Madere, R. (1994). A procedure for the separation and quantitative analysis of ascorbic acid. dehydroascorbic acid, isoascorbic acid, and dehydroisoascorbic acid in food and animal tissue. *J. Liquid Chromatogr.*, 17, 2445–2455.

Bendich, A. (1997). Vitamin C safety in humans. In: L. Packer, J. Fuchs (Eds), Vitamin C in Health and Disease. New York: Marcel Dekker Inc., 369-379.

Berger, L. & Gerson, C. D. (1977). The effect of ascorbic acid on uric acid excretion with a commentary on the renal handling of ascorbic acid. *Am. J. Med.*, 62, 71–76.

Bernasconi, P. & Massera, E. (1985). Evaluation of a new pharmaceutical form of nimesulide for the treatment of influenza. *Drugs Exp. Clin. Res.*, 11, 739-43.

Berndt, S. I.; Carter, H. B.; Landis, P. K.; Hallfrisch, J.; Rohrmann, S.; Metter, E. J. & Platz, E. A. (2005). Prediagnostic plasma vitamin C levels and the subsequent risk of prostate cancer. *Nutrition*, 21, 686–690.

Birlouez-Aragon, I.; Saavedra, G.; Tessier, F. J.; Galinier, A.; Ait-Ameur, L.; Lacoste, F.; Niamba, C.-N.; Alt, N.; Somoza, V. & Lecerf, J.M. (2010). A diet based on high-heat-treated foods promotes risk factors for diabetes mellitus and cardiovascular diseases. *Am. J. Clin. Nutr.*, 91, 1220-6.

Bishop, N. C.; Blannin, A. K.; Walsh, N. P.; Robson, P. J. & Gleeson, M. (1999). Nutritional aspects of immunosuppression in athletes. *Sports Med.*, 28 (3), 151-176.

Bjelakovic, G.; Nikolova, D.; Simonetti, R. G. & Gluud, C. (2008). Antioxidant supplements for preventing gastrointestinal cancers. *Cochrane. Database Syst. Rev.*, 3, CD004183.

Bleys, J.; Miller, E. R.; Pastor-Barrius, R.; Appel, L. J. & Guallar, E. (2006). Vitamin-mineral supplementation and the progression of atherosclerosis: a meta-analysis of randomized controlled trials. *Am. J. Clin. Nutr.*, 84, 880-7.

Block, G.; Dietrich, M.; Norkus, E. P.; Morrow, J. D.; Hudes, M.; Caan, B. & Packer, L. (2002). Factors associated with oxidative stress in human populations. *Am. J. Epidemiol.*, 156, 274–85.

Bors, W. & Buettner, G.R. (1997). The vitamin C radical and its reactions. In: Packer, L. & Fuchs, J. (eds.). Vitamin C in Health and Disease. (pp. 25–94). New York: Marcel Dekker.

Boutayeb, A.; Twizell, E. H.; Achouayb, K. & Chetouani, A. (2004). A mathematical model for the burden of diabetes and its complications. *Bio. Medical Engineering OnLine*, 3, 20.

Brites, F. D.; Evelson, P. A.; Christiansen, M. G.; Nicol, M. F.; Basílico, M. J.; Wikinski, R. W. & Llesuy, S. F. (1999). Soccer players under regular training showed imcreased oxidative stress but an improved plasma antioxidant status. *Clin. Sci.,* (Lond), 96(4), 381-385.

Brubacher, G.B. (1989). Scientific basis for the estimation of the daily requirements for vitamins. In: Walter, P.; Stähelin, H. & Brubacher, G. (Eds). *Elevated Dosages of Vitamins.* (pp. 3–11). Stuttgart: Hans Huber Publishers.

Bryant, R. J.; Ryder, J.; Martino, P.; Kim, J. & Craig, B. W. (2003). Effects of vitamin E and C supplementation either alone or in combination on exercise-induced lipid peroxidation in trained cyclists. *J. Strength Cond Res.*, 17(4), 792–800.

Bryer, S. C. & Goldfarb, A. H. (2006). Effect of high dose vitamin C supplementation on muscle soreness, damage, function, and oxidative stress to eccentric exercise. *Int. J. Sport Nutr. Exerc. Metab.*, 16, 270–280.

Bucca, C.; Rolla, G.; Oliva, A. & Farina, J. C. (1990). Effect of vitamin C on histamine bronchial responsiveness of patients with allergic rhinitis. *Ann. Allergy*, 65, 311–314.

Byerley, L. O. & Kirksey, A. (1985). Effects of different levels of vitamin C concentration in human milk and the vitamin C intakes of breast-fed infants. *Am. J. Clin. Nutr.*, 41, 665–671,.

Canestrari, F.; Buoncristiani, U.; Galli, F.; Giorgini, A.; Albertini, M.C.; Carobi, C.; Pascucci, M. & Bossu, M. (1995). Redox state, antioxidative activity and lipid peroxidation in erythrocytes and plasma of chronic ambulatory peritoneal dialysis. *Clin. Chim. Acta.*, 234, 127–136.

Carlezon, W. A. Jr; Beguin, C.; Knoll, A. T. & Cohen, B. M. (2009). Kappa-opioid ligands in the study and treatment of mood disorders. *Pharmacol. Ther.*, 123, 334–43.

Carr, A. C. & Frei, B. (1999). Toward new recommended dietary allowance for vitamin C based on antioxidant and health effects in humans. *Am. J. Clin. Nutr.*, 69, 1086-1107.

Chao, J. C.-J.; Yuan, M.-D.; Chen, P.-Y. & Chien, S.-W. (2002). Vitamin C and E supplements improve the impaired antioxidant status and decrease plasma lipid peroxides in hemodialysis patients. *J. Nutritional .Biochemistry*, 13, 653–663.

Chen, C. K.; Liaw, J. M.; Juang, J. G. & Lin, T.H. (1997). Antioxidant enzymes and trace elements in hemodialyzed patients. *Biol. Trace Elem. Res.*, 58, 149–157.

Chen, H.; Karne, R. J.; Hall, G.; Campia, U.; Panza, J. A.; Cannon, R. O.; Wang, Y.; Katz, A.; Levine, M. & Quon, M. J. (2006). High-dose oral vitamin C partially replenishes vitamin C levels in patients with type 2 diabetes and low vitamin C levels but does not improve endothelial dysfunction or insulin resistance. *Am. J. Physiol Heart Circ. Physiol.*, 290(1), H137–H145.

Chen, Q.; Espey, M. G.; Krishna, M. C.; Mitchell, J. B.; Corpe, C. P.; Buettner, G. R.; Shacter, E. & Levine, M. (2005). Pharmacologic ascorbic acid concentrations selectively kill cancer cells: action as a pro-drug to deliver hydrogen peroxide to tissues. *Proc .Natl. Acad. Sci. USA*, 102, 13604-9.

Chen, Q.; Espey, M. G.; Sun, A. Y.; Lee, J. H.; Krishna, M. C.; Shacter, E.; Choyke, P. L.; Pooput, C.; Kirk, K. L.; Buettner, G. R. & Levine, M. (2007). Ascorbate in pharmacologic concentrations selectively generates ascorbate radical and hydrogen peroxide in extracellular fluid in vivo. *Proc. Natl. Acad. Sci. USA*, 104, 8749-54.

Chen, Q.; Espey, M. G; Sun, A. Y.; Pooput, C.; Kirk, K. L.; Krishna, M. C.; Khosh, D. B.; Drisko, J. & Levine, M. (2008). Pharmacologic doses of ascorbate act as a prooxidant and decrease growth of aggressive tumor xenografts in mice. *Proc. Natl. Acad .Sci. USA*, 105, 1105-9.

Childs, A.; Jacobs, C.; Kaminski, T.; Halliwell, B. & Leeuwenburgh, C. (2001). Supplementation with vitamin C and N-acetyl-cysteine increases oxidative stress in humans after an acute muscle injury induced by eccentric exercise. *Free Radic. Biol .Med.*, 15, 745–753.

Cholewa, J.; Poprzecki, S.; Zajac, A. & Waskiewicz, Z. (2008). The influence of vitamin C on blood oxidative stress parameters in basketball players in response to maximal exercise. Impact de la supplémentation en vitamine C sur les paramètres du stress oxydatif dans le sang des basketteurs d'élite lors d'un effort maximal. *Science & Sports*, 23, 176–182.

Chong, E. W.; Wong, T. Y.; Kreis, A. J.; Simpson, J. A. & Guymer, R. H. (2007). Dietary antioxidants and primary prevention of age related macular degeneration: systematic review and meta-analysis. *BMJ*, 335, 755.

Chu, Y.-F.; Sun, J.; Wu, X. & Liu, R. H. (2002). Antioxidant and antiproliferative activities of vegetables. *J. Agric. Food Chem.*, 50, 6910-16.

Clermont, G.; Lecour, S.; Lahet, J.; Siohan, P.; Vergely, C.; Chevet, D.; Rifle, G. & Rochette, L. (2000). Alteration in plasma antioxidant capacities in chronic renal failure and hemodialysis patients: a possible explanation for the increased cardiovascular risk in these patients. *Cardiovas. Res.,* 47, 618–623.

Close, G. L.; Ashton, T.; Cable, T.; Dorana, D.; Hollowaya, C.; McArdlea, F. & MacLaren, D. P. M. (2006). Ascorbic acid supplementation does not attenuate post-exercise muscle soreness following muscle-damaging exercise but may delay the recovery process. *Br. J. Nutr.*, 95, 976–981.

Cook, N. R.; Albert, C. M.; Gaziano, J. M.: Zaharris, E.; MacFadyen, J.; Danielson, E.; Buring, J. E. & Manson, J. E. (2007). A randomized factorial trial of vitamins C and E and beta carotene in the secondary prevention of cardiovascular events in women: results from the Women's Antioxidant Cardiovascular Study. *Arch .Intern. Med.*, 167, 1610-8.

Coulter, I.; Hardy, M.; Shekelle, P.; Udani, J.; Spar, M. & Oda, K. (2003). Effect of the supplemental use of antioxidants vitamin C, vitamin E, and coenzyme Q10 for the prevention and treatment of cancer. Evidence Report/Technology Assessment Number 75. AHRQ Publication No. 04-E003. Rockville, MD: Agency for Healthcare Research and Quality, 2003.

Cross, C. E.; Halliwell, B.; Borish, E. T.; Pryor, W. A.; Ames, B. N.; Saul, R. L.; McCord, J. M. & Harman, D. (1987). Oxygen radicals and human disease. *Ann. Intern. Med.*, 107, 526- 45.

Curhan, G. C.; Willett, W. C.; Rimm, E. B. & Stampfer, M. J. (1996). A prospective study of the intake of vitamins C and B6, and the risk of kidney stones in men. *J. Urol.*, 155, 1847-51.

Curhan, G. C.; Willett, W. C.; Speizer, F. E. & Stampfer, M. J. (1999). Intake of vitamins B6 and C and the risk of kidney stones in women. *J. Am. Soc. Nephrol.*, 10, 840-5.

Davì, G.; Santilli, F. & Patrono, C. (2010). Nutraceuticals in diabetes and metabolic syndrome. *Cardiovascular Therapeutics*, 28, 216–226.

Davies, K. J. A. & Ursini, F. (1995). The oxigen paradox. Padua: CLEUP University Press.

Daviglus, M. L.; Dyer, A. R.; Persky, V.; Chavez, N.; Drum, M.; Goldberg, J.; Liu, K.; Morris, D. K.; Shekelle, R. B. & Stamler, J. (1996). Dietary beta-carotene, vitamin C, and risk of prostate cancer: results from the Western Electric Study. *Epidemiology*, 7, 472–7.

Dehoux, M.; Gobier, C.; Lause, P.; Bertrand, L.; Ketelslegers, J. M. & Thissen, J. P. (2007). IGF-I does not prevent myotube atrophy caused by proinflammatory cytokines despite activation of Akt/Foxo and GSK-3beta pathways and inhibition of atrogin-1 mRNA. *Am. J. Physiol. Endocrinol. Metab.*, 292:E145-E150.

Deneo-Pellegrini, H.; De Stefani, E.; Ronco, A. & Mendilaharsu, M. (1999). Foods, nutrients and prostate cancer: a case-control study in Uruguay. *Br. J. Cancer*, 80, 591–7.

Deruelle, F. & Baron, B. (2008). Vitamin C: is supplementation necessary for optimal health? *J. Alternative Compl. Med.*, 14 (10), 1291–1298.

Dickinson, V. A.; Block, G. & Russek-Cohen, E. (1994). Supplement use, other dietary and demographic variables, and serum vitamin C in NHANES II. *J. Am. Coll Nutr.*, 13, 22–32.

Douglas, R. M. & Hemilä, H. (2005). Vitamin C for preventing and treating the common cold. *PLoS Med.*, 2:e168.

Douglas, R. M.; Hemilä, H.; Chalker, E. & Treacy, B. (2007). Vitamin C for preventing and treating the common cold. *Cochrane Database Syst. Rev.*, 3, CD000980.

Dreher, D. & Junod, A. F. (1996). Role of oxygen free radicals in cancer development. *Eur. J. Cancer*, 32A, 30-8.

Drewnowski, A.; Rock, C. L.; Henderson, S. A.; Shore, A. B.; Fischler, C.; Galan, P.; Preziosi, P. & Hercberg, S. (1997). Serum β-carotene and vitamin C as biomarkers of vegetable and fruit intakes in a community-based sample of French adults. *Am. J. Clin. Nutr.*, 55, 1796–1802.

Durak, I.; Akyol, O.; Basesme, E.; Canbolat, O. & Kavutcu, M. (1994). Reduced erythrocyte defense mechanisms against free radical toxicity in patients with chronic renal failure. *Nephron*, 66, 76–80.

Duthie, S. J.; Ma, A.; Ross, M. A. & Collins, A. R. (1996). Antioxidant supplementation decreases oxidative DNA damage in human lymphocytes. *Can. Res.*, 56, 1291-1295.

Ederhardt, M. V.; Lee, C. Y. & Liu, R. H. (2000). Antioxidant activity of fresh apples. *Nature*, 405, 903-4.

Eichholzer, M.; Stahelin, H. B.; Ludin, E. & Bernasconi, F. (1999). Smoking, plasma vitamins C, E, retinol, and carotene, and fatal prostate cancer: seventeen-year follow-up of the prospective Basel study. *Prostate*, 38, 189 –98.

Elmqvist, L. G.; Lorentzon, R.; Johansson, C.; Langstrom, M.; Fagerlund, M. & Fugl-Meyer, A. R. (1989). Knee extensor muscle function before and after reconstruction of anterior cruciate ligament tear. *Scand. J. Rehab. Med.*, Suppl. 21, 131–139.

Ernstrom, J. E.; Kanim, L. E. & Klein, M. A. (1992). Vitamin C intake and mortality among a sample of the United States population. *Epidemiol.*, 3, 194–202.

Esmaillzadeh, A.; Kimiagar, M.; Mehrabi, Y.; Azadbakht, L.; Hu, F. B. & Willett, W. C. (2007). Dietary patterns, insulin resistance and prevalence of the metabolic syndrome in women. *Am. J. Clin. Nutr.*, 85, 910-8.

Evans, J. (2007). Primary prevention of age related macular degeneration. *BMJ*, 335, 729.

Evans, J. R. (2006). Antioxidant vitamin and mineral supplements for slowing the progression of age-related macular degeneration. *Cochrane Database. Syst. Rev.*, 2, CD000254.

Evans, W. (2000). Vitamin E, vitamin C and exercise. *Am. J. Clin. Nutr.*, 72:647–52.

Fiorillo, C.; Oliviero, C.; Rizzuti, G.; Nediani, C.; Pacini, A. & Nassi, P. (1998). Oxidative stress and antioxidant defenses in renal patients receiving regular haemodialysis. *Clin. Chem. Lab. Med.*, 36(3), 149-153.

Fogelholm, M. (2000). Vitamins: Metabolic Functions. Maughan, R. J. (Eds.). *Nutrition in Sport*. (pp. 266-280). London: Blackwell Science Ltd.

Food and Nutrition Board (2000). Dietary reference intakes for vitamin C, vitamin E, selenium and carotenoids. National Academy Press, Washington, DC.

Ford, E. S.; Will, J. C.; Bowman, B. A & Narayan, K. M. (1999). Diabetes mellitus and serum carotenoids: findings from the Third National Health and Nutrition Examination Survey. *Am. J. Epidemiol.*, 149, 168-76.

Fox, C. S.; Coady, S.; Sorlie, P. D.; D'Agostino, R. B. Sr; Pencina, M. J.; Vasan, R. S.; Meigs, J. B.; Levy, D. & Savage, P. J. (2007). Increasing cardiovascular disease burden due to diabetes mellitus: the Framingham Heart Study. *Circulation*, 115 (12), 1544-1550.

Frei, B.; England, L. & Ames, B. N. (1989). Ascorbate is an outstanding antioxidant in human blood plasma. *Proc. Natl. Acad. Sci. USA*, 86, 6377-81.

Frei, B.; Forte, T. M.; Ames, B. N. & Cross, C. E. (1981). Gas-phase oxidants of cigarette smoke induce lipid peroxidation and changes in lipoprotein properties in human blood plasma: protective effects of ascorbic acid. *Biochem. J.*, 277, 133-138.

Galli, F.; Varga, Z.; Balla, J.; Ferraro, B.; Canestrari, F.; Floridi, A.; Kakuk, G. & Buoncristiani, U. (2001). Vitamin E, lipid profile, and peroxidation in hemodialysis patients. *Kidney Int.*, 59 (Suppl 78), S148 –154.

Gandini, S.; Merzenich, H.; Robertson, C. & Boyle, P. (2000). Meta-analysis of studies on breast cancer risk and diet: the role of fruit and vegetable consumption and the intake of associated micronutrients. *Eur. J .Cancer*, 36, 636–646.

Garg, A. & Grundy, S. M. (1990). Management of dyslipidemia in NIDDM. *Diabetes Care*, 13, 153-169.

Ginter, E.; Bobek, P. & Jurcovicova, M. (1982). Role of ascorbic acid in lipid metabolism. In: P. A. Seith & B. M. Toblert (Eds.), *Ascorbic acid, chemistry, metabolism and uses*. American Chemical Society, Washington, DC, 381-393.

Giovannucci, E.; Ascherio, A.; Rimm, E. B.; Stampfer, M. J.; Colditz, G. A. & Willett, W. C. (1995). Intake of carotenoids and retinol in relation to risk of prostate cancer. *J. Natl. Cancer Inst.*, 87, 1767–76.

Goldenberg, H. & Schweinzer, E. (1994). Transport of vitamin C in animal and human cells. *J. Bioenerg. Biomembr.*, 26, 359–367.

Goldfarb, A. H.; Patrick, S. W.; Bryer, S. & You, T. (2005). Vitamin C supplementation affects oxidative-stress blood markers in response to a 30-min run at 75% VO2max. *Int. J. Sport Nutr. Exerc. Metab.*, 15, 279–290.

Goldfarb, S. (1994). Diet and nephrolithiasis. *Annu Rev Med*, 45, 235–243.

Goodman, M. N. (1991). Tumor necrosis factor induces skeletal muscle protein breakdown in rats. *Am. J. Physiol. Endocrinol. Metab.*, 260, E727–E730.

Goodman, M. N. (1994). Interleukin-6 induces skeletal muscle protein breakdown in rats. *Proc. Soc. Exp. Biol. Med.*, 205, 182–185.

Gorton, H. C. & Jarvis, K. (1999). The effectiveness of vitamin C in preventing and relieving the symptoms of virus-induced respiratory infections. *J. Manipulative Physiol. Therapeutics*, 22(8), 530-533.

Ha, T. K. K.; Sattar, N.; Talwar, D.; Cooney, J.; Simpson, K.; O'Reilly, D. St. J. & Lean, M. E. J. (1996). Abnormal antioxidant vitamin and carotenoid status in chronic renal failure. *Q. J. Med.,* 89, 765–769.

Hall, S. L. & Greendale, G. A. (1998). The relation of dietary vitamin C intake to bone mineral density: results from the PEPI study. *Calcified Tissue International,* 63, 183–189.

Halliwell, B. & Whiteman, M. (1997). Antioxidant and prooxidant properties of vitamin C. In: L. Packer & J. Fuchs (eds). *Vitamin C in Health and Disease,* (25–94).New York: Marcel Dekker.

Harats, D.; Ben-Naim, M.; Dabach, Y.; Hollander, G.; Havivi, E.; Stein, O. & Stein, Y. (1990). Effect of vitamins C and E supplementation on susceptibility of plasma lipoproteins to peroxidation induced by acute smoking. *Atherosclerosis*, 85, 47–54.

Harats, D.; Chevion, S.; Nahir, M.; Norman, Y.; Sagee, O & Berry, E. M. (1998). Citrus fruit supplementation reduces lipoprotein oxidation in young men ingesting a diet high in saturated fat: presumptive evidence for an interaction between vitamins C and E *in vivo.* *Am. J. Clin. Nutr.,* 67, 240-5.

Hardin, B. J.; Campbell, K. S.; Smith, J. D.; Arbogast, S.; Smith, J.; Moylan, J. S. & Reid, M. B. (2008). TNF-{alpha} acts via TNFR1 and muscle-derived oxidants to depress myofibrillar force in murine skeletal muscle. *J Appl. Physiol.,* 104, 694–699.

Hathcock, J. N.; Azzi, A.; Blumberg, J.; Bray, T.; Dickinson, A.; Frei, B.; Jialal, I.; Johnston, C. S.; Kelly, F. J.; Kraemer, K.; Packer, L.; Parthasarathy, S.; Sies, H. & Traber, M. G. (2005). Vitamins E and C are safe across a broad range of intakes. *Am. J. Clin. Nutr.,* 81, 4, 736-745.

Hecht, S. S. (1997). Approaches to cancer prevention based on an understanding of N-nitrosamine carcinogenesis. *Proc. Soc. Exp. Biol. Med.,* 216, 181-91.

Hellman, L. & Burns, J. J. (1958). Metabolism of L-ascorbic acid-1-C14 in man. *J. Biol. Chem.,* 230, 923-930.

Hemilä H. (2007). The role of vitamin C in the treatment of the common cold. *Am. Fam Physician.,* 76, 1111-1115.

Hemilä, H. (1994). Does vitamin C alleviate the symptoms of the common cold? A review of current evidence. *Scand. J. Infect. Dis.,* 26, 1-6.

Heron, M. (2011). Deaths: Leading causes for 2007. *National. Vital. Statistics Reports*, 59, Hyattsville, MD, U.S.A., National Center for Health Statistics.

Hochstein, P. & Ernster, L. (1963). ADP-activated lipid peroxidation coupled on TPNH oxidase system of microsomes. *Biochem .Biophys. Res. Commun.,* 12, 388- 94.

Honarbakhsh, S. & Schachter, M. (2008). Vitamins and cardiovascular disease. *Br. J. Nutr.,* 101(8), 1-19.

Huang, H. Y.; Alberg, A. J.; Norkus, E. P.; Hoffman, S. C.; Comstock, G. W. & Helzlsouer, K. J. (2003). Prospective study of antioxidant micronutrients in the blood and the risk of developing prostate cancer. *Am. J. Epidemiol.,* 157, 335– 44.

Hughes, R. E.; Hurley, R. J. & Jones, E. (1980). Dietary ascorbic acid and muscle carnitine (beta-OH-gamma-(trimethylamino) butyric acid) in guinea pigs. *Br. J. Nutr.,* 43, 385-387.

Hultqvist, M.; Hegbrant, J.; Nilsson-Thorell, C.; Lindholm, T.; Nillson, P.; Linden, T. & Hultqvist-Bengtsson, U. (1997). Plasma concentrations of vitamin C, vitamin E and/or malondialdehyde as markers of oxygen free radical production during hemodialysis. *Clin. Nephrol.,* 47, 37–46.

Hunt, C.; Chakravorty, N. K.; Annan, G.; Habibzadeh, N. & Schorah, C. J. (1994). The clinical effects of vitamin C supplementation in elderly hospitalized patients with acute respiratory infections. *Internat. J. Vit. Nutr. Res.*, 64, 212–219.

Jackson, P.; Loughrey, C. M.; Lightbody, J. H.; McNamee, P. T. & Young, I. S. (1995). Effect of hemodialysis on total antioxidant capacity and serum antioxidants in patients with chronic renal failure. *Clin. Chem.*, 41, 1135–1138.

Jacob, R. A. & Sotoudeh, G. (2002). Vitamin C function and status in chronic disease. *Nutr. Clin. Care*, 5, 66-74.

Jacques, P. F. & Chylack, L. T. (1991). Epidemiologic evidence of a role for the antioxidant vitamins and carotenoids in cataract prevention. *Am. J. Clin. Nutr.*, 53, 325S–325S.

Jacques, P. F.; Taylor, A.; Hankinson, S. E.; Willet, W. C.; Mahnken, B.; Lee, Y.; Vaid, K. & Lahav, M. (1997). Long-term vitamin C supplement use and prevalence of early age-related lens opacities. *Am. J. Clin. Nutr.*, 656, 911–916.

Johnson, C. S. (1999). Biomarkers for establishing a tolerable upper intake level for vitamin C. *Nutrition. Reviews*, 57, 71–77.

Johnston, C. S.; Corte, C. & Swan, P. D. (2006). Marginal vitamin C status is associated with reduced fat oxidation during submaximal exercise in young adults. *Nutr. Metab.* (Lond), 3, 35.

Johnston, C. S. (1996). The antihistamine action of ascorbic acid. *Subcell Biochem.*, 25, 189-213.

Johnston, C. S.; Retrum, K. R.; Srilakshmi, J.C. (1992). Antihistamine effects and complications of supplemental vitamin C. *J. Am. Diet. Assoc.*, 92, 988–989.

Johnston, C. S.; Steinberg, F. M. & Rucker, R. B. (2001). Ascorbic Acid. Rucker, R. B.; Suttie, J. W.; McCormic, D. B. & Machlin, L. J. (Eds.). *Handbook of Vitamins.* (3rd Edition, pp. 529-554). New York: Marcel Dekker, Inc.

Kallner, A.; Hartmann, D. & Hornig, D. (1981). On the requirement of ascorbic acid in man: steady-state turnover and body pool in smokers. *Am. J. Clin. Nutr.*, 34, 1347-1355.

Kallner, A.; Horing, D. & Hartman, D. (1982). Kinteics of ascorbic acid in humans. In: P. A. Seib & B. M. Tolbert (Eds.), *Ascorbic acid: Chemistry, metabolism and uses.* Advances in Chemistry Series N° 200, American Chemical Society, Washington, DC, 385-400.

Kaminski, M. & Boal, R. (1992). An effect of ascorbic acid on delayed-onset muscle soreness. *Pain*, 50, 317–321.

Kasai, H.; Crain, P. F.; Kuchino, Y.; Nishimura, S.; Ootsuyama, A. & Tanoaka, H. (1986). Formation of 8-hydroxy-guanine moiety in cellular DNA by agents producing oxygen radical and evidence for its repair. *Carcinogenesis*, 7, 1849- 51.

Knekt, P.; Ritz, J.; Pereira, M. A.; O'Reilly, E. J.; Augustsson, K.; Fraser, G. E.; Goldbourt, U.; Heitmann, B. L.; Hallmans, G.; Liu, S.; Pietinen, P.; Spiegelman, D.; Stevens, J.; Virtamo, J.; Willett, W. C.; Rimm, E. B. & Ascherio, A. (2004). Antioxidant vitamins and coronary heart disease risk: a pooled analysis of 9 cohorts. *Am. J. Clin. Nutr.*, 80, 1508-20.

Kreider, R. B.; Wilborn, C. D.; Taylor, L.; Campbell, B.; Almada, A. L.; Collins, R.; Cooke, M.; Earnest, C. P.; Greenwood, M.; Kalman, D.S.; Kerksick, C. M.; Kleiner , S. M.; Leutholtz, B.; Lopez, H.; Lowery, L. M.; Mendel, R.; Smith, A.; Spano, M.; Wildman, R.; Willoughby, D. S.; Ziegenfuss, T. N. & Antonio, J. (2010). ISSN exercise & sport nutrition review: research & recommendations. *J. Int. Society Sports Nut.*, 7, 7.

Kreider, R.; Leutholtz, B.; Katch, F. & Katch, V. (2009). *Exercise & Sport Nutrition*. Santa Barbara: Fitness Technologies Press.

Kushi, L. H.; Fee, R. M.; Sellers, T. A.; Zheng, W. & Folsom, A. R. (1996). Intake of vitamins A, C, and E and postmenopausal breast cancer. The Iowa Women's Health Study. *Am. J. Epidemiol.*, 144, 165-74.

Lee, D. H.; Folsom, A. R.; Harnack, L.; Halliwell, B. & Jacobs, D. R. Jr. (2004). Does supplemental vitamin C increase cardiovascular disease risk in women with diabetes? *Am. J. Clin. Nutr.*, 80, 1194-200.

Lee, S. H.M.; Oe, T. & Blair, I. (2001). A. Vitamin C-induced decomposition of lipid hydroperoxides to endogenous genotoxins. *Science*, 292, 2083-6.

Leutholtz, B. & Kreider, R. (2001). *Exercise and Sport Nutrition.* Nutritional Health Totowa, NJ: Humana PressWilson T., Temple N.

Leveille, S. G.; LaCroix, A. Z.; Koepsell, T. D.; Beresford, S. A.; Van Belle, G. & Buchner, D. M. (1997). Dietary vitamin C and bone mineral density in postmenopausal women in Washington State, USA. *J. Epidemiol. Comm. Health,* 51, 479–485.

Levi, F.; Pasche, C.; La Vecchia, C.; Lucchini, F. & Franceschi, S. (1999). Food groups and colorectal cancer risk. *Br. J. Cancer*, 79, 1283–1287.

Levine, M.; Conry-Cantilena, C.; Wang, Y.; Welch, R. W.; Washko, P. W.; Dhariwal, K. R.; Park, J. B.; Lazarev, A., Graumlich, J.; King, J. & Cantilena, L. R. (1996). Vitamin C pharmacokinetics in health volunteers: evidence for a recommended dietary allowance. *Proc. Natl. Acad. Sci. USA*, 93, 3704– 3709.

Levine, M.; Espey, M. G. & Chen, Q. (2009). Losing and finding a way at C: new promise for pharmacologic ascorbate in cancer treatment. *Free Radic. Biol. Med.*, 47, 27-9.

Levine, M.; Rumsey, S. C.; Daruwala, R.; Park, J. B. & Wang, Y. (1999). Criteria and recommendations for vitamin C intake. *JAMA*, 281, 1415-23.

Levine, M.; Wang, Y.; Padayatty, S. J. & Morrow, J. (2001). A new recommended dietary allowance of vitamin C for healthy young women. *Proc. Natl. Acad. Sci. USA*, 98, 9842-6.

Levine, R.L. & Stadtman, E.R. (1996) Protein modifications with aging. In: Schneider, E. L. & Rowe, J. W. (Eds). *Handbook of the Biology of Aging.* (pp. 184–197). San Diego: Academic Press.

Li, Y. & Schellhorn, H. E. (2007). New developments and novel therapeutic perspectives for vitamin C. *J. Nutr.*, 137, 2171-84.

Li, Y. P.; Schwartz, R. J.; Waddell, I. D.; Holloway, B. R. & Reid, M. B. (1998). Skeletal muscle myocytes undergo protein loss and reactive oxygen-mediated NF-κB activation in response to tumor necrosis factor α. *FASEB J.*, 12, 871–880.

Lin, R.-Y.; Choudhury, R.; Cai, W.; Lu, M.; Fallon, J. T.; Fisher, E. A. & Vlassara, H. (2003). Dietary glycotoxins promote diabeticatherosclerosis in apolipoprotein E-deficient mice. *Atherosclerosis*, 168, 213-20.

Linster, C. L. & Van Schaftingen, E. (2007). Vitamin C: Biosynthesis, recycling and degradation in mammals. *FEBSJ*, 274, 1–22.

Liu, R. H. (2003). Health benefits of fruit and vegetables are from additive and synergistic combinations of phytochemicals1–4. *Am. J. Clin. Nutr.*, 78(suppl), 517S–20S.

Lukaski, H.C. (2004). Vitamin and Mineral Status: Effects on Physical Performance. *Nutrition*, 20, 632–644.

Maramag, C.; Menon, M.; Balaji, K. C.; Reddy, P. G. & Laxmanan, S. (1997). Effect of vitamin C on prostate cancer cells in vitro: effect on cell number, viability, and DNA synthesis. *Prostate*, 32, 188 –95.

Maritim, A. C.; Sanders, R. A. & Watkins, J. B. III. (2003). Diabetes, oxidative stress, and antioxidants: A review. *J. Biochem. Mol. Toxicol.*, 17, 24-38.

McCormick, D. B. & Zhang, Z. (1993). Cellular Assimilation of Water-Soluble Vitamins in the Mammal: Riboflavin, B6, Biotin, and C. *Proc. Soc. Exp. Biol. Med.*, 202, 265–270.

Melhus, H.; Michaelsson, K.; Holberg, L.; Wolk, A. & Ljunghall, S. (1999). Smoking, antioxidant vitamins, and the risk of hip fracture. *J. Bone Miner Res.,* 14, 129–135.

Mohora, M.; Mircescu, G.; Cirjan, C.; Mihailescu, I.; Girneata, L.; Ursea, N. & Dinu, V. (1995). Effect of hemodialysis on lipid peroxidation and antioxidant system in patients with chronic renal failure. *Roman. J. Intern. Med.*, 33, 237–242.

Montilla, P. L.; & Vargas, J. F.; Tunez, I. F.; Munoz de Agueda, M. C.; Valdelvira, M. E. & Cabrera, E. S. (1998). Oxidative stress in diabetic rats induced by streptozotocin: protective effects of melatonin. *J. Pineal. Res.*, 25, 94- 100.

Morena, M.; Cristol, J. P. & Canaud, B. (2000). Why hemodialysis patients are in a prooxidant state? What could be done to correct the pro/antioxidant imbalance. *Blood Purif.*, 18, 191–199.

Mosby, T. T.; Cosgrove, M.; Sarkardei, S.; Platt, K. L. & Kaina, B. (2012). Nutrition in Adult and Childhood Cancer: Role of Carcinogens and Anti-carcinogens. *Anticancer Research*, 32, 4171-4192

Moser, U. & Bendich, A. (1990). Vitamin C. In: Machlin, L. J. (Ed.), *Handbook of Vitamins*. New York: Marcel Dekker.

Moss, A. J. (1989). Use of vitamin and mineral supplements in the United States: current users, types of products, and nutrients. Advance Data No. 174. Washington, DC: National Center for Health Statistics, Centers for Disease Control and Prevention.

Muntwyler, J.; Hennekens, C. H.; Manson, J. E.; Buring, J. E. & Gaziano, J. M. (2002). Vitamin supplement use in a low-risk population of US male physicians and subsequent cardiovascular mortality. *Arch. Intern. Med.*, 162, 1472-6.

Murase, H.; Moon, J. H.; Yamauchi, R.; Kato, K.;, Yoshikawa, T. & Terao, J. (1998). Antioxidant activity of a novel vitamin E derivative, 2-(Alpha-D-glucopyranosyl) methyl-2,5,7,8,-tetramethylchroman-6-ol. *Free Radic. Biol. Med.*, 24, 217- 25.

Myint, P. K.; Luben, R. N.; Welch, A. A.; Bingham, S. A.; Wareham, N. J. & Khaw, K. T. (2008). Plasma vitamin C concentrations predict risk of incident stroke over 10 y in 20 649 participants of the European Prospective Investigation into Cancer Norfolk prospective population study. *Am. J. Clin. Nutr.*, 87, 64-9.

Nahata, M.C.; Shim, L.; Lampman, T. & McLeod, D. C. (1977). Effect of ascorbic acid on urine pH in man. *Am. J. Hosp. Pharmacy*, 34, 1234–1237.

Naidu, K. A. (2003). Vitamin C in human health and disease is still a mystery? An overview. *Nutrition Journal*, 2, 7.

Neuhouser, M. L.; Wassertheil-Smoller, S.; Thomson, C.; Aragaki, A.; Anderson, G. L.; Manson, J. E.; Patterson, R. E.; Rohan, T. E.; van Horn, L.; Shikany, J. M.; Thomas, A.; LaCroix, A. & Prentice, R. L. (2009). Multivitamin Use and Risk of Cancer and Cardiovascular Disease in the Women's Health Initiative Cohorts. *Arch. Intern. Med.*, 169(3), 294-304.

Osganian, S. K.; Stampfer, M. J.; Rimm, E.; Spiegelman, D.; Hu, F. B.; Manson, J. E. & Willett, W. C. (2003). Vitamin C and risk of coronary heart disease in women. *J. Am. Coll Cardiol.*, 42, 246-52.

Padayatty, S. J. & Levine, M. (2006). Vitamins C and E and the prevention of preeclampsia. *N. Engl. J. Med.*, 355, 1065.

Padayatty, S. J. & Levine, M. (2009). Antioxidant supplements and cardiovascular disease in men. *JAMA*, 301, 1336.

Padayatty, S. J.; Riordan, H. D.; Hewitt, S. M.; Katz, A.; Hoffer, L. J. & Levine, M. (2006). Intravenously administered vitamin C as cancer therapy: three cases. *CMAJ*, 174, 937-42.

Padayatty, S. J.; Sun, H.; Wang, Y.; Riordan, H. D; Hewitt, S. M.; Katz, A.; Wesley, R. A. & Levine, M. (2004). Vitamin C pharmacokinetics: implications for oral and intravenous use. *Ann. Intern. Med.*, 140, 533-7.

Paul, J.L.; Sall, N. D.; Soni, T.; Poignet, J.L.; Lindenbaum, A.; Man, N. K.; Moatti, N. & Raichvarg, D. (1993) Lipid peroxidation abnormalities in hemodialyzed patients. *Nephron*, 64, 106–109.

Pauling, L. (1971). The significance of the evidence about ascorbic acid and the common cold. *Proc. Natl. Acad. Sci. USA*, 68, 2678-81.

Peake, J. M. (2003). Vitamin C: effects of exercise and requirements with training. *Int J Sport Nutr. Exerc. Metab.*, 13, 125–51.

Peppa, M.; He, C.; Hattori, M. McEvoy, R.; Zheng, F. & Vlassara, H. (2003). Fetal or neonatal low-glycotoxin environment prevents autoimmune diabetes in NOD mice. *Diabetes*, 52, 1441-8.

Peters, E. M.; Goetzsche, J. M.; Grobbelaar, B. & Noakes T. D. (1993). Vitamin C supplementation reduces the incidence of postrace symptoms of upper-respiratory-tract infection in ultramarathon runners. *Am. J. Clin. Nutr.*, 57, 170-4.

Peters, E. M.; Goetzsche, J. M.; Joseph, L. E. & Noakes, T. D. (1996). Vitamin C as effective as combination of anti-oxidant nutrients in reducing symptoms of URTI in ultramarathon runners. *S. Afr. J. Sports Med.*, 4, 23-7.

Peuchant, E.; Delmas-Beauvieux, M-C.; Dubourg, L.; Thomas, M-J.; Perromat, A.; Aparicio, M.; Clerc, M. & Combe, C. (1997). Antioxidant effects of a supplemented very low protein diet in chronic renal failure. *Free Radic. Biol. Med.*, 22, 313–320.

Podmore, I. D.; Griffiths, H. R.; Herbert, K. E.; Mistry, N.; Mistry, P. & Lunec, J. (1998). Vitamin C exhibits pro-oxidant properties. *Nature*, 392, 559.

Polidori, M. C.; Mecocci, P.; Stahl, W.; Parente, B.; Cecchetti, R.; Cherubini, A.; Cao, P.; Sies, H. & Senin, U. (2000). Plasma levels of lipophilic antioxidants in very old patients with type 2 diabetes. *Diabetes Metab. Res. Rev.*, 16, 15-9.

Qiao, Y. L.; Dawsey, S. M.; Kamangar, F.; Fan, J. H.; Abnet, C. C.; Sun, X. D.; Johnson, L. L.; Gail, M. H.; Dong, Z.-W.; Yu, B.; Mark, S. D. & Taylor, P. R. (2009). Total and cancer mortality after supplementation with vitamins and minerals: follow-up of the Linxian General Population Nutrition Intervention Trial. *J. Natl. Cancer Inst.*, 101, 507-18.

Ramon, J. M.; Bou, R.; Romea, S.; Alkiza, M. E.; Jacas, M.; Ribes, J. & Oromi, J. (2000). Dietary fat intake and prostate cancer risk: a case-control study in Spain. *Cancer Causes Control*, 11, 679–85.

Riccioni, G.; Bucciarelli, T.; Mancini, B.; Corradi, F. Di Ilio, C.; Mattei, P. A. & D'Orazio, N. (2007). Antioxidant vitamin supplementation in cardiovascular diseases. *Ann. Clin. Lab. Sci.*, 37, 89–95.

Ripple, M. O.; Henry, W. F.; Rago, R. P. & Wilding, G. (1997). Prooxidant-antioxidant shift induced by androgen treatment of human prostate carcinoma cells. *J. Natl. Cancer Inst.*, 89, 40–8.

Risberg, M. A.; Holm, I.; Steen, H.; Eriksson, J. & Ekeland, A. (1999). The effect of knee bracing after anterior cruciate ligament reconstruction: a prospective, randomized study with two years' follow-up. *Am. J. Sports Med.*, 27, 76–83.

Rose, R. C.; Choi, J. L. & Koch, M. J. (1988). Intestinal transport and metabolism of oxidized ascorbic acid (dehydroascorbic acid). *Am. J. Physiol.*, 254, G824–G828.

Rosenberg, T. D.; Franklin, J. L.; Baldwin, G. N. & Nelson, K. A. (1992). Extensor mechanism function after petallar tendon graft harvest for anterior cruciate ligament reconstruction. *Am. J. Med.*, 20, 519–526.

Rosenblat, M. & Aviram, M. (2002). Oxysterol-induced activation of macrophage NADPH-oxidase enhances cellmediated oxidation of LDL in the atherosclerotic apolipoprotein E deficient mouse: inhibitory role for vitamin E. *Atherosclerosis*, 160(1), 69-80.

Rumsey, S. C. & Levine, M. (1998). Absorption, transport, and disposition of ascorbic acid in humans. *J. Nutr. Biochem.*, 9, 116–130.

Rumsey, S.C.; Kwon, O.; Xu, G.; Burant, C. F.; Simpson, I. & Levine, M. (1997). Glucose transporter isoforms GLUT1 and GLUT3 transport dehydroascorbic acid. *J. Biol. Chem.*, 272, 18982–18989.

Sabuncu, T.; Vural, H.; Harma, M. & Harma, M. (2001). Oxidative stress in polycystic ovary syndrome and its contribution to the risk of cardiovascular disease. *Clin. Biochem.*, 34, 407-13.

Sandu, O.; Song, K.; Cai, W.; Zheng, F.; Uribarri, J. & Vlassara, H. (2005). Insulin resistance (IR) and type 2 diabetes (T2D) in high fat-fed mice are linked to high glycotoxin, rather than high fat intake. *Diabetes*, 54, 2314-9.

Sargeant, L. A.; Wareham, N. J.; Bingham, S.; Day, N. E.; Luben, R. N,; Oakes, S.; Welch, A. & Khaw, K. T. (2000). Vitamin C and hyperglycemia in the European Prospective Investigation into Cancer–Norfolk (EPIC-Norfolk) study: a population-based study. *Diabetes Care*, 23, 726–32.

Sauberlich, H. E (1985). Bioavailability of vitamins. *Prog. Food Nutr. Sci.*, 9, 1-33.

Sauberlich, H. E. (1990). Ascorbic acid. In: M. L. Brown (Ed.), *Present knowledge in Nutrition*. Nutrition Foundation, Washington DC.

Schrauzer, G. N. & Rhead, W. J. (1973). Ascorbic acid abuse: effects of long term ingestion of excessive amounts on blood levels and urinary excretion. *Int. J. Vitam Nutr. Res.*, 43, 201–211.

Schuurman, A. G.M; Goldbohm, R. A.; Brants, H. A. & van den Brandt, P. A. (2002). A prospective cohort study on intake of retinol, vitamins C and E, and carotenoids and prostate cancer risk (Netherlands). *Cancer Causes Control.*, 13, 573– 82.

Sen, C. K. & Hanninen, O. (1994). Physiological antioxidants. In: Sen, C. K.; Packer, L. & Hanninen, O. (Eds). *Exercise and Oxygen Toxicity*. (pp. 89–126). Amsterdam: Elsevier Science.

Sesso, H. D.; Buring, J. E.; Christen, W. G.; Kurth, T.; Belanger, C.; MacFadyen, J.; Bubes, V.; Manson, J. E.; Glynn, R. J. & Gaziano, J. M. (2008). Vitamins E and C in the prevention of cardiovascular disease in men: the Physicians' Health Study II randomized controlled trial. *JAMA*, 300, 2123-33.

Shahidi, F. & Naczk, M. (1995). Food phenolics: an overview. In: Shahidi, F. & Naczk, M. (eds.). *Food Phenolics: Sources, Chemistry, Effects, Applications.* 1–5. Lancaster, PA: Technomic Publishing Company Inc.

Shekelle, P.; Hardy, M. L.; Coulter, I.; Udani, J.; Spar, M.; Oda, K.; Jungvig, L. K.; Tu, W.; Suttorp, M. J.; Valentine, D.; Ramirez, L.; Shanman, R. & Newberry, S. J. (2003). Effect of the supplemental use of antioxidants vitamin C, vitamin E, and coenzyme Q10 for the prevention and treatment of cancer. Evidence Report/Technology Assessment Number 75. AHRQ Publication No. 04-E003. Rockville, MD: Agency for Healthcare Research and Quality.

Shibata, A.; Paganini-Hill, A.; Ross, R. K. & Henderson, B. E. (1992). Intake of vegetables, fruits, beta-carotene, vitamin C and vitamin supplements and cancer incidence among the elderly: a prospective study. *Br. J. Cancer*, 66, 673–9.

Shurtz-Swirski, R.; Mashiach, E.; Kristal, B.; Shkolnik, T. & Shasha, S. M. (1995). Antioxidant enzymes activity in polymorphonuclear leukocytes in chronic renal failure. *Nephron.*, 71, 176–179.

Sinclair, A. J.; Taylor, P. B.; Lunec, J.; Girling, A. J. & Barnett, A. H. (1994). Low plasma ascorbate levels in patients with type 2 diabetes mellitus consuming adequate dietary vitamin C. *Diabet. Med.*, 11, 893-8.

Singh, R. B.; Niaz, M. A.; Agarwal, P.; Begom, R. & Rastogi, S. S. (1995). Effect of antioxidant-rich foods on plasma ascorbic acid, cardiac enzyme, and lipid peroxide levels in patients hospitalized with acute myocardial infarction. *J. Am. Diet Assoc.*, 95, 775–780.

Sobal, J. & Marquart, L. F. (1994). Vitamin/mineral supplement use among athletes: a review of the literature. *International. Journal of Sport Nutrition*, 4, 320-334.

Song, Y.; Cook, N. R.; Albert, C. M.; Van Denburgh, M. & Manson, J. (2009). Effects of vitamins C and E and b-carotene on the risk of type 2 diabetes in women at high risk of cardiovascular disease: a randomized controlled trial. *Am. J. Clin. Nutr.*, 90, 429–37.

Stein, H. B.; Hasan, A. & Fox, I. H. (1976). Ascorbic acid-induced uricosuria. *Ann. Intern. Med.*, 84, 385–388.

Steinmaus, C. M.; Nuanez, S. & Smith, A.H. (2000). Diet and bladder cancer: a meta-analysis of six dietary variables. *Am. J. Empidemiol.*, 151, 693–702.

Subar, A. F. & Block, G. (1990). Use of vitamin and mineral supplements: demographics and amounts of nutrients consumed. *Am. J. Epidemiol.*, 132, 1091–1101.

Suchitra, M. M.; Pallavi, M.; Sachan, A.; Reddy, S. V.; Bitla, A. R. & Rao, S. P. V. L. N. (2011). Lipid peroxidation measured as serum malondialdehyde and vitamin-C as oxidative-antioxidative biomarkers in type II diabetic patients. *IJBAR*, 2, 378-388.

Sun, F.; Iwaguchi, K.; Shudo, R.; Nagaki, Y.; Tanaka, K.; Ikeda, K.; Tokumaru, S. & Kojo, S. (1999). Change in tissue concentrations of lipid hydroperoxides, vitamin C and vitamin E in rats with streptozotocin-induced diabetes. *Clin. Sci.*, 96, 185- 90.

Sun, J.; Chu, Y.-F.; Wu, X. & Liu, R. H. (2002). Antioxidant and antiproliferative activities of fruits. *J. Agric. Food Chem.*, 50, 7449–54.

Tavan, E.; Maziere, S.; Narbonne, J. F. & Cassand, P. (1997). Effects of vitamin A and E on methylazoxymethanol-induced mutagenesis in Salmonella typhimurium strain TA100. *Mutat. Res.*, 377, 231-7.

Taylor, E. N.; Stampfer, M. J. & Curhan, G. C. (2004). Dietary factors and the risk of incident kidney stones in men: new insights after 14 years of follow-up. *J. Am. Soc. Nephrol.*, 15, 3225-32.

Taylor, P. R.; Li, B.; Dawsey, S. M.; Li, J. Y.; Yang, C. S.; Guo, W. & Blot, W. J. (1994). Prevention of esophageal cancer: the nutrition intervention trials in Linxian, China. Linxian Nutrition Intervention Trials Study Group. *Cancer Res.*, 54 (7 Suppl), 2029s-31s.

Thompson, D.; Williams, C.; Garcia-Roves, P.; McGregor, S. J.; McArdle, F. & Jackson, M. J. (2003). Post-exercise vitamin C supplementation and recovery from demanding exercise. *Eur. J. Appl. Physiol.*, 89, 393–400.

Thompson, D.; Williams, C.; McGregor, S. J.; Nicholas, C. W.; McArdle, F.; Jackson, M. J. & Powell, J. R. (2001). Prolonged vitamin C supplementation and recovery from demanding exercise. *Int. J. Sport Nutr. Exerc. Metab.*, 11, 466–481.

Toborek, M.; Wasik, T.; Drozdz, M.; Klin, M.; Magner-Wrobel, K. & Kopieczna-Grzebieniak, E. (1992). Effect of hemodialysis on lipid peroxidation and antioxidant system in patients with chronic renal failure. *Metab. Clin. Exp.*, 41, 1229–1232.

Vaksh, S.; Pandey, M.; Zingade, U. S. & Reddy, V. S. (2013). The effect of vitamin-C therapy on hyperglycemia, hyperlipidemia and non high density lipoprotein level in type 2 diabetes. *Int. J. Life Sc. Bt & Pharm. Res.*, 2(1), 290-295.

van der Beek, E. J. (1992). Vitamin supplementation and physical exercise performance. In: C. Williams, J. Devlin (eds). *Foods, Nutrition and Sports Performance*. London: E & FN Spon, 95-112

van Leeuwen, R.; Boekhoorn, S.; Vingerling, J. R.; Witteman, J. C.; Klaver, C. C.; Hofman, A. & de Jong, P. T. (2005). Dietary intake of antioxidants and risk of age-related macular degeneration. *JAMA*, 294, 3101-7.

Vasankari, T.; Kujala, U.; Sarna, S. & Ahotupa, M. (1998). Effects of ascorbic acid and carbohydrate ingestion on exercise induced oxidative stress. *J. Sports Med. Phys. Fitness*, 38(4), 281–5.

Vlassara, H.; Cai, W.; Crandall, J.; Goldberg, T.; Oberstein, R.; Dardaine, V.; Peppa, M. & Rayfield, E. J. (2002). Inflammatory mediators are induced by dietary glycotoxins, a major risk factor for diabetic angiopathy. *Proc. Natl. Acad. Sci. USA*, 99, 15596-601.

Voorrips, L. E.; Goldbohm, R. A.; Verhoeven, D. T.; van Poppel, G. A.; Sturmans; F.; Hermus, R. J. & van den Brandt PA. (2000).Vegetable and fruit consumption and lung cancer risk in the Netherlands Cohort Study on diet and cancer. *Cancer Causes and Control*, 11,101–115.

Vural, H.; Aksoy, N.; Arslan, S. O. & Bozer, M. (2000). Effects of vitamin E and selenium on lipid peroxidation and antioxidant enzymes in colon of methylazoxymethanol treated rats. *Clin. Chem. Lab. Med.*, 8(10), 1051-3.

Vural, H.; Sabuncu, T.; Arslan, S.O. & Aksoy, N. (2001). Melatonin inhibits lipid peroxidation and stimulates the antioxidant status of diabetic rats. *J. Pineal. Res.*, 31, 193-8.

Wandzilak, T. R.; D'Andre, S. D.; Davis, P. A. & Williams, H. E. (1994). Effect of high dose vitamin C on urinary oxalate levels. *J. Urol.*, 151, 834–837.

Weber, P. (1999). The role of vitamins in the prevention of osteoporosis—a brief status report. *Inter. J .Vit. Nutr. Res.*, 69, 194–197.

Will, J. C.; Ford, E. S. & Bowman, B. A. (1999). Serum vitamin C concentrations and diabetes: findings from the Third National Health and Nutrition Examination Survey, 1988-1994. *Am. J. Clin. Nutr.*, 70, 49-52.

Willcox, B. J.; Curb, J. D. & Rodriguez, B. L. (2008). Antioxidants in cardiovascular health and disease: key lessons from epidemiologic studies. *Am. J. Cardiol.*, 101, 75D-86D.

Williams, M. H. (1999). *Nutrition for Health, Fitness, and Sport*. Dubuque, IA: ACB/McGraw-Hill.

Williams, M.H. (1986). *Nutritional Aspects of Human Physical and Athletic Performance*. Charles C. Thomas, Springfield, IL.

Wintergerst, E. S.; Maggini, S. & Hornig, D. H. (2006). Immune-enhancing role of vitamin C and zinc and effect on clinical conditions. *Ann. Nutr. Metab.*, 50, 85-94.

World Cancer Research Fund/American Institute for Cancer Research (2007). *Food, Nutrition, Physical Activity, and the Prevention of Cancer: a Global Perspective*. Washington, DC, U.S.A., American Institute for Cancer Research.

Ye, Z. & Song, H. (2008). Antioxidant vitamins intake and the risk of coronary heart disease: meta-analysis of cohort studies. *Eur. J. Cardiovasc Prev .Rehabil.*, 15, 26-34.

Yoshida, M.; Takashima, Y.; Inoue, M.; Iwasaki, M.; Otani, T. & Sasaki, S. (2007). JPHC Study Group. Prospective study showing that dietary vitamin C reduced the risk of age-related cataracts in a middle-aged Japanese population. *Eur. J. Nutr.*, 46, 118-24.

Zhang, S.; Hunter, D. J.; Forman, M. R.; Rosner, B. A.; Speizer, F. E.; Colditz, G. A.; Manson, J. E.; Hankinson, S. E. & Willett, W. C. (1999). Dietary carotenoids and vitamins A, C, and E and risk of breast cancer. *J. Natl. Cancer Inst.*, 91, 547-56.

Zouhal, H.; Jacob, C.; Delamarche, P. & Gratas-Delamarche, A. (2008). Catecholamines and the effects of exercise, training and gender. *Sports Med.*, 38, 401-23.

Zysk, S. P.; Fraunberger, P.; Veihelmann, A.; Dorger, M.; Kalteis, T.; Maier, M.; Pellengahr, C. & Refior, H. J. (2004). Tunnel enlargement and changes in synovial fluid cytokine profile following anterior cruciatae ligament reconstruction with petallar tendon and hamstring tendon autografts. *Knee Surg. Sports Traumatol. Arthrosc.*, 12, 98–103.

In: Vitamin C
Editor: Raquel Guiné

ISBN: 978-1-62948-154-8
© 2013 Nova Science Publishers, Inc.

Chapter 13

VARIABILITY IN THE VITAMIN C CONTENT OF BAOBAB (*ADANSONIA DIGITATA* L.) FRUIT PULP FROM THREE AFRICAN SAHELIAN COUNTRIES

Charles Parkouda[1,], Jan Svejgaard Jensen[2] and Bréhima Diawara[1]*

[1]Département Technologie Alimentaire /IRSAT/CNRST, 03 BP7047 Ouagadougou
Burkina Faso
[2]Planting and Landscape Majsmarken, Billund, Denmark

ABSTRACT

The Baobab (*Adansonia digitata* L.) tree is one of the most widely used wild trees providing food, medicine and fodder in West Africa. The most valuable product from Baobab fruit for the international market is the pulp and is accepted in Europe as a novel food ingredient. Indeed the pulp has found to have a high content of calcium, phosphorus and high levels of vitamin C. Undertaken studies reported a significant variation in vitamin C content within and among Baobab populations in three African Sahelian countries including Burkina Faso, Mali and Niger. The content of vitamin C was ranged from 397 to 575m g/100g. There was a significant correlation between annual precipitation of the origin site and vitamin C content (r = -0.296, P < 0.001). No relation was found between pulp or bark colour and vitamin C content. Based on the vitamin C content, Baobab has a potential to improve nutrition for millions people in West Africa. The variation for vitamin C within sites is an indication that valuable gains could be made by selection of good varieties.

1. INTRODUCTION

In several countries including African countries, natural tree fruits constitute an important part of population diets and are also an important source of income for these populations (Parkouda et al., 2007). Mainly crudely consumed, they improve the daily food ration as an

---

* Email: cparkouda@yahoo.fr.

energy source and through their content in micronutrients.The Baobab (*Adansonia digitata* L.) tree is one of the most widely used wild trees providing food, medicine and fodder (Sidibe & Williams, 2002).The most valuable product from Baobab fruit for the international market is the pulp (Chadare et al., 2009). The dried Baobab fruit pulp has indeed been accepted by the European Union (EU) commission as a novel food ingredient under Regulation (EC) N° 258/97 of the European Parliament and of the Council. The pulp has found to have a high content of calcium and phosphorus and high levels of vitamin C (Diop et al., 2005; Osman, 2004).

Several studies have reported variation in Baobab taxonomy, distribution, agronomy, agroecology as well as variation in Baobab fruits nutrient content including vitamin C in pulp (Assogbadjo et al., 2008; Chadare et al., 2009; Parkouda et al., 2012; Scheuring et al., 1999; Sidibe et al., 1996).

The present chapter aim is to highlight the variationof vitamin C content of Baobab fruit pulp from three African Sahelian countries (Burkina Faso, Mali and Niger).

2. THE BAOBAB TREE

2.1. Description and Geographical Distribution

The Adansonia genus called the Baobab tree in both English and French is a multipurpose tree belonging to the family Bombacaceae. The genus includes eight species, namely *Adansonia grandidieri, A. madagascarensis, A. perrieri, A. rubrostipa, A. suarezensis, A. za, A. gibbosa* and *A. digitata* L. The first six species are endemic in the island of Madagascar and *A. gibbosa* is only located in the north-west of Australia. *Adansonia digitata* is present on the African mainland and is the most widespread and the best described species (Alverson et al., 1999; Diop et al., 2005; Sidibe & Williams 2002).

A. digitata L. is very characteristic of the Sahelian region. It grows naturally and is a typically scattered tree in the savannah and is often associated with human settlements (De Caluwe et al., 2009). The tree is very massive, with a very large trunk (up to 10 m diameter). It can grow up to 25 m in height and may live for hundreds or thousand years under suitable conditions (Diop et al., 2005). It has been introduced to areas outside Africa and grown successfully (Sidibe & Williams, 2002). Investigations revealed that *A.digitata* tree can be propagated by seeding, grafting or vegetative multiplication (Ishii & Kambou, 2007).

The form of the trunk varies. In young trees it is conical; in mature trees it may be cylindrical, bottle shaped or tapering with branching near the base (Gebauer et al., 2002). The trunk ramifies at the top in several short and broad branches, often irregular. The bark is smooth, reddish brown or greyish with a purplish tinge or rough and wrinkled (Figure 1A).

The leaves reach up to 20 cm in diameter and present 3 to 6 oblong leaflets (Figure 1B). The flowers are white but sometime greenish or brownish; they measure 8 to 20 cm in diameter and are suspended with a peduncle of about 15 cm or more in length (Figure 1C).

The fruit is generally ovoid, but it can also present a spherical form, very lengthened or club-sharped. The fruit is covered by a woody shell up to 50 cm in length and up to 10 cm in diameter (Figure 1D), which is covered by brownish or greenish felted hair. Moreover the shell contains numerous hard, brownish seeds, round or ovoid, up to 15 mm long which are embedded in a yellowish-white pulp (Figure 1E and 1F).

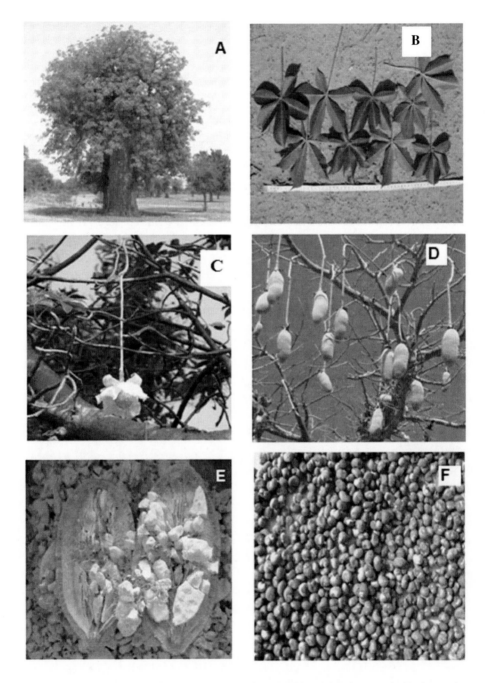

Figure 1. A: Baobab (*Adansonia digitata*) tree. B: Leaves. C: Flower on the tree. D: Fruits on the tree. E: Pods broken showing seeds embedded in pulp. F: Cleaned seeds. (Own pictures).

2.2. Importance of the Baobab (*Adansonia digitata* L) Tree

*A. digitata*is a widely-used plant species with medicinal properties and numerous food and non-food uses (Diop et al., 2005). The leaves of *A. digitata* tree are a staple food for many populations in many parts of Africa. Young leaves are commonly used as a vegetable in soups or cooked and eaten as spinach. Dried green leaves are used throughout the year, mostly in soups served with the staple dish of millet (Gebauer et al., 2002). Strangely, it is only in West Africa that Baobab leaves contribute to diets in a major way; Eastern and Southern Africa have the tree but seldom consume the leaves (NRC, 2006; NRC, 2008). Leaves are generally harvested during the rainy season when they are fresh and tender. During the last month of the rainy season, leaves are harvested in great abundance and are dried for domestic use and for marketing during the dry season. Thousands of tons are consumed annually in Africa, and Baobab greens are a commonplace in the markets as well as the daily meals (NRC, 2006, Yazzie et al., 1994). Nordeide et al. (1996) reported that the leaves are important protein sources in complementing the amino acid profile and thereby improving the protein quality of the diet.

The fruit of the Baobab tree is an ovoid pod containing about hundred seeds embedded in a pulp (Diop et al., 2005). The pulp has been found to have a high content of calcium and phosphorus and high levels of vitamin C (Afolabi & Popoola, 2005; Obizoba & Amaechi, 1993; Diop et al., 2005; Osman, 2004). The fruit pulp is used to prepare several kinds of beverages in rural areas and has recently become a popular ingredient in ice products, sweets and cakes in urban areas (Sidibe et al., 1996). Whole fruits can be stored for months under dry conditions and the pulp powder is extracted and stored in polyethylene bags which protect it against ambient moisture (Sidibe et al., 1996).

Baobab seeds are a rich source of nutrients. Nkafamiya et al. (2007) reported that Baobab seeds contain 21.75, 5.01, and 6.71 g/100 g of protein, ash and fiber, respectively. Whole seeds are pounded into a coarse meal and added to soups and other dishes as thickening agent (Dirar, 1993).

In some areas, roasted seeds are used as a coffee substitute (NRC, 2006). When fermented, they are used to enhance the flavour of many dishes. Although the seeds contain some antinutritive factor such as oxalate, phytate, saponin and tannin, Nkafamiya et al. (2007) reported that concentration of these components are below established toxic levels (oxalate, phytate, saponin and tannin representing 10.31, 2.00, 7.16, and 2.84% of seeds respectively), and the toxicant components can even be more reduced when seeds are processed before consumption especially when seeds are soaked and fermented. Addy et al. (1995) reported degradation of trypsin inhibitor whilst Nnam et al. (2003) reported a reduction of the antinutrients, phytate and tannins during fermentation of Baobab seeds.

3. REGIONAL VARIABILITY OF BAOBAB FRUITS CONTENT IN VITAMIN C

Baobab fruit pulp content in vitamin C has been reported by several studies (Nour et al., 1980; Becker, 1983; Arnold et al., 1995, Diop et al., 2005; Parkouda et al., 2012) which revealed the variability of this content. Indeed, several studies have reported varying levels of

Baobab fruit pulp vitamin C content with mean values between 337 mg/100g (Nigeria), 300 mg/100g (Sudan), 150-500 mg/100g (Senegal), 280 mg/100g (Mali) and 74-163 mg/100g (South Africa) (Nour et al. 1980; Becker 1983; Ighodalo et al. 1991; Arnold et al. 1995; Sidibe et al. 1996; Manfredini et al. 2002; Diop et al. 2005).

Parkouda et al. (2012) reported an average level of 478 mg/100g with values ranged from 397 to 575 mg/100g (Table 1). Tree-to-tree variability in the vitamin C contents of the fruit pulp, also ranging from 150 to 500 mg/100g was reported by Scheuring et al. (1999). As also seen by Parkouda et al. (2012) the coefficient of variation (CV) within populations varied from 18 to 26 %, except for the Toulfé site (Burkina Faso) which had a particularly low variation (9 %) and showed a vitamin C content (476 mg/100g) slightly lower than the average of all sites (478 mg/100g). Significant variation between populations vitamin C (P = 0.0064) and fruit pulp weight (P < 0.001) was also reported during this study (Parkouda et al., 2012). During their investigations, Parkouda et al. (2012) reported that there was more variation within populations than among populations. The highest levels of vitamin C were found in the two populations with lowest precipitation (450 mm year) of Mansila in Burkina Faso (575 mg/100g) and Komodiguili (554 mg/100g). The site Koumadioba with highest precipitation had a low vitamin C content of 416 mg/100g.

Several parameters can explain this variability including sol type, genetic, precipitation, etc. Indeed, as reported by Parkouda et al. (2012) there was a positive correlation between vitamin C content and latitude indicates that vitamin C content increased towards the north, and the weak negative correlation between vitamin C and longitude indicates that vitamin C content was slightly higher in the eastern part of the sample region; A strong relationship between average precipitation and vitamin C content was observed (Table 2). The vitamin C content was highest at the dry sites.

Table 1. Vitamin C content of fruits pulp from Baobab in 11 populations in Burkina Faso, Mali and Niger. The data are arithmetic means. The coefficients of variance (CV %) express the relative standard error between trees in % of the mean value (Parkouda et al., 2012)

Country	Site	Number of trees	Fruit weight (g)	Pulp weight (g)	Vitamin C (mg/100g DW)	Vitamin C CV%
Mali	Samé	18	130	21.0	466	24
Mali	Kourougue	20	321	48.7	480	23
Mali	Nabougou	14	259	50.0	463	24
Mali	Koumadiobo	20	250	34.9	416	26
Mali	Zambougou	19	285	51.7	397	22
Mali	Komodiguili	20	220	26.3	554	18
Burkina Faso	Nankoun	10	338	58.2	491	19
Burkina Faso	Toulfé	17	201	28.2	476	9
Burkina Faso	Mansila	6	369	58.3	575	23
Niger	Torodi	17	358	69.5	504	22
Niger	Park W	17	496	94.0	442	23
	Mean		293	49.2	478	
	SD		98	21	53	

NB: nutritional composition is expressed on a dry weight basis, DW: dry weight, SD: Standard Deviation.

Table 2. Spearman-rank correlations based on mean tree values of vitamin C, sugar, fruit weight, latitude (positive direction north to south), longitude (positive direction east to west) and precipitation (Parkouda et al., 2012)

	Sugar	Fruit Weight	Precipitation	Longitude	Latitude
Vitamin C	0.029[NS]	-0.004 [NS.]	-0.296***	-0.151**	0.224**

Significance levels: Ns: non-significant, * $P < 0.05$; ** $P < 0.01$; *** $P < 0.001$.

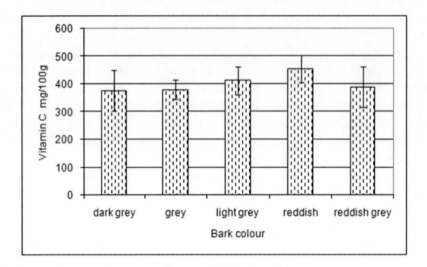

Figure 2. Variation of vitamin C content related to the tree bark colour (Trees from Mali).

Baobab trees from Burkina Faso and Mali are generally divided in five morphologique according to bark colour including dark grey, grey, light grey, reddish and reddish grey. Sidibe et al. (1996) showed that the vitamin C content is not related to the tree bark colour as generally thought by the farmer; this has been confirmed by Parkouda et al. (2012) who reported no significant correlations between the bark colour and the content of vitamin C (Figure 2).

The pulp samples were divided in white and cream coloured pulp samples and there were no significant correlations between the two pulp colour types and vitamin C.

CONCLUSION

Baobab is a Pan-African tree species and the fruit pulp possesses extremely valuable food properties and there is a large nutritional potential of vitamin C within its natural range.From different fruits pulp collected in different populations representing various climatic conditions, several investigations showed low variation on vitamin C content within population but high variation between populations. Based on the pulp vitamin C content Baobab has a potential to improve nutrition for millions of people in West Africa.

ACKNOWLEDGMENTS/REVISION

The present chapter has been reviewed by:

- Donatien Kaboré (PhD), Département Technologie Alimentaire/IRSAT/CNRST Ouagadougou, Burkina Faso.
- Fatoumata Ba/Hama (PhD), Département Technologie Alimentaire/IRSAT/CNRST Ouagadougou, Burkina Faso.

REFERENCES

Addy, E.O.H.; Salami, L.I.; Igboeli, L.C. & Remawa, H.S. (1995). Effect of processing on nutrient composition and anti-nutritive substances of African locust bean (*Parkia filicoidea*) and baobab seed (Adansoniadigitata). *Plant Foods for Human Nutrition* 48, 113-117.

Afolabi, O.R. & Popoola T.O.S. (2005). The effects of baobab pulp powder on the micro flora involved in tempe fermentation. *European Food Research and Technology,* 220, 187-190.

Alverson, W.S.; Whitlock, B.; Nyffeler, R.; Bayer, C. & Baum D.A. (1999). Phylogeny of the core Malvales: evidence from ndhF sequence data. *Am. J. Bot.,* 86, 1474-1486.

Arnold, T.H.; Well, M.J. & Wehmeyer, A.S. (1995). Koisan food plants: taxa with potential for economic exploitation. In, Plants for Arid Lands, ed. by Wickens GE, Goodin JR and Field DV, London: 69-86.

Assogbadjo, A.E.; GlèlèKakai, R.; Chadare, F.J.; Thomson, L.; Kyndt, T.; Sinsin, B. & Van Damme, P. (2008). Folk classification, perception, and preferences of baobab products in West Africa: Consequences for species conservation and improvement. *Econ. Bot.,* 62,74-84.

Becker B. (1983). The contribution of wild plants to human nutrition in the Ferlo (Northern Senegal). *Agro for Syst.,* 1, 252–267.

Chadare, F.J.; Linnemann, A.R.; Hounhouigan, J.D.; Nout, M.J.R. & Van Boekel, M.A.J.S. (2009). Baobab Food Products: A Review on their Composition and Nutritional Value. *Crit. Rev. Food Sci. Nutr.,* 49, 254-274.

De Caluwé, E.; De Smedt, S.; Assogbadjo, A.E.; Samson, R.; Sinsin, B. & Van Damme, P. (2009). Ethnic differences in use value and use patterns of baobab (*Adansonia digitata* L.) in northern Benin. *African Journal of Ecology,* 47, 433–440.

Diop, A.G. ; Sakho, M. ; Dornier, M., Cisse, M. & Reynes, M. (2005). Le baobab Africain (*Adansonia digitata* L.): principales caractéristiques et utilisations. *Fruits,* 61, 55–69.

Gebauer, J.; El-Siddig, K. & Ebert G. (2002). Baobab (*Adansonia digitata* L.): A review on a multipurpose tree with promising future in the Sudan. *Gartenbauwissenschaft,* 67, 155-160.

Ighodalo, C.E.; Catherine, O.E. & Daniel, M.K. (1991). Evaluation of mineral elements and ascorbic acid contents in fruits of some wild plants. *Plant Foods Hum. Nutr.,* 41, 151-154 (1991).

Ishii, K. & Kambou, S. (2007). In vitro culture of an African multipurpose tree species: *Adansonia digitata* L. *Propagation of Ornamental Plants,* 7, 62–67.

Manfredini, S.; Vertuani, S.; Braccioli, E. & Buzzoni, V. (2002). Antioxidant capacity of *Adansonia digitata* fruit pulp and leaves.*ActaPhytotherapeutica,* 2, 2-7.

Nkafamiya, I.I.; Osemeahon, S.A.; Dahiru, D. & Umaru H.A. (2007). Studies on the chemical composition and physicochemical properties of the seeds of baobab (*Adasonia digitata*).*African Journal of Biotechnology,* 6, 756-759.

Nnam, N.M. & Obiakor, P.N. (2003). Effect of fermentation on the nutrient and antinutrient composition of baobab *Adansonia digitata,* seeds and rice Oryza sativa, grains. *Ecology of Food and Nutrition,* 42, 265–277.

Nordeide, M.B.; Hatløy, A.; Følling, M.; Lied, E. & Oshaug, A. (1996). Nutrient composition and nutritional importance of green leaves and wild food resources in an agricultural district, Koutiala, in Southern Mali. *International Journal of Food Sciences and Nutrition, 47, 455–468.*

Nour, A.A.; Magboul, B.I. &Kheiri, N.H. (1980). Chemical composition of baobab fruit (*Adansonia digitata*).*Tropical Science,* 22, 383-388.

NRC (National Research Council), (2006). Lost Crops of Africa. Volume II: Vegetables. The National Academies Press, Washington, DC 378 p

NRC (National Research Council)(2008). Lost Crops of Africa. Volume III: Fruits. The National Academies Press, Washington, DC 380 p

Obizoba, I.C. &Amaechi, N.A. (1993). The effect of processing methods on the chemical composition of baobab (*Adansonia digitata* L.) pulp and seed. *Ecology of Food and Nutrition,* 29, 199–205.

Osman, M.A. (2004). Chemical and nutrient analysis of baobab (*Adansonia digitata*) fruit and seed protein solubility. *Plant Foods Hum. Nutr.,* 59, 29–33.

Parkouda, C. ; Diawara, B. ; Ganou, L. & Lamien, N. (2007). Potentialités nutritionnelles des produits de 16 espèces fruitières locales au Burkina Faso. *Science et Technique, Sciences appliquées et Technologies,* 1, 35-47.

Parkouda, C.; Sanou, H.; Tougiani, A.; Korbo, A.; Nielsen, D.S.; Tano-Debrah, K.; Ræbild, A.; Diawara, B. & Jensen, J.S. (2012). Variability of Baobab (*Adansonia digitata* L.) fruits' physical characteristics and nutrient content in the West African Sahel. *Agroforestry Systems,* 85, 455-463.

Scheuring, J.F.; Sidibé, M. & Frigg, M. (1999). Malian agronomic research identifies local baobab tree as source of vitamin A and Vitamin C. *Sight and Life, Newsletter,* 1, 21-24.

Sidibe, M.; & Williams, J.T. (2002). Fruits for the Future 4 – Baobab – (*Adansonia digitata* L) Monograph. International Center for Underutilised Crops, Southampton, UK, 96 p.

Sidibe, M.; Scheuring, J.F.; Tembely, D.; Sidibé, M.M.; Hofman P. & Frigg, M. (1996). Baobab – homegrown vitamin C for Africa. *Agroforestry today,* 8, 13-15.

Yazzie, D.; VanderJagt, D.J.; Pastuszyn, A.; Okolo, A. & Glew, H. (1994). The Amino Acid and Mineral Content of Baobab (*Adansonia digitata* L.) Leaves. *Journal of Food Composition and Analysis,* 7, 189-193.

INDEX

C

D

E

F

J

K

L

M

O

P

Q

R

S

T

U